Occupational Therapy in Childhood

Occupational Therapy in Childhood

CHIA SWEE HONG, MA, DIP COT, CERT ED, SROT

and

LYNNE HOWARD, MSC, DIP COT, ILTM, SROT
*both of the School of Occupational Therapy and Physiotherapy,
University of East Anglia*

Consulting Editor in Occupational Therapy
Clephane Hume

W

WHURR PUBLISHERS
LONDON AND PHILADELPHIA

© 2002 Whurr Publishers
First published 2002 by
Whurr Publishers Ltd
19b Compton Terrace, London N1 2UN, England and
325 Chestnut Street, Philadelphia PA 19106, USA

British Library Cataloguing in Publication Data
A catalogue record for this book is available from the
British Library.

ISBN: 1 86156 252 7

Printed and bound in the UK by Athenaeum Press Ltd,
Gateshead, Tyne & Wear

Contents

Preface

This book has been written to present current principles and practice underlying occupational therapy intervention with children. It is designed for use by students and newly qualified occupational therapists. However, other professionals in education and social care, and parents, may also find it of value to gain an understanding of the role of occupational therapy with children.

The book is divided into four parts:

Part I sets the context for practice
Part II reviews application models that are currently used in practice
Part III examines the needs of children with a variety of conditions
Part IV provides an example of an evaluation of practice.

We have invited a number of specialists to write individual chapters, and thus there are variations in the use of terminologies and the style of writing, but all address similar issues. In Part III, for example, they examine the impact of the condition on the child's occupation and review assessment and management procedures.

We envisage that the final chapter will promote interest in evidence-based practice and hope that future publications will have more of a research base.

Chia Swee Hong
Lynne Howard

Acknowledgements

Although every effort has been made, it has not been possible to trace or contact all sources of material cited in this book, and we therefore regret any inadvertent omission of acknowledgement where it is due.

We would like to thank all the children whose photographs or case histories appear in this book, and their parents for giving permission for these to be used.

We are grateful for the patience, assistance and encouragement from our families, contributors, and colleagues, in particular Robbie Meehan who also helped with the typing of the manuscript.

List of contributors

Fiona Carnegie, *Senior Occupational Therapist* Roehampton Rehabilitation Centre, Queen Mary's Hospital, Roehampton Lane, London

Chia Swee Hong, *Lecturer in Occupational Therapy* School of Occupational Therapy and Physiotherapy, University of East Anglia, Norwich

Sidney Chu, *Community Occupational Therapy Service Coordinator* Middlesex

Shona Comben, *Senior Occupational Therapist* Family Consultation Centre, Huntingdon, Cambs

Becky Durant, *Head Occupational Therapist Clinical Specialist* Bethel Child and Family Centre, Norwich

Caitlin Goggin, *Clinical Specialist Occupational Therapist* Burns and Plastic, Health Waikato, Hamilton, New Zealand

Dido Green, *Specialist Head Paediatric Occupational Therapist* Newcomen Centre, Guy's Hospital, London

Janine Hackett, *Senior Occupational Therapist* Childhood Arthritis and Rheumatic Diseases Unit, Birmingham Children's Hospital NHS Trust, Birmingham

Lindsay Hardy, *Clinical Specialist, Paediatric Occupational Therapy* Royal Free Hospital, London

Philippa Harpin, *National Occupational Therapy Adviser* Muscular Dystrophy Campaign, Newcastle General Hospital, Newcastle upon Tyne

Susan Henderson, *Occupational Therapist, Special Needs Coordinator* The Children's Centre, Chelmsford, Essex

Lynne Howard, *Lecturer in Occupational Therapy* School of Occupational Therapy and Physiotherapy, University of East Anglia, Norwich

Betty Hutchon, *Head Occupational Therapist* The Royal Free Hospital, London

Heather Last, *Director* PACE Centre, Aylesbury, Bucks

Jo Lloyd, *Acting Head Occupational Therapist* The Children's Trust Tadworth, Tadworth, Surrey

Sue Middleton, *former Head Occupational Therapist* The Children's Trust Tadworth, Tadworth, Surrey

Joan O'Rafferty, *Occupational Therapist* formerly at Child Development Centre, Warrington

Christine Peck, *Clinical Audit, Research and Development Manager* Wenlock House, Enfield, Middlesex

Sue Price, *Senior Occupational Therapist* Occupational Therapy and Sensory Services, Seymour House, Cambridge

Terry Robinson, *Neuro-Muscular Family Care Officer* Addenbrooke's Hospital, Cambridge

Carolyn Simmons Carlsson, *Occupational Therapist* Specialist Education Services, Auckland Central, New Zealand

Jenny Tucket, *Paediatric Occupational Therapy Service* Gwent Community Health NHS Trust, Abergavenny, Gwent

Part I
The Context for Practice

Chapter 1
Occupational therapy and children with disabilities

CHIA SWEE HONG AND LYNNE HOWARD

Since the pioneering work by Stow (1946), the practice of occupational therapy with children has continued to develop and be influenced by:

- The impact of twentieth-century technology on diagnosis, treatment and care of children
- The longer life expectancy of children with multiple disabilities
- The improved provisions for children with disabilities
- Increased recognition of the role of occupational therapy
- Legislative acts

Current practice

A coherent structure for occupational therapy

A current debate within occupational therapy is the need for a framework that is flexible to incorporate the philosophical, theoretical and practical aspects of the discipline. Such a framework would include a global view of the philosophy of the profession, the different schools of thought, and the models used to translate theory into practice. Hagedorn (1997) pointed out that, although the terminologies are used as synonyms, the concepts that are used for illustration are not necessarily the same.

Kortman (1995) proposed four major types of models. First, a professional model is applicable across various clients with different needs and practice settings, and is often considered as a professional 'blueprint'. Second, a delineation model identifies principles and seeks to identify occupational therapy approaches with specific groups of clients, while, third, an application model describes specific assessment and therapeutic techniques, and is linked closely to a delineation model. In our opinion,

3

delineation and application models are similar to 'frames of reference' (Kramer and Hinojosa, 1993), which organise theoretical material in occupational therapy and translate it into practice through a functional perspective. Fourth, a personal model acts as a filter, which occupational therapists use before translating the other models into practice.

The occupational therapy process

The following processes are generic to occupational therapy practice (Figure 1.1):

- Referral
- Assessments
- Establishment of relationship
- Goal-setting

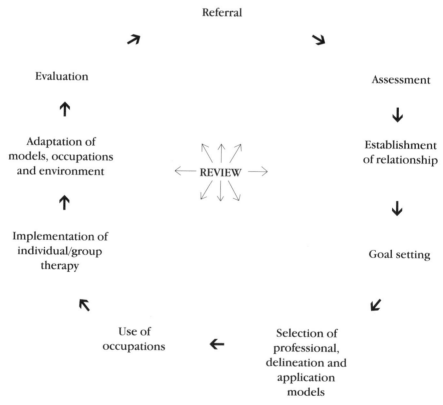

Figure 1.1: Processes generic to occupational therapy practice.

- Selection of professional, delineation and application models
- Use of occupations
- Implementation of individual/group therapy
- Adaptation of models, occupations and environment
- Evaluation
- Review

Referral

According to the College of Occupational Therapists (2000), 'Occupational therapists shall accept referrals which they deem to be appropriate and for which they have the resources'.

Occupational therapists are increasingly involved in screening programmes to identify children who may be in need of therapy. Inglis (1990) asked parents and teachers of 258 children to indicate by questionnaire whether their children were experiencing difficulty in daily living skills, handwriting/perceptual skills, and general upper limb function and coordination. The results showed that there were 77 children who were experiencing difficulties in one or more of the above areas, and the parents and teachers of 92 per cent of these children indicated that they felt that occupational therapy would be of benefit.

Young et al. (1995) carried out a study to identify whether there was a need for some children in an independent special school to receive occupational therapy. They found that, overall, there was a high demand for occupational therapy among pupils' parents, teachers, care and senior staff.

Assessments

Assessments form an integral component in the occupational therapy process. A paediatric assessment involves two essential features: an observational study of a child carrying out specific tasks and the use of the data to make a decision concerning an aspect or several aspects of the child's life.

Briefly, the aims are to:

- identify the general level of development of each child
- establish a baseline of present occupational performance skills (sensorimotor, cognitive and psychosocial) and occupations (self-maintenance, productivity and leisure) both qualitatively and quantitatively, and the impact of the environment on the child
- identify areas of occupational strengths and need(s) as identified by the child, his or her parents and the therapist
- contribute data for differential diagnosis, if appropriate

- decide on appropriate models for therapy
- help in selecting goals for a programme of therapy in order to help the children to learn or relearn skills needed to perform the occupations
- provide a measure of progress (Reed and Sanderson, 1983; Peck and Hong, 1994).

Various assessment methods are used by paediatric occupational therapists to fulfil different purposes. Chia (1997a) found that the following types of assessment methods were employed: interviewing, non-standardised and standardised tests, and unstructured and structured observations.

Interviewing helps the therapist to gain a global picture of the child's performance in a non-structured manner. Penso (1987) considered that subjective comments made by children and their parents constitute important parts of any assessment, particularly when they are used together with the objective evidence elicited by the occupational therapist.

Another common method of assessment is using observations and non-standardised tests. Although they may have specific procedures for presentation, timing and scoring, they have not been standardised on the normal population. Pratt and Allen (1989) suggested that skilled observation requires therapists to use all their senses and record the assessment.

Assessments that are non-standardised are usually flexible in terms of procedures or settings and in the manner in which they are administered. They are valuable for addressing, in particular, the functional ability of the child, the qualitative aspects of a child's performance, and the dynamics of the child and his family. Clancy and Clark (1990) cautioned against assessments that rely on therapists making personal judgements, even when the therapists are experienced. Chow (1989) raised the ethical question of making therapeutic decisions based on questionable assessment data.

Standardised tests are used to identify the child's developmental level as well as his or her general performance, strength and needs. These assessments have been standardised on a large population and have specific methods of presentation, timing and scoring. Clancy and Clark (1990) recommended the use of standardised assessments because they increase the value of the findings. De-Clive Lowe (1996) added that standardised assessments are basically one more potentially useful tool in the repertoire of assessments.

According to a survey (Chia, 1997a), there are eight commonly used standardised tests:

1. Bruininks–Oseretsky Test of Motor Proficiency (Bruninks, 1978).
2. Developmental Test of Visual–Motor Integration (Beery and Buktenica, 1989).
3. Goodenough–Harris Drawing Test (Goodenough and Harris, 1963).
4. Miller Assessment for Pre Schoolers (MAP) (Miller, 1988).
5. Developmental Test of Visual Perception (2nd edn, DTVP-2) (Hammill et al., 1993).
6. Motor Free Visual Perception Test (Revised) (Colarusso and Hammill, 1995b).
7. Movement Assessment Battery for Children (Henderson and Sugden, 1992).
8. Test of Visual Perceptual Skills (Gardner, 1982).

Despite the increasing usage of standardised tests, a number of concerns have been raised by occupational therapists (Chia, 1997a). Some occupational therapists felt that they needed more training in the selection, implementation and interpretation of tests, as well as in understanding the psychometric properties of the assessments. Most of the tests listed above were standardised on samples that are not representative of the British population. Apart from MAP, none of the tests has been developed by occupational therapists.

The usefulness of any assessments depends on the experience, perceptiveness and clinical judgement of the occupational therapist who administered the assessment. It is, however, essential that the findings made by the occupational therapist can withstand critical analysis from the therapist, the multidisciplinary team and the child's parents. De-Clive Lowe (1996) added:

> Ideally, standardised assessment should be just one part of your continuing clinical relationship with the client so that, in interpreting the numerical results, you are able to form and test hypothesis based on a holistic approach to the client.

A growing focus is the development of a client-centred approach. Sumsion (2000) defined client-centred occupational therapy as 'a partnership between client and the therapist that empowers the client to engage in functional performance and fulfil his or her occupational roles in a variety of environments'. The initial step in client-centred assessment is for the occupational therapist to listen to the client's concerns. The therapist and the client subsequently establish a partnership to enable the achievement of the individual's goals. For some clients, this will be an easy task; for others, the identification or resolution of a problem may be difficult to achieve.

The involvement of clients in the assessment process is fundamental because it:

- recognises the client as the expert on his or her unique problem, enabling the client to be at the centre of any decision-making process;
- encourages autonomy, giving the client a sense of control of him- or herself;
- enables the client to be involved in making decisions about the nature and direction of therapy.

There are, however, barriers to the implementation of client-centred practice, e.g. children with severe cognitive difficulties may not be able to participate fully in the process. These barriers are discussed in Law (1998) and Sumsion (1999).

Relationship

The establishment of a relationship is basically an interaction of the child, his family and the occupational therapist with the principal aim of the latter to assist the former to meet his or her needs. The focus of the relationship is the establishment of trust and exploration of the child's feelings, needs and aspirations within a supportive environment. Hagedorn (1997) remarked that occupational therapy is not 'talking therapy', but it is 'doing therapy'. Consequently, although the establishment of a relationship can be a powerful tool for positive change, the use of occupations should be the focus and structure for continuing interactions between the therapist and the child.

Goal-setting

After the assessment, the next important considerations involve the identification of both long- and short-term goals that are realistic and achievable, and written in measurable terms, so that changes in the child's progress can be easily documented. The child and the parents are involved in identifying and setting long- and short-term goals. Goals are often used interchangeably with aims and objectives. Aims are general statements of the direction of therapy, e.g. to develop independence in self-help skills. Objectives are much more specific than aims, stating in clear terms the precise level of performance to be achieved.

Selection of professional, delineation and application models, and use of occupations

Professional model

According to our observations, many paediatric occupational therapists base their practice on the work of Reed and Sanderson (1983). They suggest that an individual adapts through the use of various occupations. By occupations is meant those activities and tasks that an individual does as part of daily life and that engage his or her time, energy and attention. Such adaptation should be viewed as two directional. Through occupations, an individual may adapt to the environment or the environment may be adapted to the individual. Both provide the means for successful integration that will meet the individual's needs and provide satisfaction. According to Reed and Sanderson (1983), occupations can be divided into three areas – self-maintenance, productivity and leisure – which in turn are made up of three skill components: sensorimotor, cognitive and psychosocial.

Delineation and application models

According to observations made by a group of occupational therapy students (Chia, 1996b), the following models are used either singly or in combination:

- behaviour modification
- Bobath concept
- conductive education
- creative approaches
- perceptual–motor function
- play therapy
- sensory integration
- sensory motor stimulation

In contrast, Howard (2000) found that the following were the models most commonly used in Britain:

- sensory integration
- Bobath concept
- biomechanical model

Occupations

The current trend is for occupational therapists to select appropriate delineation/application models and occupations depending on the needs and interests of the child. Occupations can facilitate change because they enable a child to acquire new skills, develop interests and learn to use time effectively (Bruce and Borg, 1993). The interaction of the occupational therapist, the child and the occupation within a supportive environment is an essential component of the therapeutic process.

Play is the primary occupation of children (Bundy, 1993; Morrison et al., 1996). Bundy describes children's playfulness in terms of three critical elements: intrinsic motivation, internal control and suspension of reality.

Implementation of individual/group therapy

After the assessment, the next step in the occupational therapy process is the organisation, implementation and evaluation of a programme of therapy that is within the domains of occupational therapy. Recent publications from the American Occupational Therapy Association (AOTA, 1994) have recommended occupational therapists to be much more focused on domains of concern which consist of sensorimotor components, including sensory and perceptual processing, neuromuscular abilities and motor skills. Cognitive components underlie the child's ability to perceive, attend to and learn from the environment. Psychosocial skills refer to the child's underlying abilities to interact with others, to cope with new or difficult situations, and to manage his or her behaviours in socially appropriate ways. Performance areas of the child are self-care, play, and school and work activities.

This may involve the child receiving individual therapy or group therapy or advice.

The decision of whether to treat a child individually or in a group is complex. In Lawlor and Henderson's study (1989) of American paediatric occupational therapists, they found that 41 per cent provided individual therapy only and 50 per cent provided combinations of individual and group treatment. The remainder treated groups only or did no direct therapy.

Davies and Gavin's paper (1993), which compared individual and group treatments for pre-school children with developmental delay, found no statistically significant difference between the two methods on a number of assessments. However, they suggest that the results merit closer inspection and further research. Given that estimates suggest that group treatment decreases labour costs by one-third (Trahey, 1991), this makes it the more cost-effective method of treatment. Evidence suggests that, in paediatrics, children with developmental coordination disorder (Howard, 1997) and those receiving sensory integrative therapy (Duncombe and Howe, 1994) are most frequently treated in groups.

According to Penso (1993), occupational therapists tend to work on two basic concepts. In the activity-based approach, the activity in which the child is having difficulty is practised on a regular basis. This approach suggests that continuing practice of a skill may result in the achievement of the skill. Normally, such activities are broken down into smaller steps, each step being taught and practised separately, e.g. if the child has difficulties with undressing, he is taught initially to remove his socks from his toes. The next stage will involve him removing his socks from his ankles, etc. In the function-based approach, the occupational therapist focuses on the underlying functional abilities that are necessary to achieve specific activities, not on the activities themselves, e.g. if the child has difficulties with undressing, he may be involved in pre-dressing activities involving body awareness. This approach suggests that these functions can be taught and generalised into the real-life setting.

Individual therapy

In individual therapy, the child is seen for intensive input on a regular basis. Just how frequent this should be depends on the therapist's judgement and the presenting characteristics of the individual child. Jenkins and Sells' (1984) work found that they could demonstrate no difference in overall outcome for the child depending on the frequency of direct therapy. It would seem that the child needs time to consolidate the intervention and perhaps practise the skills gained in his or her own play or educational settings, before advancing further. Giving parents or teachers guidance on practising a skill introduced during treatment can be valuable to the child.

There is much to be said for individual therapy and some of the advantages include the following:

- It enables the development of a one-to-one therapeutic relationship, which may have benefits over and above that of the therapy alone, in making the child feel valued, supported and understood.
- It gives more time and input to the child who lacks concentration and is easily distractible, for whom the group setting is intolerable.
- It is particularly useful for certain activities such as teaching attention control, and early sensory and perceptual motor skills. Here the child needs to be closely watched and guided in very specific tasks, which require the therapist to give the child his or her undivided attention.

Group therapy

Finlay (1999) considers that the practice of group work in occupational therapy includes elements of both psychotherapy and psychoeducation.

All the groups share the use of 'activity' and a focus on 'occupational performance', i.e. how individuals function in their daily work, leisure and domestic/personal activities. Traditionally, there has been a division of psychotherapeutic from activity-oriented groups, indicating a separation of task and verbal elements. Within occupational therapy, however, most groups can be considered to combine the two aspects. Occupational therapists tend to work in three types of group: those that are predominantly activity based, those that are support based and those that are a mixture of the two. In general terms, activity groups emphasise the task and end-product of the group, whereas support groups value sharing and group process dimensions.

In group therapy, the children are seen together at the same time in a group. The advantages include the following:

• It provides opportunities for interaction, social skills and learning skills, such as taking turns and working together.
• It eases the pressure on children who may find one-to-one interaction too intense.
• It enables a wider range of games and activities to be used.
• It enables the children to practise and generalise skills taught on a one-to-one basis and give them the opportunity to achieve by tackling challenges.

Mosey (1986) considered activity groups as laboratories for learning because they provide opportunities for individuals to try out and practise ways of dealing with others in a relatively safe environment. The importance of belonging to a group and the cohesiveness achieved cannot be overestimated (Falk-Kessler et al., 1991). The development of trust and belonging that the group engenders may be as important to children as it has been proved to be for adults (Yalom, 1985).

Activity groups involve a doing process. The activity helps to focus the groups' attention and provides a structure and organisation that many children need. Howe and Swartzberg (1986) found that, with adults, activity or task groups were more effective than verbal groups at improving social skills, and this is even more likely to be so with children who may have fewer verbal skills.

The size of the group will depend on a number of factors, including the number of staff available and the size of the facilities. Duncombe and Howe (1994) found that six was the most common group size for manageability. They also found that sensory motor groups were the most commonly cited group involving children, and that these tended to be small, closed and long term in nature.

Adaptation of models, occupations and the environment

The environment includes the physical environment, the biopsychological environment and the sociocultural environment (Reed and Sanderson, 1983).

To help children with physical disabilities become more independent, occupational therapists assess for, and may recommend, major adaptations to the environment, e.g. a ramp at school or the provision of a ground-floor bathroom and bedroom at home. Changes such as these may ease the role of the carers. The occupational therapist is also involved in the provision of adapted equipment, such as a spoon or a special chair. Such equipment is widely available and of many different kinds. The experienced therapist will be familiar with what is suitable for particular children and representatives of the manufacturers are available to bring large pieces of equipment to the child's home to assess its comfort, safety and convenience. The therapist may have a stock of smaller equipment for the child to try or this may be available from the local Department of Social Services.

The occupational therapist may also be involved in designing an environment that offers varied opportunities for the child to engage in age-appropriate activities.

Evaluation

Occupational therapists could never function adequately without the combination of knowledge of psychological and medical subjects, of methods of assessment, of social interaction and conditioning, and of various occupations and skills. They must have the capacity to use certain facets of their own personalities in the treatment situation, to evaluate the use of a variety of other interventions and to develop their work on increasingly scientific lines. At the same time, they must not exclude the intuitive approach, which should in turn be analysed, criticised and evaluated.

The evaluation of the service that they provide is becoming increasingly important to occupational therapists. It must be shown to be of a certain standard and the outcomes of treatment measured to show that the service represents value for money.

A good deal has now been written about how to assess the quality of therapy services (Wright and Whittington, 1992; Ellis and Whittington, 1993; Howard, 1994a, 1994b, 1994c) and the occupational therapy manager should have little difficulty in instigating quality measurements of the service. Outcome measures are less well developed. More standardised tests are being produced for use in paediatric therapy services, but there is still some way to go before we can prove that input of occupational therapy treatment definitely produces a measured outcome (Howard, 1997). This is particularly true in paediatrics, where the child's natural growth and development may influence outcomes to a large degree. As more therapists evaluate their services and publish the methods or results, our ability to monitor what we are doing effectively should improve.

A method of service evaluation used successfully by one paediatric occupational therapy department is recorded by Howard and Leeson (1999).

Schooling

The 1981 Education Act was an important landmark. It indicated that children with special educational needs should be identified and that the local education authority (LEA) would have the responsibility of preparing a statement of those needs and how they were to be met.

Anyone concerned about some aspect of the child's education can suggest that a child may need statementing. Around 50 per cent of statements are because of medical conditions and such children tend already to be known to the health services.

A meeting is called where all concerned with the child, including the parents, report on his or her progress, level of development or physical state, for example. An educational psychologist, as a representative of the LEA, is usually present.

A child with a severe disability may start school at 2 years of age, so the statementing process begins early. The recommended time to prepare a statement is 6 months, but in many cases it is longer.

All those involved with the child prepare a document stating their present involvement and what their continuing intervention will be.

Parents then see the statement and have a set time to respond to it by agreeing or disagreeing that it meets their child's needs. Appeal can be made to a local panel set up by the LEA if the parents disagree.

When all parties agree, the recommendations can be instituted and the statement produced; this should be reviewed annually for changes. It is mandatory to review it when the child is 14 years old (under the Disabled Persons Act 1986) in order to plan for the child's future after the age of 16.

The Audit Commission of 1990 found that statementing was not being carried out as efficiently as it might be, and so it made recommendations on ways of overcoming these difficulties. This process was further addressed in the 1993 Education Act.

A new code of practice, which was enforced from 1 September 1994, made statementing into a five-stage process: stages 1–3 are school based, and 4 and 5 are the shared responsibility of the school and LEA.

Stage 1: the child is identified as having a problem of any kind. Each school has a special education needs coordinator (SENCO) who works closely with the child in the classroom, and parents are consulted. The child is monitored and reviewed.

Stage 2: if the child is still not progressing, an individual education plan is formulated. The SENCO works alongside the child's teacher.

Stage 3: if there is still a problem, specialists from outside the school (e.g. occupational therapists) are called in when school cannot meet the child's need unaided. Strategies for the classroom setting are drawn up and are incorporated into the individual education plan.

Stage 4: if the problem is still not solved, the LEA considers carrying out a statutory assessment. There is now a set timetable for this:
- 6 weeks – considering whether a statement is necessary
- 10 weeks – making the assessment
- 2 weeks – drafting the proposed statement or note in lieu
- 8 weeks – finalising the statement
- total = 26 weeks.

Stage 5: the LEA issues the statement, with arrangements to monitor and review the position. If a note in lieu is issued, it means that the LEA has considered the statement and has decided not to issue it, but rather suggests that the child's needs can be met in school.

Parental choice

Parents should have a choice about where their child goes to school under this system. Ideally this should be where other children in the neighbourhood go. Realistically, however, severely physically handicapped children have to go to a mainstream school that has been specially adapted because financially the LEA cannot adapt every school.

Benefits of mainstream versus special schools

The child may have limited experiences at a special school and may gain in self-confidence and independence in a mainstream one. There is also the opportunity to have a more varied social life with non-disabled friends.

However, the special school offers smaller classes and experienced staff, familiar with the impact of the disability, who can draw up and implement individual programmes of work. In addition, there is usually more intensive therapy available. Hickling (2000) pointed out that, although inclusion allows children to attend their local mainstream schools, therapists may have only one child at each of the schools in the area. Consequently, the intensity of therapy that each child receives may be reduced because the therapist may experience practical difficulties in visiting the children in all the schools. The child who attends a special school with children of similar needs had a therapist on site with a high level of therapeutic input.

Education after the age of 16

Pupils with severe learning difficulties may remain in school until they are 19, usually in a 'leavers unit' where the accent is on preparation for independent living.

After 19 they may attend adult training centres; there is usually one in each local authority (LA) which can cater for those with very high dependency.

In the case of physically handicapped pupils, at least one sixth-form college in each LA is adapted for those with mobility or other problems. The student may then progress on to a job, another course or university, for example.

For those with moderate learning difficulties there may be life skills courses at the local college of further education, which gives the students help with reading and writing, form filling, cookery and budgeting, for 2–3 years. After this some may get jobs, but many are unemployed.

For young people with emotional or behavioural difficulties or autism, the ideal is supportive housing with structured activity and further learning outside the home.

In practice many return to their family.

Once people leave school or reach 19, they are no longer the responsibility of hospital paediatric units.

The role of the occupational therapist, in addition to therapy, is particularly important in schools that have not had disabled pupils before.

- Explain the child's condition and how it affects his or her learning.
- Reassure parents and teachers that the child will be able to cope in the school.
- Provide equipment and plan any necessary adaptations to the environment.
- Train non-teaching assistants to help with the child.
- Review and monitor the child's progress.

Conclusion

In this chapter, the process of occupational therapy with children who have disabilities has been outlined. The basic philosophy for practice, the current trends in assessment and models used, and some of the issues that impinge on the practice of occupational therapy have been described.

Part II
Review of Application
Models

Chapter 2
Behavioural approaches (or acquisitional frame of reference)

CHIA SWEE HONG AND CHRISTINE PECK

According to Royeen and Duncan (1999), occupational therapists' use of the acquisitional frame of reference flourished in the late 1960s and early 1970s. Mosey (1986) described the acquisitional frame of reference as the linking of learning theories prominent at this time, focusing on the mastery of specific skills required for optimal performance within the environment. Intervention is provided with this focus in mind, and activities given solely for the purpose of acquiring specific skills. Mastery of each skill (or subskill within an activity) is the primary goal.

Theoretical basis

The behavioural approach is based on the theory of operant learning (Atkinson et al., 1990) and is complex yet logical in application. Its use requires acceptance of the view that behaviours (both good and challenging) are learned and that consequently manipulating the learning process can change behaviours.

Operant learning is one of two main types of conditioned learning, the other being classical conditioning/learning. Classical conditioning occurs when an association is formed between a conditioned stimulus (i.e. one that has no previous connection with the response) and an existing behaviour (unconditioned response) that can already be elicited by another stimulus (unconditioned stimulus). By repeated association, the conditioned stimulus becomes linked with the unconditioned response, and can produce a response that is very similar, if not identical, to the original unconditioned response; this new learned response is called a conditioned response. This process is clearly seen through Pavlov's experiments with dogs (Atkinson et al., 1990). Pavlov observed that dogs salivated at the sight and smell of food (unconditioned response) and, by associating a

19

bell (conditioned stimulus) with the delivery of food, he was able to produce salivation to the sound of the bell alone (conditioned response). Both the unconditioned and conditioned stimuli produced the same response.

Operant conditioning is similar in some ways to classical conditioning, but it changes behaviours by reinforcing or rewarding desired behaviours after they have occurred. Classical conditioning elicits certain behaviours in response to a presented stimulus; operant conditioning does not require any stimulus to be present to produce the desired behaviour, but relies on the subsequent reinforcement/reward to teach new responses (e.g. a dog salivates in response to food, but does not usually beg for it). Skinner (cited in Atkinson et al., 1990) demonstrated operant learning with rats kept in a box that was completely empty apart from a lever with a food dish beneath it. In the process of wandering around the box, the rats would occasionally press the lever, causing a pellet of food to drop into the food tray. The lever-pressing behaviour was reinforced by the food and gradually the rats learned to press the lever specifically to get food.

In daily life, the two types of learning usually occur concurrently, but in formal learning situations they are often separated. Operant learning is particularly useful in solving specific learning or behavioural problems because change occurs through the positive manipulation of interaction and environment and the behavioural approach makes full use of this as a teaching technique. The behavioural approach has two main principles:

1. The reaction to any behaviour determines the likelihood that behaviour is repeated.
2. Behaviour is defined as anything that can be seen/perceived, described and measured.

Behaviours can be divided into challenging behaviours and skill-related behaviours. Challenging behaviours usually refer to previously learned inappropriate behaviours, whereas skill-related behaviours usually refer to performance areas where the child needs to progress developmentally. Examples of challenging behaviours might be physical aggression, screaming or running away, but would not be frustration, anger or boredom. Challenging behaviours associated with frustration, anger or boredom can indeed occur, but only the physical manifestation of such feelings can be defined as 'behaviour' in this context, e.g. boredom could be measured only subjectively but verbal abuse, self-harm or falling asleep (which may be symptomatic of boredom) can be seen/perceived, measured and described more objectively. Examples of skill-related behaviours are usually functional, e.g. manual dexterity, eating and drinking, or dressing.

Assessment and intervention techniques

The environment

The environment in which the intervention takes place is crucial to the success of this approach, and behaviours must always be considered in the context of the environments in which they occur. There is little point in using an intensive training programme for any child if the general environment in which the child lives and works restricts opportunities to use and practise the skills being taught. Equally, it is also pointless to use a specific training approach if reorganising or changing the environment might obtain the same results. Many inappropriate behaviours first develop in response to inadequate environments and, although the behavioural approach can be very successful in reducing or eliminating inappropriate behaviours, the best approach (if possible) is to work to prevent their initial development. The ideal environment is one that prompts and reinforces appropriate responses and behaviours, and offers varied opportunities for the child to engage in acceptable and appropriate activities. The environment should also be stimulating and interesting, and actively encourage children to initiate and explore. Achieving an ideal environment is made easier when living and working groups are small.

Teaching areas may need to be more specifically structured to allow staff to alter the arrangement of resources to meet differing needs. Generally, the more able the child, the more visual stimuli can be included in a teaching room, but a child whose concentration is poor initially benefits from being taught in a small, functional area. When skills have developed in specific settings, the environment then needs to be changed to allow the child to tolerate progressively more stimulating environments and ultimately cope with any situation.

Observing behaviours

Detailed observation of behaviour is most commonly found in relation to the incidence/frequency of challenging behaviours, whereas information about functional problems tends to be gathered by planned assessment. However, the principles of observation apply to both types of observation scenario.

Once behaviour has been identified as needing intervention, it must be precisely defined so that information about its characteristics and frequency can be gathered. Exceptions to this may occur when there is disagreement about the particular nature and/or antecedents of a problem behaviour. In this situation, initial observations should be gathered on a chart in which each individual records details of the problem in their own words; this then becomes the basis for a discussion about the behaviour and how to manage it. Once agreement is reached about the way forward, precise definitions can be used to observe and record a baseline of frequency and/or severity.

When a behaviour has been defined, the data collected from observation are useful only if there is a high level of consistency in those responsible for recording it. It is possible to measure consistency and this is called inter-rater reliability. Generally, the more detailed the description, the better the inter-rater reliability, but detail should always be balanced against brevity in order to make recording charts as effective as possible. The easiest method of checking inter-rater reliability is to ask several people to watch a video or observe a demonstrated behaviour, and then ask them to fill in a record chart using the initial definition of a behaviour. An agreement of more than 85 per cent is usually seen as satisfactory, but if there is less than 85 per cent agreement the definition of the behaviour to be observed needs to be more accurately described. For example, the definition 'verbally abusive' would probably lead to less than 85 per cent accuracy, whereas 'verbally abusive, i.e. swears, verbally threatens and/or shouts abuse for more than 10 seconds' is likely to get a higher level of inter-rater reliability.

Once the behaviour has been adequately defined, and inter-rater reliability established, the method of gathering the information must be decided. Usually the more discretely the information is gathered, the more accurate it is likely to be; observations that require written recording are always obvious, but more discrete recording methods are available, e.g. using wrist counters, body microphones or even micro-surveillance cameras, if recording can be based on numerical rather than descriptive information. There are various methods of gathering information, some of which are described below.

Continuous recording

This involves recording everything a child does within a specific period of time, which in practice is very difficult to carry out. Videotaping evidence is not the main problem, although that in itself requires a commitment of time and resources; the main cost to this type of observation is the time needed to view and analyse the recorded material. Nevertheless, continuous recording can be useful in establishing the frequency of a range of behaviours in certain children, as long as staffing levels can be temporarily increased either to observe and record manually, or to analyse the video-taped evidence. One disadvantage is that staff keeping manual records, or even staff who are not comfortable being video-taped, are very easy to spot by both children and visitors, and this can result in 'staged' or 'provoked' incidents. There are also issues about consent for children, staff, relatives and visitors which need to be carefully considered.

Event recording

This involves recording every occurrence of a defined behaviour over a given period of time. This is useful in comparing initial frequency with frequency after a period of intervention, and can usually be managed within normal staffing levels because data can be collected numerically.

Duration recording

Some types of behaviours are not separate events but are continuous, e.g. crying or the time taken to complete a task without help. Duration recording measures when these behaviours occur and the length of time for which they last. This then provides a baseline for measuring whether a problem behaviour is decreasing in duration or a new skill is being completed in less time.

Interval recording

This is used to discover when behaviours occur within a given period. The period (e.g. 10 min or 1 h) is divided into equal intervals (e.g. single minutes or 10-min blocks), and the observer then records whether or not the designated behaviour occurs within that period, irrespective of the number of times that it may have occurred. Again, this requires a high staff input and can be obvious to the children who are being observed.

Time sampling

In time sampling, regular times are chosen (e.g. every 15 min) and at those times the observer records whether or not the defined behaviour is occurring. The defined behaviour can have occurred between these times, but if it is not occurring at the chosen time it is not recorded. This method is economical of staff time and can be useful in toilet training programmes, but may not always yield sufficiently detailed information.

After a suitable period of observation the data are analysed and used to help make decisions about management of the behaviour.

Reinforcement

Reinforcement is the agent of change in the behavioural approach and can be either given to increase the frequency of behaviour, or temporarily withheld or withdrawn to decrease the frequency of behaviour. Giving reinforcement in response to desired behaviour is easily understood but the withholding of reinforcement must be carried out in an environment where, for most of the time, appropriate behaviours are demonstrated and programmes are structured to allow the child a reasonable chance of receiving reward.

Reinforcement need not always involve things that are generally seen as pleasant, enjoyable or purposeful. Unpleasant responses can often become reinforcing because of their association with something pleasurable, e.g. if a child discovers that he can get more attention by being naughty than by being good, then he may eventually (through association) find being told off (or even punished) desirable, and ultimately find this negative interaction reinforcing in itself. Many stereotyped responses can be traced back to inappropriate associations.

Reinforcement can be divided into two types: positive and negative. Positive reinforcement describes any interaction where something pleasurable is given in direct response to a desired behaviour. It is often the preferred method of reinforcement because of the following:

- It makes the teaching environment and the teaching experience more pleasant and motivating.
- The rewarding response always happens after the action has been completed.
- It stops the teaching session from becoming aversive.
- It is much easier to understand and use, which is an important consideration when many people may participate in carrying out programmes.

Negative reinforcement also describes a situation where something pleasurable is given in response to a desired action, but the pleasurable response usually takes the form of escaping from, or stopping, something that is disliked. For example, the positive reinforcement for making eye contact could be a cuddle or a drink or something else liked by the child; in negative reinforcement the child would have to work in the presence of something they disliked (e.g. loud noises) and then make eye contact in order for the noise to be switched off. Another name for negative reinforcement is escape training, because it teaches children to carry out certain actions in order to escape into a more preferred activity (Premack's principle). Negative reinforcement provides much more control over the learning situation, but it equally requires much more specific use.

Premack's principle is often used automatically in training activities because it involves a commonsense approach to motivation. Basically, it says that individuals will carry out activities that are not particularly attractive to them in order to gain access to more pleasurable activities. So, a child who must finish his or her homework (a less preferred activity) before watching television or meeting friends (a more preferred activity) will probably produce more work than a child who watches television or meets his or her friends before doing his or her homework.

Reinforcers are actual items, events or responses that are pleasurable and rewarding. Reinforcers can be classified in various ways but the most usual are shown below.

Primary reinforcers

These are things that satisfy basic human needs, e.g. food and drink. They are the most immediately effective form of reinforcer because their value does not have to be taught, and because the giving of food and drink is a regular event. They are particularly useful for children who have a small range of enjoyed activities or events. Physical contact can also be seen as a primary reinforcer.

Secondary reinforcers

This type of reinforcer has no value in itself and cannot satisfy basic needs but the reinforcers acquire value through their association with more pleasurable items, i.e. they are conditioned reinforcers. For example, tokens or money gain value because they can either be used to purchase desired items or lead to desired social interaction. This type of reinforcer can be very effective, although the value often has to be taught by pairing the secondary reinforcer with a primary reinforcer, followed by the fading out of the latter.

Social reinforcers

These reinforcers require the highest conceptual ability because their value depends on an understanding of abstract ideas and social values. Like secondary reinforcers, they are conditioned reinforcers. Verbal praise is the most common reinforcer, and is the one reinforcer that should be used alongside all others. The ultimate goal of using reinforcement is to teach behaviour and then maintain it with the minimum support; verbal praise is the best medium of maintaining previously learned behaviours. Also, by pairing verbal praise with an existing reinforcer, verbal praise becomes a conditioned reinforcer. Other types of social reinforcer, e.g. respect or compliments, rely on the child wishing to be seen positively by others.

Variety is essential when choosing reinforcers for training purposes, because repetitive use of one or two reinforcers can actually work against the training goals as a result of the boredom or satiation that is created. This is particularly true when using food and drink as reinforcers; size of reinforcer is also important. Primary reinforcers, i.e. food and drink, should have marked texture and/or taste, and should be given in small quantities that can be quickly consumed. As a guide, pieces of food should be approximately the size of a raisin and drinks given at approximately 5 ml at a time. These amounts may be small, but if used repeatedly during a training session, the amount of food or drink taken can mount up, and reinforcers should whet the appetite for more, not satiate it!

Secondary reinforcers should be measured in terms of number or access time. If the reinforcer is access to a preferred activity, then the reinforcer needs to be measured in time; if the reinforcer is money or tokens, then it is easy to measure the reward numerically. As social reinforcers reflect a child's desire to be part of a social group, no firm guidelines can be given, except that the size of the reinforcer should avoid over-praising or under-praising expected levels of behaviour.

When selecting reinforcers, information can be gathered by talking to people who know the child, by testing the child's reactions to various reinforcers, or by measuring the difference various reinforcers make to the performance of an existing skill. The administration of reinforcers needs to be done very carefully to avoid reinforcing the wrong behaviours. A reinforcer must therefore be given:

• Clearly, i.e. its value/significance must be obvious to the child.
• Immediately, i.e. it must occur directly after the desired behaviour.
• Contingently, i.e. it must be given only for the complete desired behaviour.
• Consistently, i.e. it must be given every time the desired behaviour occurs.

If reinforcers are administered poorly, other less desirable behaviours may be encouraged, e.g. if a child is reinforced correctly every time a Makaton sign is copied, signing skills are likely to develop, but if between demonstrating the sign and receiving the reinforcement the child screams, then screaming will be reinforced, and probably increase in frequency.

Initially, reinforcement should be given each time the desired behaviour occurs, but once learning has taken place this level of reinforcement should be reduced. Stopping all reinforcement immediately is not effective, because the original behaviour reappears relatively quickly (although this is more usual with challenging behaviours than with skill-related behaviours). The frequency of reinforcement is gradually reduced/faded out; initially this might mean reinforcing every other occurrence of the defined behaviour, then every third occurrence, and so on, and would eventually lead to a random frequency of reinforcement. By making the frequency of the maintenance reinforcement variable, the child is unsure of when reinforcement will be forthcoming and, as long as a reasonable level of reinforcement is maintained, the child will continue to be motivated by the possibility of a reward. If a combination of reinforcers is used, the primary and/or secondary reinforcers should be faded out completely before making verbal praise random.

Intervention techniques

Skill building

In the behavioural approach, specific techniques are often necessary to teach new skills. Generally, most skill-building techniques use positive reinforcement, whereas many of the intervention techniques for behaviour management use negative reinforcement. Very few of the techniques described below are used individually, and most can be carried out either within formal teaching programmes or as part of an informal management approach.

Modelling

Modelling teaches new behaviours by prompting the child to copy and is therefore also called imitation. The therapist modelling the new skills needs to be someone as much like the child as possible, or someone who is particularly liked or respected by the child. Ideally, the model should demonstrate the desired behaviour while another person leads the teaching and prompts the child, but, if this is not possible, then good results can be obtained by positively reinforcing other children who model desired behaviours in front of the child being taught.

Children must be able to perceive the modelled behaviour accurately, and be able to achieve or reproduce it. This means that the child must be able to concentrate for appropriate periods of time and be able to imitate. Individuals who find it hard to imitate may initially respond better to a combination of modelling and shaping.

In specific programmes, the child sits or stands opposite or next to the model. The model demonstrates part or all of the task, and asks the child to copy the action; if the child can independently copy the action, reinforcement is given straight away, but, if the child needs help, the desired action is prompted before reinforcement is given. General use of modelling is based on the assumption that children will copy the behaviours of people with whom they work. This means that staff need to be conscious of the importance of modelling desirable attributes in appearance, attitude to work and attitude to others, and manners and interactions. It also implies that modelling should be a continual, but informal, training process.

Prompting

Prompting is a frequently used technique, and one that is common in daily life. It encourages children to perform actions by using various levels of support and encouragement. There are three types of prompts.

Physical prompts

This is physical guidance given in varying degrees to help the child complete an action. Physical prompts may be used, for example, to help encourage feeding or any other functional activity, and can vary from a full physical prompt to a very slight touch. Physical prompts are even more effective when used in combination with verbal and/or gestural prompts.

Gestural prompts

This type of prompt uses gesture to indicate a course of action. A gestural prompt should mimic the movement required, e.g. pointing to a ball and then pointing to the person to whom it should be given, and to be really effective they should be used together with verbal prompts.

Verbal prompts

A verbal prompt is simply a reminder to do something that includes relevant information, yet remains concise and succinct. Verbal prompts are often identical to key phrases used in teaching programmes, e.g. 'Give the ball to Tom', and they should always be paired with gestural and/or physical prompts.

Prompting as a single technique is most successful in teaching simple skills with one- or two-component parts. However, it can be used in combination with other teaching techniques to encourage a wide variety of skills. Once a new behaviour has been established, the amount of prompting given should be reduced in a process known as fading. However, prompts need to be faded out carefully: if faded too quickly, the child may miss the regular reinforcement and fail to complete the task, but if faded out too slowly, the child could become over-dependent on the reinforcers used. Practically, the last part of any prompt should be faded first.

There are two methods of fading physical prompts. First, support can be reduced throughout the whole task (while maintaining constant physical contact), by moving the point of prompt further away from the original position, e.g. in a feeding programme, initially a full hand prompt may be used but, as the child progresses, the position of this prompt may change to a half-hand prompt, then over to the wrist and the forearm, before finally fading out completely. The second type of fading out involves maintaining the same prompt position throughout the task, but breaking the physical contact at certain points. Using feeding again as an example, the whole task would be prompted by a full hand prompt, although the prompt would gradually be removed for parts of the process. Initially this might mean removing the prompt during the downward (gravity-assisted) movement from mouth to bowl, and then replacing it once the cutlery was in the bowl; gradually more of the task would be completed with the prompt removed, until eventually the child could carry out the whole task. The choice between the two types of fading depends on the child and on the task. Gestural prompts are usually faded by reducing the size and quality of the gestures, whereas verbal prompts are usually only reduced in frequency.

Chaining

Chaining is a very powerful teaching technique because it allows complex skills to be broken down into component parts, and constantly reinforces previously learned elements. Prompting is also an essential element in any chaining programme. To use chaining, the task first has to be broken down into its component parts with the size, range and difficulty of each part varying according to the needs of the child. After this stage, two methods of teaching are available – forward and backward chaining.

Forward chaining takes the component parts of the task and begins by teaching the first stage. Once the first stage has been learned, the second stage is introduced and is practised immediately after the first stage; the same procedure happens with each subsequent component until the whole task has been taught. Backward chaining takes the same task, and teaches the last stage first. Once this part has been learned, the previous stage is introduced and practised before the learned component is completed; this process is repeated until the whole task has been taught. So, in a four-part task where 1 is the first stage and 4 is the last stage, the difference in teaching order between the two types of chaining could be expressed as:

Forward   = 1 ... 1 + 2 ... 1 + 2 + 3 ... 1 + 2 + 3 + 4
Backward = 4 ... 3 + 4 ... 2 + 3 + 4 ... 1 + 2 + 3 + 4

Both types of chaining can be effective, but the differences between them make each of them suitable for teaching different skills. In both types of chaining reinforcement occurs at the end of the task, but in forward chaining there is always a point between the previously learned stage and the new stage at which reinforcement is currently being given. In effect, this means that a child will always reach a point where further work is required to achieve the same level of reinforcement. Backward chaining, however, places the newly introduced stage in front of previously learned stage(s), so that, once the child has worked through a new component, the remainder of the task is instantly recognisable as the start of a procedure that leads to reinforcement. Reinforcement is always given at the same point (i.e. on completion of the activity), which not only underlines important concepts, but also makes giving reinforcement easier (giving reinforcement in forward chaining can fragment the task). Backward chaining also allows the child to take over from the trainer, thus reinforcing independence, whereas, in forward chaining, the trainer ultimately has to intervene and prompt new skills, which can emphasise dependence. Backward chaining is consequently the method of first choice.

Once a behaviour or skill is firmly established, the ability to maintain the skill becomes intrinsically reinforced. In other words, performing the behaviour or skill correctly in and by itself becomes self-reinforcing.

Behaviour management

The best way to reduce problem behaviours is to eliminate the conditions that encourage them. All intervention techniques assume that problem behaviours have developed because they have been inappropriately or inadvertently reinforced, and these techniques therefore describe methods of ensuring that access to whatever is reinforcing behaviour is strictly controlled. Many techniques assume that attention is the reinforcing agent, and withhold that attention until appropriate behaviours are demonstrated. With any techniques of this kind, withdrawing or withholding attention inevitably makes the frequency of the behaviour increase, as the child repeatedly tries to gain attention through previously successful methods. With any intervention technique that is successfully used, problem behaviours may worsen for a few weeks, after which there should be a noticeable reduction in the level of the problem. If, however, the intervention programme is stopped during the period of worsening behaviour, there is a real possibility that the child will maintain the worsened level of behaviour permanently. This is an important factor to consider when using intervention techniques such as extinction, reinforcement of incompatible behaviours, restitution and over-correction, because all staff must be willing and able to cope with the temporary increase in problem behaviour until improvement occurs. Records need to be kept to chart progress and assess the degree of change that has occurred in relation to the use of any intervention technique. Record sheets should provide brief but informative details about the administration of any programmes.

It is always advisable to consult clinical psychologists for management of challenging behaviours.

Relationship between the application model and occupational therapy

Early papers commented on the close relationship between the behavioural approach and the teaching role of occupational therapy. As Ethridge (1970) commented, this can often make therapists complacent, thinking that they already know enough about the behavioural approach to be expertly carrying it out in their routine practice, whereas in reality they have just enough knowledge to apply the approach only in general terms. Such over-confidence can lead to very poorly applied teaching methodologies and poor outcomes, and inevitably to a poor evaluation of the value of the behavioural approach.

A common criticism of the behavioural approach is that it deals with small, specific behaviours and fails to tackle the major issues. In fact, this is a complete misconception and the behavioural approach is an excellent vehicle for making major changes in any type of behaviour. The reasons for the misperception probably lie in the fact that the behavioural approach does not usually set out to change major behaviours in a single move, because by its very nature it prefers to analyse major behaviours into component parts and then deal with each component progressively. In an ideal world, each child would respond quickly and positively to each component part of the behavioural intervention, but in the real world change often takes longer than the therapist and family expect. It is easy to lose sight of the original goal or overall behaviour to be changed; this is even more common if the therapists involved in setting up the original programme leave and their successors do not have access to full records of why and how the programme was started. Ethridge (1970) supports this view, when commenting that gains achieved quickly are usually attributed to miracles or prayer, whereas gains achieved through the application of science are usually made up of small discrete steps towards the end goal.

Chia (1978) found the following similarities between occupational therapy and behaviour modification techniques:

- Undertaking assessments;
- Formulating the baseline before intervention;
- Analysing and breaking tasks down into small manageable steps in order to help the child to succeed.

There are, however, aspects of behaviour modification techniques that may prove useful to occupational therapists:

- Importance of objective assessments
- Emphasis on recording
- Systematic method of teaching a skill
- Systematic reinforcement.

Royeen and Duncan (1999) concluded that many aspects of the behavioural approach are an integral part of occupational therapy, particularly in the way in which therapists use both positive and negative reinforcement automatically to help a child progress appropriately. They felt that the behavioural approach fitted well as both a background skill for the occupational therapist, and an area where particular expertise can be acquired and applied.

Review of practice

As a therapeutic strategy, behaviour modification is thoroughly investigated and well supported in the literature, e.g. Yule and Carr (1990). In the field of learning disability, this approach forms the core of much systematic instruction, particularly in teaching self-care skills to individuals with profoundly multiple disabilities (Gates, 1997). Some researchers have documented successful teaching of adaptive behaviour skills in individuals with learning disabilities: eating (Matson et al., 1980), grooming (Vollmer et al., 1992), communications skills (Wacker et al., 1990), social skills (Bradlyn et al., 1983) and play skills (Wehman et al., 1976) have all been studied.

The behavioural approach has critics who see it as manipulative and coercive. Stein and Cutler (1998) support the view that the approach itself is neither good nor bad, but simply a tool or method with potential to help children to become more independent and learn new skills.

The basic theory of the behavioural approach is common in daily life, and it is easy to forget that the behavioural approach is specifically used only with children who have problems in achieving behavioural change in daily life. Bruce and Borg (1993) describe how behaviourism has influenced the use of reinforcement and modelling in learning situations, and see it as an approach that has inspired others to investigate the processes of cognition and social learning. However, they also argue that therapists should balance the use of the behavioural approach with the need to encourage creativity and curiosity, and caution about the use of any approach to the extent that a child is deprived of access to the normal, fun activities of growing up.

This last point is supported by Jones (1995) who suggests that, where the behavioural approach is used to teach skills, it is difficult to ensure continuity of antecedents and consequences from one situation to another because the complex web of norms, values and expectations can be truly experienced only in the natural setting.

The therapist's responsibilities in using the behavioural approach are considerable. Marvin (1999) particularly draws attention to the way in which the precision and specificity of the behavioural approach can create an active–passive relationship between the therapist and child. This is particularly valid with very disabled children, where the therapist is initiating a set of circumstances for the benefit of the child. Marvin cautions that this can stifle any possibility of the therapist responding spontaneously to an unexpected (but positive) action or communication initiated by the child. Ware (1996) also supports this point. Marvin suggests adapting the approach so that the child is more of an equal partner, and is able to develop through taking control.

This adapted approach is supported by Smith (1991), who refers to research that indicates that the best results are achieved through a mixture of methods. This links to advice from McCue (1993) that any intervention using the behavioural approach should be based on a combination of factors, including the individual needs and wishes of the child.

The appropriateness of what is taught is highlighted by Lindsay and Michie (1995). They are particularly concerned that therapists should ensure that the skills taught are age and situation appropriate, citing specifically social interaction, training, leisure and work skills.

The needs of the individual are highlighted in a different way in MacKay (1993), who identifies difficulties in both matching reinforcers to goals and fading out those reinforcers once the child has achieved the goal. MacKay advises that building individual control into the fading-out process is important if the child is to gain sufficient reinforcement from the satisfaction of having achieved something, and avoid the child being reliant on reinforcement provided by others.

The meaning of the term 'challenging' is interpreted in different ways. Some definitions are broad in scope whereas others are narrower, specifying danger to self or others. According to Swain et al. (1999), the whole issue of challenging behaviour is one of controversy rather than answers, and their definition includes behavioural, humanistic and social viewpoints. Many more recent approaches to challenging behaviours emanate in general terms from a humanistic perspective. This viewpoint, in comparison to behavioural approaches, focuses on the person as a unique and valued individual rather than the source of a problem, and the meaning and behaviour rather than behaviour itself. Gentle Teaching

(McGee et al., 1987; McGee, 1992) emphasises a humanising and respectful positive approach towards individuals with severe learning difficulties. Specific techniques include ignoring challenging behaviour, redirecting the person with learning difficulties to another activity, and rewarding the person by simply remaining with them rather than rejecting them. Cheseldine (1991) also preferred to focus on teaching the person rather than changing the behaviour, and saw the teaching process as one of mutual changes in which teachers spend as much time analysing their own values as those of the people they are teaching.

Challenging behaviours are produced by individuals with very severe learning disability as a response to the forces that are affecting their lives. Hewett (1998) suggests a stance of understanding as the best starting point in terms of the attitudes, i.e. of viewing the behaviours that the child produces as a natural, normal response. His model for the living and working atmosphere in which we place children and adults who present challenging behaviours includes consideration of the individual's feelings and attitudes, and of what quality of life is like from that person's point of view. The moral and ethical implications of using strategies involving unpleasant circumstances and reinforcers have been dealt with by Gates (1997), and in a number of publications by the British Institute of Mental Handicap (1981) and by Presland (1989).

Conclusion

The success of the behavioural approach lies in the consistency with which it is used by everyone involved. Terminology and techniques need to be understood to avoid confusion, and clear and relevant records need to be kept. The behavioural approach can be rejected as having failed to work when in fact its principles have been misunderstood and misapplied. The most common problems are:

- Using a technique incorrectly
- Using, but not understanding the reasons behind, a technique
- Misunderstanding of the components of each technique
- Inappropriate use of techniques
- Inadequate teaching programmes
- Fear or reservations about using techniques.

Many people think that the behavioural approach can be used only to change challenging behaviours, but do not also see its application as a method of teaching new skills. In fact the behavioural approach is used more frequently to teach new skills than it is to reduce challenging behaviours.

Chapter 3
The Bobath concept

CAROLYN SIMMONS CARLSSON

The Bobath/neurodevelopmental treatment (Bobath/NDT) approach is respected and widely used in the therapeutic world by physiotherapists, occupational therapists and speech–language therapists (Sasad, 1998; Higgins, 1999). Berta Bobath's concept, or rather original philosophy, has remained constant for more than 50 years. Despite this, however, the practice model has not remained stagnant. Instead it has evolved and changed over the years to reflect and integrate new concepts and theoretical thinking. For instance, the way constructs related to theory and treatment are explained today reflects emerging knowledge of neurophysiology and nervous system functioning, as well as theories of motor control and learning (Bryce, 1991; Mayston, 1992, 2000a, 2000b, 2001; Bobath Centre, 1997; Mayston et al., 1997; Bly, 2000). The importance of the child's active participation in meaningful occupation has become a central focus of treatment. The way that many of the tools of treatment are applied in practice has evolved to reflect advances in theoretical thinking, as well as the changes seen in clinical practice with client groups. Yet, in essence, the Bobath concept continues to be a 'way of thinking' based on a problem-solving approach. It is an approach to the treatment and management of children with cerebral palsy (CP) and allied neurological conditions, which equally emphasises the importance of the therapist's skills of observation and analysis (Bryce, 1991; Mayston, 1992), the importance of working towards functional goals, the importance of the child's parents and caregivers in intervention (Bobath Centre, 1997), and the importance of the contexts that enfold each individual child's life (Mayston, 2001).

Historical and current view of the Bobath concept

The Bobath concept was pioneered by the late Berta Bobath, a physiotherapist and remedial gymnast, in close association with her husband

Dr Karel Bobath, a physician and psychiatrist. Bobath believed that it was possible to achieve change in the child with CP during a point in time when there was little realisation, or acceptance, that spasticity/hypertonus had the potential to be changed. Through astute observation and sensitive handling skills, Bobath's clinical experimentation led to the discovery that abnormal degrees of postural (muscle) tone, which resulted in abnormal patterns of posture and movement, could be influenced and modified through the use of specialised techniques of handling. Furthermore, the change achieved in tonus, and subsequently patterns of movement, in turn assisted the client to move in a 'more normal' and thereby more functional way, despite the presence of spasticity. This, in turn, allowed the possibility for improved postural alignment and postural control – improved quality of functional movement. Bobath found that the risk of contracture, asymmetry and deformity could also be influenced/ minimised by the handling techniques. These postulates formed some of the cornerstones of the concept. Dr Bobath researched the literature of the time to answer his wife's clinical questions, and together they developed their ideas to apply in the treatment and management of adults with hemiplegia, and children with CP and allied neurological conditions, thus establishing an innovative practice model that continues to be practised worldwide today.

Influences, changes and misconceptions

> Since we began our treatment in 1943 we have been learning constantly, and experience has taught us to change our approach and our emphasis on certain aspects of treatment. However, the basic concept has not changed . . . we have been guided by the child's reactions to our handling . . . improved our knowledge . . . tried to avoid repeating mistakes. We have learned to test the value of a particular technique by the child's response to it, and . . . on the close interplay between child and therapists.
>
> Bobath and Bobath (1984, p. 7)

Dr Bobath drew from 'accepted' bodies of knowledge of the time to form the theoretical constructs to underpin his wife's clinical findings. The neuroscientific data available on nervous system functioning, pathology and normal and abnormal motor control in those days was, however, incomplete and relatively limited, and included: Sherringtonian physiology (classic reflex theory of motor control); Magnus, Schaltenbrand and Weisz's work on normal postural reflex mechanism; and Hughlings Jackson's hierarchical theory of motor control (cited in Bobath Centre, 1997). These patriarchal theories of the pre-1950s have led to much misinterpretation of the concept (Bobath Centre, 1997; Mayston et al., 1997;

Mayston, 2001). Today the Bobath concept is articulated in terms of emerging neurophysiology and theories of motor control and motor learning (Mayston, 2001) in line with other contemporary models of practice.

Bodies of knowledge from different disciplines and theorists have influenced the evolution of the Bobath concept, including: Kabat, Knott and Voss (importance of providing proprioceptive information to build up/regulate tone); Rood and Goff (tactile stimulation techniques) (cited in Bobath Centre, 1997); and Petö (treatment of children with athetosis) (Bobath and Bobath, 1984). Disciplines, such as occupational therapy and speech–language therapy, have contributed greatly to the ongoing development of the concept through interdisciplinary discourse and their teaching on Bobath courses, reflecting the strong interdisciplinary philosophy of the treatment approach. This has enhanced the focus of treatment on a functional task-oriented approach. In the 1970s, 'changes in the understanding of the development of postural control and skill against gravity' (Mayston et al., 1997) led to a review of the perspective of motor development and its application in treatment, in recognition that development did not always proceed in a definite sequence, as stated in the developmental schedules (Bobath and Bobath, 1984). The role of reflexes was de-emphasised in recognition that their presence 'did not explain the patterns of posture and movements observed in the child with CP' (Mayston et al., 1997). The original strict adherence to a cephalocaudal progression in treatment was de-emphasised, in recognition of the reciprocal interacting relationship between proximal–distal and caudocephalocaudal dimensions of development. Recognition of sensorimotor development and its influence on the development of perceptual–cognitive abilities has also intensified in the last decade. The premise of 'preparation for function' has been expanded upon.

Latterly, there has been a strong movement towards acknowledgement and recognition of the role of sensation, in particular the role of feedback and feed-forward mechanisms in postural control (Bly, 1996, 1999; Bobath Centre, 1997; Simmons Carlsson, 1997, 1999a; Schoen and Anderson, 1999). The significance of working towards a meaningful functional goal or outcome and the need for active participation of the child during problem-solving, plus the context in which tasks are practised and performed, have all been integrated as key components of the approach (Mayston, 2000a, 2000b, 2001).

The changed clinical picture of CP that resulted from advances in neonatal technology (see Stanley, 1987; Hagberg et al., 1989, 1993, 1996; Stanley and Watson, 1992) has influenced clinical reasoning and treatment application. The way that handling techniques are explained and applied

(Mayston et al., 1997) has been modified: first, in recognition that the development of surviving extreme low birthweight and pre-term infants, and infants with severe asphyxiation, begins from a 'different point of postural tone and control' (Mayston et al., 1997, p. 2); second, to accommodate the different combinations of hypotonia, hypertonia and secondary weakness now more commonly observed in the CP population; and, third, to increase the emphasis of sensory processing, sensation and perception on postural control (The Bobath Centre, London, 1996; Simmons Carlsson, 1999a, 1999b, 2000).

Theoretical advances in motor control, motor learning, movement science theory and neurophysiology have greatly influenced the Bobath concept, allowing therapists, researchers and educators alike to review and redefine the theoretical underpinnings of the concept (Bly, 2000; Mayston, 2001), and to use/integrate contemporary theories to provide a more evidence-based scaffold for practice. For example, a systems view of the CNS is taken rather than Dr Bobath's original premise based on a hierarchical, reflexive view of the nervous system. The premise that active participation in goal-directed meaningful tasks potentially drives neuroplastic adaptation is recognised. The interaction of the nervous system and the musculoskeletal system, both being equally important for meeting the demands of the environment (internal and external), is highlighted in clinical reasoning and treatment.

Table 3.1 summarises the changes related to the understanding of postural tone and subsequent changes in the way techniques of handling are labelled and described.

Bobath/NDT terminology has proved an ongoing source of misinterpretation. Table 3.1 (Mayston, 2000b, 2001; Mayston, 1998, personal communication) provides a summary of the changes. The term 'inhibition' was first introduced by Bobath to explain tone reduction commensurate with the idea that hypertonus was produced by abnormal tonic reflex activity – 'a view which no longer can be supported' (Mayston, 2001). The use of the term 'inhibition' is also being questioned. In treatment, the Bobath/NDT perspective of inhibition relates to the following: reducing hypertonus, 'loosening' up, adaptation, elongation, mobilisation, preparation for function. This is not the same in physiological terms. Physiologically, inhibition is associated with counteraction of synaptic excitation, a shaping of a firing pattern of action potentials or depression of transmitter release. The term 'facilitation' in treatment means to make possible, to make easier. Physiologically, it is associated with enhancement of synaptic transmission/transmitter release. This is more in keeping with the term 'stimulation' as used in the Bobath concept/NDT (Mayston, 1998, personal communication).

Table 3.1: Summary of the changes related to the understanding of postural tone and subsequent changes in the way techniques of handling are labelled and described

Abnormal postural tone	Handling technique	Aim of use of the technique	Comment
Released tonic reflexes	Reflex inhibiting postures (RIPs) (Bobath and Bobath, 1940s)	Inhibition of tonic reflexes	Static – little or no movement
Abnormal tonic (postural) reflex activity	Reflex inhibiting postures (RIPs) (Bobath and Bobath, 1970s)	Simultaneous inhibition and facilitation (and stimulation)	Emphasis on automatic postural reactions; dynamic nature of handling
Neural (reflex) and non-neural components	Tone influencing patterns (TIPs) (Dr Mayston, 1995 to present)	Inhibition, facilitation, stimulation and biomechanical influence	Influences both the control of posture and task performance

Reprinted with permission by courtesy of Dr Margaret J. Mayston, 1998, The Bobath Centre, London (Mayston, 2001).

The current Bobath/NDT perspective on tone recognises that tone is made up of both neural and non-neural components. Both central *and* peripheral nervous system factors are acknowledged as important in efficient motor task execution. Bobath's early ideas on postural tone focused on released tonic reflexes, such as the tonic labyrinthine reflex, or symmetrical tonic neck reflex (Mayston, 1998, personal communication). Handling techniques of static positioning – termed 'reflex inhibiting postures' (RIPs) – were applied to 'inhibit' these reflexes (Table 3.1) in postures that were the opposite to the pattern of spasticity; however, Bobath found that they were too static. The focus shifted to postural activity, with handling becoming more dynamic to facilitate postural reactions, based on the hypothesis that, if the postural reactions were equivalent to 'more normal' motor coordination, it followed that task performance would become 'more normal' when based on the assumption that voluntary and automatic movements were coordinated in the same way. The terminology changed to reflex inhibiting patterns, which enable simultaneous inhibition/facilitation and stimulation, with the emphasis placed on facilitation.

Currently, Mayston (2000a) states that the Bobath-trained therapist should not claim to inhibit abnormal reflexes, facilitate postural reactions, or categorically prevent the child from moving in ways that will increase abnormal tone. Handling techniques are hypothesised as enabling inhibition, facilitation and stimulation, largely by influencing the biomechanical aspects of postural tone and the term 'tone influencing patterns' (TIPs) reflects this shift in thinking (Mayston, 1995, 1996, 2000b). It is hypothesised that TIPs may have a large effect on the plasticity of muscle, thereby enabling improved alignment for more efficient force production. In treatment, TIPs are more readily adapted to functional activities, and allow the therapist to 'work for optimal length and activity of muscles in a functional context' (Mayston, 2000a).

In addition, Mayston (2000a, 2001) and colleagues (Davies, 1996 – cited in Edwards, 2001; Mayston, 2001) have begun to question and clarify for therapists some of the issues in Bobath/NDT treatment related to 'spasticity'/'hypertonus', and the use of the term 'inhibition'. Therapists 'must divide true spasticity from other elements of hypertonia in order to prescribe appropriate intervention. Spasticity affects the neural component of tone, the non-neural components are secondary to this' (Mayston, personal communication, 5 October 2000). Clinical reasoning must therefore encompass the question of whether the therapist is managing spasticity, hypertonia or both. Dr Bobath's (1984) caveat, 'The Bobath Concept is unfinished. We hope it will continue to grow and develop in the years to come', continues to be followed. Theoretical constructs and application in practice continues to evolve in response to expanding knowledge, theories, understanding and clinical findings (Mayston, 1995). Contemporary bodies of knowledge have helped to clarify and modify the Bobaths' earlier theoretical debate, as well as provide support for the concept (Mayston, 1995, 2001).

Core assumptions and principles

Bobath philosophy encompasses a commonsense, realistic way of seeing the child/young person/adult as a 'whole' entity. Parent and caregiver participation is paramount to ensure realistic and successful carry-over of appropriate handling and functional activities into the daily routines of home, school and/or community environments. The focus is on enhancing the individual child's best possible recovery and potential. According to Mayston (2000a), citing Bobath, the child's potential is that which he is able to do with a little help.

As a practice model, Bobath/NDT is forward looking, working towards not only short-term functional goals, but also long-term functional outcomes, along the individual's life-span continuum, within the individual's given environments. Bobath/NDT therapists are cognisant of the fact that children with CP grow up to be adults. The parent/caregiver (and client) collaboration is therefore vital for long-term intervention planning. The concept advocates an interdisciplinary and/or transdisciplinary (Case-Smith et al., 1996; Dunn, 2000) basis for teamwork, and individualised planning and treatment. Treatment outcomes focus on function, whether to (1) extend skills and improve the quality of functional ability, (2) retain skills and maintain function and/or (3) make management easier and/or possible for parents/caregivers (Mayston et al., 1997). Bobath/NDT lends itself to being combined with other approaches, such as the biomechanical frame of reference, or sensory integration model (Blanche et al., 1995; Farrington and Pruzansky, 1999). Although the concept continues to maintain that 'quality' of movement is desirable, it does not assert this as mandatory nor is it the only focus of intervention; rather 'concern for quality of movement needs to be realistic' (Mayston, 2001).

Figures 3.1 and 3.2 summarise past and current views of the Bobath concept (Mayston et al., 1997). Originally, Bobath explained the development of postural control against gravity in terms of the normal postural reflex mechanism (NPRM) (Figure 3.1). This was based on a hierarchical theory of the nervous system, and handling techniques aimed at addressing postural reflexes and eliciting automatic righting and equilibrium reactions. This caused much misinterpretation, despite Bobath's intention that the word 'reflex' referred to the 'sum of activity occurring in all neural pathways at any stage of the task, whether anticipatory or accompanying the task, to suggest that movement is the result of muscles working together' (Bobath Centre, 1997), not postural reflexes. Reinterpretation of tone (neural and non-neural components) has led to redefining of the NPRM in terms of the normal postural control mechanism (NPCM) (Figure 3.2) and better reflects the modified understanding of the theoretical basis of the concept. Reflexes are not responsible for the control of posture and movement (Mayston et al., 1997).

The Bobath concept is based on the recognition of two factors. First, a lesion of the brain affects an immature, or rather a developing, central nervous system (CNS), leading to delay or arrest of motor development. Second, this results in the presence of abnormal patterns of posture and movement as a consequence of a disordered postural control mechanism – postural tone, reciprocal innervation and variety of movement are all affected to varying degrees and in various combinations. A third factor – associated conditions including sensory–perceptual disorders – historically has always been recognised and acknowledged by Bobath; however, these aspects had not been given as much relevance as they have in the last decade. To summarise so far, the Bobath concept provides a systematic framework for observing and thinking about the abilities and disabilities of the child with CP. It offers a dynamic system for individual analysis and management of the multitude of conditions that each child with CP may face, within the context of occupational performance, performance components and performance contexts. The clinical nature of the framework allows treatment tools and techniques to evolve, based on ongoing clinical findings, and emerging theory and knowledge about neuroplasticity, neurophysiology, motor control and motor learning. These help to guide, modify and support Bobath-based hypotheses and clinical reasoning.

The normal postural control mechanism

Like all other practice models, the Bobath concept is hypothetical in nature (Mayston, 1992) and describes the problems of abnormal postural tone and abnormal coordination in relation to the NPCM, which gives the prerequisites for automatic and voluntary movement. Upper motor neuron (UMN) lesions are hypothesised to cause a disturbance of the NPCM and, as one consequence, abnormal postural tone leading to abnormal patterns of posture and movement may result, as well as disordered reciprocal interaction of muscles and disturbed automatic background activity. The degree and severity will depend on the site and extent of the lesion, the impact of cognitive–perceptual deficits on motor

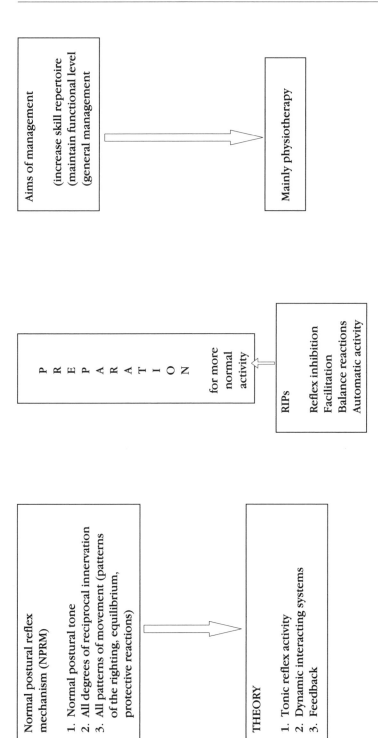

Figure 3.1: Model of the Bobath concept based on clinical practice. (Reprinted with permission by courtesy of Dr Margaret J. Mayston, 1997, The Bobath Centre, London.)

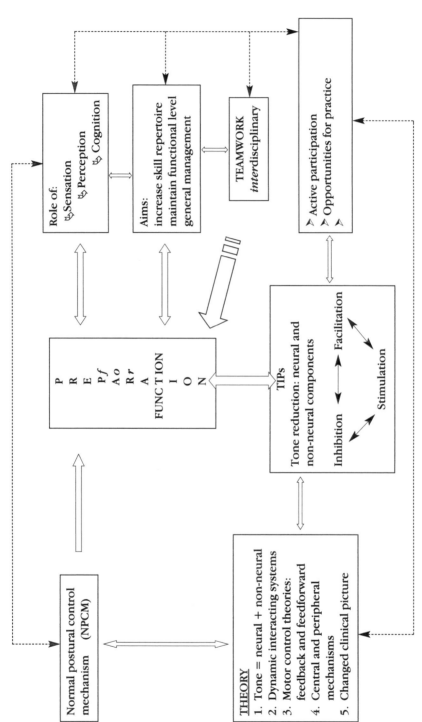

Figure 3.2: Model of the Bobath concept based on clinical practice and emerging theory and knowledge (Mayston et al., 1997, 2000a, 2000b). (Reprinted with permission by courtesy of Dr Margaret J. Mayston, 1997, The Bobath Centre, London, with adaptations.)

control and learning, and the nervous system's potential for plastic adaptation. These factors all impact on functional movement, and thus on functional performance.

The Bobath concept rests on the belief that postural tone underlies the coordination of posture and movement, both normal and abnormal, and that tone may be 'changed' through specialised techniques of handling – tone is changeable, not only in relation to activity and moods, but also in response to handling (Bobath Centre, 2000). In keeping with the current understanding about tone, it is proposed that handling cannot change spasticity when the stiffness is related to velocity-dependent hyperreflexia; however, handling may be the most appropriate and effective intervention strategy to apply when stiffness is related more to muscle weakness and associated changes in viscoelastic properties of muscles, resulting in increased tone/contracture over time. It is the active engagement of the child in 'more optimal and meaningful ways, within the limits of the CNS damage' that leads to the potential reduction of the negative effects of spasticity which, in combination with handling, allows the therapist to teach the child to move more efficiently during functional tasks (Mayston, 2001).

There are three components to the NPCM. The first component addresses the issue of postural tone. To move efficiently and effectively, we need a degree of normal postural tone for maintaining posture and movement. Postural tone needs to be high enough to withstand gravity, yet low enough to allow movement. Postural tone provides the dynamic inter-play between stability with mobility and mobility with stability – in associa-tion with other body systems and structures, e.g. the skeletal system – arousal and the action–perception system, and the functional task and environmental dimensions. Abnormal postural tone may manifest as 'too much stability with not enough movement', as in the case of spasticity/hypertonia, or 'too much mobility and not enough stability', as may be observed in the child who has athetosis or ataxia; alternatively, a combination of both aspects may manifest, as in the case of the premature child with CP who may present with proximal hypotonia, distal hypertonia and flexor spasms at the hips. The Bobath concept refers to postural tone rather than 'muscle tone', to reflect the construct that the CNS activates muscles in groups, or rather patterns of activity/movement. Although the notion of tone itself is a controversial one, the concept currently defines postural tone in keeping with Brooks (1986) (the resistance offered by muscles to continuous stretch), Basmajian and De Luca (1985) (at complete rest a muscle has not lost its tone, even though there is no neuromuscular activity in it), and Kandel et al. (1991) (normal tone can be defined as a slight constant tension of healthy muscles). Neural aspects of tone include reflex activity, level of arousal, and feedback and feed-forward mechanisms. Non-neural aspects include, for example, the passive–elastic properties of muscles, and the length–tension relationship of muscles and range of motion (Bobath Centre, 1997).

The second component of the NPCM relates to the normal reciprocal interactions of muscle groups. This allows for synergic fixation proximally, which in turn allows for distal mobility, e.g. a stable trunk may serve as the point of reference for distal head/limb function, or head control as a basis for selective eye movements. Alternatively, there may be situations where distal points of stability will provide for proximal mobility, e.g. moving the trunk over a weight-bearing arm, or using grasp as a point of fixation/stability for truncal activity. Reciprocal interactions of muscle groups give us our automatic postural adaptations and graded control of agonist and antagonist to give normal co-contraction – timing, grading, force and direction of movements. Disturbed patterns of movement as a result of the disturbance of reciprocal innervation may lead to a limited variety of movement patterns, difficulty in the organisation of movements with movement in more total/stereotypical patterns and reduced selectivity of movement (Bobath Centre, 1997).

The third component of the NPCM relates to all the various movement patterns that are common to humans, which form the background against which all movements take place. Postural background adjustments encompass the many dynamic postural reactions that work together to maintain balance and adjust posture before (feed-forward), during and after (feedback mechanisms) movement, and include the righting reactions, equilibrium reactions and protective reactions. Righting reactions work to assist with orientation in space via visual and vestibular mechanisms, as well as to restore normal alignment after rotation (de-rotation). Equilibrium reactions help to maintain and restore balance during activities. They overlap and work in tandem with righting reactions. Protective reactions form the link between righting and equilibrium reactions, and give the individual a last line of defence when the body is displaced beyond the capabilities of the first two mechanisms (Bobath Centre, 1997).

Understanding the nature of cerebral palsy

Application of the Bobath concept is grounded in therapists' understanding of CP as a neurodevelopmental and sensory–perceptual–motor disorder. The child with CP has a developing nervous system, so the nature of the movement disorder must be understood in order that effective treatment strategies may be planned and used; appropriate functional goals that maximise the child's potential for functional independence may be set, and each child assisted to achieve his or her potential, within a family-centred model (Simmons Carlsson, 1999a; Mayston, 2001). CP is a descriptive umbrella term for a group of disorders of posture and movement that manifest in a multitude of sensory and motor signs and symptoms, and associated sensory–perceptual–cognitive functions. It is defined as 'a permanent impairment of movement and posture resulting from a non-progressive brain disorder due to hereditary factors, or events occurring during pregnancy, delivery, neonatal period, and the first two years of life' (cited in Bobath Centre, 1997). Cerebral palsy is, however, progressive in nature (Bobath Centre, 1997). Although the originating 'brain' damage itself is non-progressive, the resulting disability, or rather the impairments, are permanent and these do change over time, further compounding neuromuscular and musculoskeletal limitations/restrictions on function, learning and participation. In children, the potential for a progressive picture is highlighted because the damage has occurred to a developing nervous system and brain, and in general the lesion tends to interfere with the child's overall development. Thus, CP may be best described as an evolving and changing condition that results from the changing clinical, and functional, picture which evolves as the child develops and matures. These changes occur with age and growth, in response to the increasing environmental and psychosocial demands placed on a child, such as gravity, and its influence on tone, the functional task and/or cognitive effort demands, and factors such as the way the child is managed and what he or she actually does when participating in given environments.

Cerebral palsy captures a broad spectrum of types and mixtures (Palisano et al., 1997). Intervention may be provided for a range of ages – from neonate to adult. Types of CP manifest in different distributions of abnormal postural tone, typically described as quadriplegia (whole body involvement), diplegia (primarily lower half of the body, although the trunk may be involved) or hemiplegia (one side of the body). Although the predominant distribution of abnormal tone is recognised, intervention also takes account of the potential resultant 'abnormality' in the so-called non-involved body parts, and the impact of the child's altered body image as a result of the nature of the condition. Tonus quality may manifest as spasticity/hypertonia, hypotonia, fluctuating or ataxia, and includes combinations thereof. The degree of involvement (in terms of tonus quality) may vary and range from mild to moderate to severe degrees. This may change from one level to the next, depending on the postural demands of the task and/or environment, which is influenced by the amount of excitation and effort of functional performance, e.g. hypertonia in the child with hemiplegia may increase from a moderate to severe degree on the hemiplegic side/extremity during play with objects that require skills that are bilateral, fine and manipulative. A second descriptor related to the severity level of the disability itself is often used; however, care must be taken to distinguish this descriptor clearly from the descriptor relating to abnormal tonus quality, e.g. one child with hemiplegia may have a relatively mild level of disability despite the presence of moderately severe degrees of spasticity/hypertonia. Conversely, another child may have a mild–moderate degree of spasticity, but a severe level of motor and cognitive–perceptual disability as a result of the influence of his or her associated conditions on motor control and learning. Readers should note that the Bobath/NDT classification of CP uses the first descriptor to highlight the child's degree and quality of abnormal tone, not the 'severity' level of the child's disability.

Cerebral palsy is a multitude of conditions (Badawi et al., 1998) and includes a wide range of associated primary and/or secondary impairments. Distinguishing between what are primary impairments resulting from the CNS lesion, and what are secondary impairments resulting, for example, from biomechanical restrictions, is crucial to treatment planning and intervention. Motor disorders may also impact on the child's learning and behaviour. Poverty or lack of movement may place limitations on the child's opportunity to explore and actively participate in learning experiences. Premature children with CP may have a primary disorder of sensory modulation concurrent with their movement disorder and will require treatment to be combined with another approach that would better address sensory modulation disorders (Simmons Carlsson, 1997). The child's environment, his exposure to a range of life experiences, the home and learning contexts, and cultural aspects all impact on the child's functional disability and potential for functional opportunities. These factors must all be considered in clinical reasoning and the overall management plan for the child and family. Berta Bobath believed that children with CP cannot be treated in the same way – each child/young person is an individual and as such has individual needs. Each child deserves and requires an individual intervention/management plan.

Bobath/NDT classification

The existence of many types of CP highlights the importance for Bobath/NDT therapists to use a systematic classification system in order to treat. No two children are the same as a result of: the complexity of the brain; the timing, nature and extent of the brain damage; and the ecological contexts in which the child will grow up. Therefore, no two intervention plans should be the same. Palisano et al. (1997) and colleagues (Wood and Rosenbaum, 2000) have presented the need for a valid and reliable standardised system of classification for children with CP. The Gross Motor Function Classification System (GMFCS; Palisano et al., 1997), which is based on current concepts of disability and functional limitation, provides a framework to assist therapists and doctors to classify CP according to the child's gross motor function. As such, the GMFCS is proving useful in research (Knox, 2000). The Bobath concept classifies CP on the basis of the quality, distribution and degree of involvement of postural tone, not the severity of the disability itself. This is combined with other classification tools such as the GMFCS (Knox, 2000). Classification based on clinical judgement provides a common language for diagnosis (Palisano et al., 1997) and for predicting potential outcomes and prognosis. The Bobath/NDT classification system is used to achieve a common language and more importantly to paint a 'micro-picture' of the child. In this sense the classification can point to treatment – 'we classify in order to treat' rather than to place a diagnostic label on the condition (Bobath Centre, 1997). Medical-model diagnostic classification/labelling is frequently insufficient and at times can be misleading as a guide to clinical decision-making and intervention planning, so therapists may re-classify the child in Bobath/NDT terms in order to treat. A case example is useful to illustrate this point.

Case example 1 – Jack

Jack is a 13-month-old twin who was born at 30 weeks' gestation. His paediatrician has diagnosed him as having CP, spastic diplegia. After assessment by a Bobath-trained therapist, Jack has been re-classified with 'moderate–severe spastic diplegia of prematurity; right side more than left; with truncal hypotonia'. This classification based on Bobath/NDT analysis communicates to the Bobath/NDT-trained therapist the following: the quality of Jack's postural tone may vary from moderate to severe degrees of spasticity/hypertonus, depending on what he is doing; how alert/excited he is; and/or how he is feeling. The term 'of prematurity' signals to the therapist that Jack's postural tone will not be 'typical' in terms of what is expected of spasticity/hypertonia. From the classification, the Bobath-trained therapist could ascertain that, although Jack's lower half may be 'more involved' and he may have arm support, he is likely to present with more whole body involvement and asymmetry. The right side is 'stiffer' than the left, suggesting potential risk of further asymmetry when Jack begins to become more active against gravity. Truncal hypotonia (weakness/inactivity) is likely to be present and be accompanied with distal (in the extremities) hypertonia, including the limb girdles, especially when Jack is active as he attempts to compensate for the lack of central stability. This, in turn, may further increase his asymmetry and further restrict his functional movements, which, in turn, would reduce his ability to participate in play activities and to move on the floor in order to explore his environment. In addition, the knowledge that Jack was born prematurely signals to the therapist that primary and/or secondary sensory–perceptual conditions may accompany his movement disorder, e.g. visual–perceptual dysfunction and/or difficulties with sensory processing. This is especially important because these factors would play a major role in Jack's potential for not only motor learning, but also his overall learning and behaviour. Clinical reasoning, assessment, analysis, treatment/management plans will therefore encompass all of the above aspects of Jack's Bobath/NDT classification.

Analysis of normal/abnormal movement and 'typical' child development

Bobath/NDT therapists develop high-level skills and knowledge in analysing normal movement (Mayston, 2000a). This is one of the core platforms for basing clinical reasoning and intervention planning. The therapist's knowledge and understanding of child development, in particular motor development, and how this is visible in functional movement abilities and skills are vital. Development is seen as a process that results from the multi-dimensional interaction of developmental areas, and as such it is an adaptive process that is horizontal, sequential and upward spiralling. Treatment plans 'should consider that many motor activities develop simultaneously, and in fact they overlap' (Bobath and Bobath, 1984, p. 11), and are interrelated with other aspects of development, such as hand function, motivation and cognition. The influence of the environment (physical, social, cultural) on development must also be acknowledged. This has been given a much greater emphasis as person–environment–occupation, motor control and motor learning postulates are integrated into the concept (Bobath Centre, 1997; Mayston, 2001). Motor development requires a sound awareness and understanding of the components of normal movement (Bly and Whiteside, 1997) and includes kinesiological factors, as well as the role of the therapist, the environment, treatment tools and the adaptive equipment that the therapist may use to facilitate active posture and movement. Fundamental to analysis and treatment planning is: the interplay between stability and mobility to give dynamic functional movement; the effects of the NPCM; kinesiological considerations including range of motion, postural alignment, base of support and dissociation and the development of postural control in the three planes of space – sagittal (extension and flexion against gravity), frontal (lateral righting) and transverse (dissociation and rotation); and sequences and variety of movement. Also fundamental is the child's sensorimotor development, the influence of associated conditions on motor learning, and the dynamics of the environment, functional task and the child (Bly and Whiteside, 1997; Bobath Centre, 1997).

Bobath/NDT intervention also requires grounded understanding of abnormal motor development (Bobath and Bobath, 1975) and current theories of abnormal motor control and activity in order to analyse and understand the child's condition. Knowledge of 'abnormal' motor coordination encompasses kinesiological components, abnormal non-neural properties of muscles, including any structural deformity and/or soft tissue contracture, because secondary impairments resulting from musculoskeletal limitations/restrictions may negatively impact on the child's potential for functional participation. Similarly, the influence that associated problems, or perceptual–cognitive and sensory–perceptual disorders, may have on movement control must be recognised and understood, including any potential long-term risks for learning and behaviour.

Sensory influences on motor control

The interplay of the sensory and motor systems has long been acknowledged: we do not learn movements, but the sensation of movement (Bobath and Bobath, 1984, p. 10); we learn as we do and we do only as well as we have learned (Brooks, 1986); and 'how we move influences how we sense and in turn how we sense influences how we move' (Shumway-Cook and Wollacott, 1995, p. 136). Understanding the sensory mechanisms related to postural control is vital in the application of the Bobath concept (Bly, 1996). Movement arises from the interaction of multiple processes, including sensory–perceptual, cognitive and motor systems (Shumway-Cook and Woollacott, 1995) and this must be understood by the Bobath/NDT therapist. The 'importance of perception and processing of sensory information' cannot be emphasised enough 'not only for learning, but for the efficient execution of a required task' (Mayston, 2001). When this factor is missed in clinical reasoning one has seriously to question the logic and direction of Bobath/NDT intervention (Simmons Carlsson, 1997). Principles of neuroplasticity underpinning skill learning (Mayston, 2001) to apply the practice model knowledgeably with children who have CP, and/or allied neurological conditions, must also be understood.

Berta Bobath recognised that postural control was a sensorimotor task. She also recognised the sensory effects that 'hands-on' therapy had on the child's systems during handling. Abnormal patterns of movement may be influenced, or modified by altering/modifying the sensory input to the CNS via specialised handling techniques, which, when combined with the active participation of the child in the context of goal-directed, meaningful, functional activities, provides a medium to allow learning to take place (Bobath Centre, 1997; Schoen and Anderson, 1999; Mayston, 2001). The 'hands-on' approach allows the therapist to 'transmit' externally to muscles and joints, indirectly sending feedback messages to the brain, in conjunction with those facilitated via the child's active engagement in functional tasks. The skilled Bobath/NDT therapist handles responsively in a 'silent dance' that guides and mirrors the child's activity, responding to the child's actions and responses as he or she moves and plays, and being guided by the child's reactions to handling and the task. Guidance primarily includes 'hands-on' tactile–proprioceptive-based handling techniques, and also verbal, other sensory-based and environmental cueing. Most importantly, the therapist must be sensitive to the child's own active control – withdrawing guidance as the child takes over control and becomes active, and guiding only when necessary – to teach the child how to move as he or she is 'doing' an activity/task. Sensory input acts as a means of bringing about change (Bly and Whiteside, 1997; Schoen and Anderson, 1999), and when given 'effectively and often enough can expand sensory areas of the cortex', providing some support for therapeutic intervention. Although it is recognised that 'sensory information is not necessary for tasks to occur, it is important for fine-tuning and learning motor/postural tasks' (see Mayston, 2001). Careful orchestration of functional tasks and the environment is necessary and is a complementary tool to handling to provide the 'just-right' challenge and input.

The role of inhibition in the control of posture and movement

Physiological inhibition is important for the development of selective and graded movement for function. It is active at every level of the CNS where the balance between excitation and inhibition during movement controls speed, range and direction, and efficiency. Inhibition modifies and controls actions to achieve coordination (Mayston, 1992). The Bobath concept/NDT uses handling as a tool to modify and/or influence that which is outwardly observed as abnormal, i.e. abnormal postural tone and abnormal patterns of posture and movement; however, handling itself does not inhibit spasticity in the neurophysiological sense. By handling, the therapist can enable the child to gain 'improved muscle length to allow for more efficient muscle activation', so that the child may be helped to 'move actively in more optimal and meaningful ways within the limits of [his or her] CNS damage' (Mayston, 2000a). This notion of activation is a key component in motor learning, a concept that has long been recognised in the Bobath approach. Bobath referred to this in 1965 when she stressed, in her teachings, that unless the therapist makes the child active through her or his handling she basically will 'have done nothing at all' (Mayston, 2000a, citing Bobath, 1965).

Specialised techniques of handling

Handling techniques, now conceptualised as tone influencing patterns (TIPs) (Mayston, 2000b) are only tools of practice, and form only part of the Bobath concept. TIPs are dynamic techniques of handling, which are guided by the child's reactions to handling and the environment. They are aimed at influencing the child's postural tone, thus enabling the child to achieve more normal patterns of posture and movement for functional use (Bobath Centre, 1997). TIPs involve normal patterns of movement used to modify abnormal patterns of movement, to reduce/prevent hypertonus, and to prevent abnormal patterns of activity occurring when trying to build up tone (Mayston et al., 1997). The following case example illustrates this point.

Case example 2 – Jason

Jason is a 5-year-old boy with right hemiplegia. When he plays with a ball his right arm tends to stiffen and 'pull' into a pattern of internal rotation, forearm pronation, ulnar deviation of the wrist and semi-fisted, with an adducted thumb; his pelvis is retracted on the right side and the right knee is hyperextended. During a bilateral ball-catching activity, the therapist applies a TIP to the upper limb to counteract the pattern of abnormal hypertonus and at the same time to facilitate a more normal pattern of external rotation, forward reach, forearm supination to midposition, thumb abduction/extension, and fingers open with semi-extension of the wrist. This specific preparation for catching the ball in standing may include elongation of the right side of Jason's trunk, mobilisation of the scapula against the chest wall, elongation of the chest flexors to free the arm, alignment of the pelvis to counteract retraction, and activation of bilateral weight bearing through the legs, while counteracting hyperextension in the knees.

Tone influencing patterns allow inhibition, facilitation and stimulation, and are applied via key points of control (KPCs). These involve specific parts of the body from which one can effectively guide and change patterns of activity in other parts of the child's body; they are used during handling as a point from which to influence/reduce abnormal tone, as well as simultaneously to facilitate more normal postural reactions/movement. KPCs may be proximal, e.g. the shoulder girdle, or distal, e.g. the elbow or leg. They may also be used in combinations. KPCs change as the child changes in response to handling, the functional task demands and/or the environment. Through KPCs the therapist is able to help to align body parts, stabilise body parts, initiate movement and/or prevent movement in a part of the body (Bly and Whiteside, 1997). Thus, handling via KPCs allows the therapist effectively to direct, guide and change the patterns of activity in other parts of the body.

Specialised handling techniques are hypothesised as acting as an external medium which guides neural plasticity by enhancing synaptic pathways through demanding a change in activity – from abnormal patterns of activity to 'more normal' patterns of movement. The child's active participation is necessary in the problem-solving, performing and practising of the goal-oriented task. In treatment handling, techniques are used to prepare the child systematically for function and they are used during participation in functional tasks. As the child becomes more active, they may be altered and/or gradually withdrawn. This is monitored by the therapist through sensitive handling, observation and continual analysis of what she 'feels and sees' as she guides the child through movement, or creates the 'just-right' challenges via task/environment set-up. Handling techniques affect both excitatory and inhibitory synaptic activity in addition to influencing the passive–elastic properties of the muscles themselves (Bobath Centre, 1997); they assist the child to learn new, or rather 'more normal' motor programmes for functional performance (Bly, 2000). However, 'it is essential to recognize that these techniques can only bring about change if there is the potential for long-term adaptability of the CNS, the cognitive ability to recognize these changes as beneficial, as well as the required perceptual abilities' (Mayston et al., 1997, p. 2), and the child must be an active participant.

Berta Bobath left therapists a legacy – the power of sensitive handling when combined with astute observational skill and systematic clinical reasoning. When handling, the therapist's hands must be placed with care, respectfully and purposefully, on the child's body. Further, her hands shape/mould to the contour of the body part/KPC, and the fingers do not grab at the child. The palms of the hands provide much of the control for the desired movement pattern. Alternatively, a less hands-on approach may be required, e.g. the use of only the therapist's fingertips, and/or intermittent handling. Handling should not cause any discomfort to the child, or push, pull at or lift the child (Bly and Whiteside, 1997), and the child should not be overly aware of the therapist's hands. The therapist's task is to 'read and respond positively to the subtle messages' that arise in the child's body, changing her handling in response to what she observes, feels and hears. This highlights the importance of the therapist's own need consciously to use her body in synchrony with the child's movements (Bly and Whiteside, 1997), e.g. when the child shifts weight the therapist will also shift her weight to that same side and/or forwards. Hand placement will vary depending on the child and his potential for postural control. At times the therapist may place her hands over joints, which may be proximal or distal or both, and/or over muscles. The therapist learns to change the pressure, timing, speed and direction, amount and point of contact and pressure from her hands, as she engages in a 'dance' with the child's body, gradually withdrawing her hands as and when the child takes over active control of his body part(s), or the component or sequence of functional movement. The following continuation of case example 1 illustrates one possible scenario of the application of handling.

Case example 1 – Jack (continued)

Jack primarily prefers to be held in his mother's arms, and/or be placed momentarily on the floor on his back; however, he is unable to roll and therefore becomes frustrated in this position as he cannot get to his toys, or move towards his mother, or sibling Molly. When he is placed sitting on the floor and propped up with pillows, he is unable to move in or out of the position and his attempts to play with his toys result in his legs extending out; his right side begins to stiffen and flex as he tries not to fall and his tone further increases. As a result, he ends up falling to the side and backwards and he cannot save himself. For Jack's mother, neither position is helpful because Jack is dependent on her to help him get his toys and stay in a stable sitting position. For Jack, both positions are fraught with frustration and he has quickly learnt that being held in mummy's arms gives him the best options for security, stability and play opportunities. This, however, means that Jack's mother is unable to leave him to play independently in a variety of positions while she gets on with her own activities around the home.

In collaboration with Jack's mother the therapist decides to work on floor mobility and positioning, so that Jack may learn to play happily and independently on the floor for short periods of time. In addition, the therapist problem-solves with Jack's mother to determine solutions for seating Jack appropriately, so that he may sit and play. They agree that his high chair would be one suitable option, with minor adaptations to the seating.

During treatment Jack's therapist decides to begin handling him in supine so that she may maintain visual contact with him. She plays peek-a-boo with Jack and sings his favourite nursery rhymes. As they interact she begins to prepare Jack for rolling into prone, first elongating his trunk, in particular the right side, using the pelvis and shoulder girdle as the KPCs. The therapist also uses the pelvis as a KPC to mobilise the pelvis, by using small inner-range upward and downward motions of the pelvis with rotation, to gain pelvic mobility and extension of the hips. While handling Jack the therapist encourages him actively to reach up to tussle her hair, play tickle with his tummy and find features on their faces. In this way, the therapist prepares Jack for the sequence of rolling. The therapist feels through her handling and observes that Jack has gained alignment of his trunk and head and that he is able to reach upwards with little influence of hypertonia. She moves her KPC more distally to Jack's feet to counteract the hypertonus that manifests in a pattern of plantar flexion, with hyperextension at the knees and handles to 'break' this pattern up. She continues to engage Jack in age-appropriate reciprocal social interactions. As the therapist feels Jack's quality of tone alter under her handling, she strategically introduces Jack's favourite musical pop-up toy on his left side slightly above his eye level and, as Jack begins to attempt to roll over that side to reach for the toy with his right hand, she deftly alters her KPCs to the left knee and pelvis, simultaneously facilitating the rolling sequence over onto his tummy, and uses these KPCs to counteract the pull into flexion that could occur on the right side and at his hips, with the effort/initiation of rolling.

Thus, the therapist facilitates the 'more normal' sequence of rolling while counteracting the abnormal pattern of internal rotation/flexion at the hips and especially through his right side, which would typically occur without handling. Ordinarily, when Jack attempts to roll he will achieve only side lying momentarily in a relatively flexed position. In prone, Jack is unaware of the therapist's handling, plays for minutes with his toy in prone with forearm support and when he is ready the therapist helps to facilitate rolling back into supine, and then back into prone, working on rolling over both the right and the left sides. The session continues in this way for the time that Jack is busy playing with his toy and enjoying the sequence of movement that allows him to practise rolling. With each successive rolling sequence, the therapist aims to withdraw her hands as she feels that Jack is taking over the control; however, she is ready to re-intervene at any time, if and when she observes that the quality of his movement deteriorates to a point of immobility and/or frustration. While handling, the therapist also ensures that Jack has several opportunities to problem-solve and self-correct his own activity.

Opportunities for practice and repetition

Throughout the chapter, it has been stressed that the active participation of the child in the problem-solving process is vital for motor learning to occur. Engaging the child in meaningful goal-directed activities provides opportunities for taking in both external and internal feedback. In this way the child gains knowledge of results (external feedback) and performance (internal feedback), both of which help in the planning and anticipation of the next movement (feed-forward mechanism). Children learn through practice and repetition while engaged in meaningful, purposeful, goal-directed activities in a variety of contexts. As the infant/child grows and develops – actively engaging in increasingly complex interactions with his/her world – the internal representations (foundations) of past experience are laid. Treatment should aim to foster this and carry these principles over into the varying contexts of the child's daily life (Bobath Centre, 1997; Simmons Carlsson, 1999a).

Sensory information is integrated so that output can be meaningful; however, it is only meaningful with a normal past experience, and with perception of the task/function. The 'CNS operates in a task or goal directed way' (Mayston, 2001). This helps the brain to learn the most efficient/effective 'programme' through the parametric specifications of the task and environmental context, via practice and repetition. Practice and repetition of the task reinforce learning, and include factors such as the grading of movement, force, speed, timing and visuomotor coordination, for example (Recordon, 1998). Bobath/NDT hypothesises that the use of abnormal patterns is reflected by the neuromuscular system, and thus the child's internal representations, or rather the learnt programmes, are those of abnormal, stereotypical patterns and the abnormal sensations of posture and movement. Treatment aims to 'break'/interrupt/influence and/or modify the abnormal cycle of motor learning that has been established as a result of a CNS lesion (in a sense, programme differently/re-programme) and to 'force', or bring about neuromuscular adaptation. In other words, the therapist aims to train the client in the least effortful, more normal pattern (Recordon, 1998) and to build a basis for more automatic control through the use of feed-forward and feedback techniques. Bobath discovered in her clinical experimentation that, in order to break this cycle, something needed to be done about the abnormal patterns, such as abnormal postural tone, and that one could not simply attempt to superimpose normal movement on a basis of abnormal postural tone and abnormal patterns of posture and movement. Thus, specific preparation is necessary as part of the intervention process. This may occur before, during and after function.

Preparation for function

Preparation for function involves a process of mobilisation, active muscle lengthening or activation, and practice of parts or whole movement components (Bobath Centre, 1997). Preparation is not a 'treatment' in itself. It is of no value on its own and must be incorporated into useful activity (Mayston, 2001). Case example 1 is continued here to illustrate aspects of preparation.

Case example 1 – Jack (continued)

Jack's therapist has found that Jack is able to sit with support if he is held at the pelvis and upper trunk when placed on the floor in long sitting. However, when the support is removed from the upper trunk, Jack pulls into a pattern of flexion with his arms, his legs extend stiffly and he falls backwards, to the right side, and he is fearful. As previously mentioned, Jack is unable to be left in this position for play, even if his mother tries to prop him up with cushions, or against furniture.

Through her observations and analysis gained from playing with and handling Jack in this position, Jack's therapist determines that, in order to help Jack learn to sit and play in a more efficient/functional way on the floor, she must first 'prepare' Jack for sitting and reaching with his arms. Jack's inability to sit alone is partially related to truncal weakness and lack of efficient coactivation of the trunk muscles for anti-gravity activity and an inadequate base of support. As a result of this, Jack tends to use abnormal patterns of hypertonus as a strategy to stabilise himself over a precarious and small base of support; however, this only manifests in an abnormal postural pattern of flexion at the shoulder girdle with flexion at the hips and right side, and semi-adduction/extension of the legs with feet plantar flexed, and he hyperextends at the neck to try to stay upright. All of these are unsuccessful compensatory strategies on his part.

To 'prepare' Jack for sitting, the therapist selects to work/play/interact with Jack in prone position over one of her thighs, with his upper trunk across the thigh, arms propped forwards. In this position, the therapist's thigh acts as a roll and provides the KPC via Jack's shoulder girdle. The therapist handles Jack using the pelvis as the KPC to facilitate Jack actively to prop on his extended arms, and at the same time to reach up, slightly out-to-the-side and forwards with the right hand for his toy, whilst actively weight-bearing through the lower body as the base of support. This 'prepares' Jack for sitting by counteracting the hypertonus (pull-down) on the right side, as well as to elongate/lengthen and align Jack's trunk, plus gaining active extension of the upper body spine and hips. Encouraging Jack to reach up actively for his most favourite small toy helps him to feel what it is like to be active in his trunk, without the influence of hypertonus in a position where the postural control demands are relatively less than in unsupported floor sitting. Propping on his extended arms also helps to counteract the hypertonus through active weight bearing and small weight shifts, because Jack's own 'more normal' activity has an 'inhibitory' (i.e. reduces/counteracts) effect on hypertonia. Depending on Jack's play, progression of treatment may incorporate facilitation of rolling from prone to supine and supine to prone, and eventually leads to Jack being facilitated into sitting where the activity gained on the floor is translated into postural activity up against gravity. Jack continues to reach for and play with his toys.

When Jack is in sitting position, the therapist may continue to handle him using the pelvis, knees and/or feet as KPCs to continue to facilitate activity/control in Jack's trunk. The therapist is mindful of the degree of postural control demand and grades the play level accordingly to match his ability, but also to challenge his postural activity and play interactions. As the therapist feels that Jack is becoming more active she reduces her handling, using the pelvis and lower trunk as a KPC, specifically directing her handling so that Jack feels the effect of an appropriate base of support for sitting while he is active in the upper part of his body. The therapist continues to observe vigilantly and feel for changes in tone, and may provide further 'preparation' such as encouraging Jack to reach up and out to the side for his toy. Specific preparation for the right upper limb may need to be incorporated at times and may include the right elbow as a KPC to gain better elongation/extension in the right side and arm.

Focus on function

The aim of Bobath/NDT is function. The goal of handling is to enable the child to achieve more efficient functional movement, to enable him or her to move in a more effective, less effortful way to interact meaningfully with his or her environment. Short- and long-term goals also encompass reducing/counteracting/minimising the risk of secondary impairments, such as contracture and deformity, which typically ensue as a result of abnormal postural tone and patterns of posture and movement, and which inevitably place further limitations/restrictions on the acquisition of functional abilities. Instructing and guiding parents and caregivers is of great importance (Bobath and Bobath, 1984; Bobath Centre, 1997; Simmons Carlsson, 1999a), so that they may become equally competent with handling techniques during carrying and transfers, as well as during the routine activities of daily living, such as dressing and undressing, eating and drinking, bathing and toileting. This enables parents to carry-over handling into the child's daily life. Assisting parents to understand the nature of their child's CP and any associated conditions is of equal importance (Finnie, 1997; Erhardt, 1999), so that they may be empowered and understand why and how their child is functioning/could potentially function.

Systematic analysis of movement limitations/restrictions and how these impact on participation leads to intervention, which focuses on finding ways to enable the child to incorporate what is achieved in therapy into their daily lives. The importance of considering and using the occupations of childhood in treatment is vital. Childhood occupations serve not only as a tool to achieve a motoric aim, but more importantly allow the therapists/parents/caregivers to tap the child's inherent motivation by engaging the child in tasks that are individually meaningful to him. In turn this also helps to ensure that treatment becomes goal-oriented towards function rather than purely movement. Participation in exploration, play and school activities, leisure/recreational or self-care activities, or being able to communicate one's likes/dislikes, or being able to move from one place to another, become the goals of intervention, rather than the motor outcome itself.

The drive for emphasising goals that are related to function and issues of treatment versus management continue. Functional goals must become the pivotal point of individually tailored, top-down, holistic, management plans, which are function focused, rather than bottom-up, motor-component-focused intervention. Scrutton (1984) reflected on this almost two decades ago: 'however good the immediate effect [of treatment], the carry-over into out-of-treatment life is often small . . . the long-term outcome by no means impressive' (p. 51). This has become the challenge for all treatment approaches – to achieve top-down function-focused intervention strategies that activate the child in meaningful ways, rather than to be so concerned with 'changing tone' at the expense of active participation and to ensure motor learning. There is 'no good evidence to show that stopping a person from being active will prevent spasticity' (Mayston, 2000a). Bobath-trained therapists continue to be at risk of over-emphasising the motor components in treatment, rather than placing the emphasis on functional end-results. The greatest challenge for therapists is therefore to take what is effective in treatment and functionally embed this into the child's life, with his/her family and caregivers, within his/her contexts, by providing daily management programmes that are realistic, functional and relevant to the child's day (Mayston, 2000a). The following case example provides examples of a range of functional goals for one child.

Case example 3 – James

James is a 5-year-old boy with choreoathetosis who is independently mobile with the aid of a powered mobility aid. James is able to walk with handling for short distances, and sit alone on the floor in w-sitting for short periods of time before overbalancing backwards. His school-related goal is to draw with a pencil like his schoolmates and to be part of the ball games at breaks. James's parents would like him to have opportunities to play alone at the dining table at home, and they would like to find ways of managing his dressing and undressing so that it is not so time-consuming. They are interested in exploring a means for James to walk independently and would also like James to be able to feed himself. James's teacher would like him to be able to participate more actively in some of the manipulative maths activities when he is at school, and to be able to partic-ipate actively during news time. In addition, although he has access to a computer for written communication at school, it is not well used and the teacher is unsure of how James should access it and what subjects to use it for.

Team work as a basis for carry-over

The Bobath concept is suited to both the interdisciplinary and transdisci-plinary (see Case-Smith et al., 1996; Dunn, 2000) team approaches and aims to teach therapists, parents/caregivers and other professionals such as teachers and doctors to view the child from a similar perspective. Such an approach to teaming, serves to foster team relationships and create realistic role release among the various professionals involved with the child, in the best interests of the child and his or her family. This is especially useful in times when funding constraints threaten increas-ingly to restrain services in the next decade. The child is at the centre of his or her circle of parents/family, caregivers and professionals within the broader context of societal, cultural and political factors. Parents are a vital part of the team and know their child best. Embracing concepts of family-centred practice (see Case-Smith, 1998; Law et al., 1998) allow Bobath/NDT interventionists to collaborate with parents/caregivers, to address their main concerns and to aim for common, shared, realistic goals, and to ensure a shared focus and understanding of each child's individual abilities and disabilities. Parents are part of the team and have a central role in planning services for their child and thus should be part of the decision-making process. They bring their unique and valuable perspective to treatment which helps to guide the therapist to address what is 'real', and potentially the realistic functional goals for their child.

Assessment

Bobath/NDT uses the process of dynamic assessment. Assessment is primarily based on the therapist's knowledge and skills in clinical observation and analysis. Treatment and assessment are seen as a dynamic, continuous, circular process – the therapist assesses in order to treat, and in turn treats in order to assess. Assessment is an ongoing process – from moment to moment during a treatment session and from session to session over the course of intervention. Assessment begins wherever and in whatever position and/or context the therapist finds the child. In other words, assessment will commence as the child comes in the door, when the child is playing on the floor, with the child's first communication/interaction with the therapist, in standing, or during undressing, etc. Clinical analysis and problem-solving follow a flexible yet systematic set of clinical questions, which begin by focusing on what the child is able and/or unable to do. This includes observation and analysis of how he or she is moving/performing functional activities. Clinical observations include the child's postural control and functional movements, the responses to being moved and, when moving, the response to handling, and the types of play and interactions seen. No standardised evaluations specific to Bobath/NDT have been developed as yet; however, a range of standardised tools is applicable for use with children with CP (DeMatteo et al., 1992; Hayley et al., 1992; Russell et al., 1993; Miller and Roid, 1994; Palisano et al., 1997; Coster et al., 1998). Occupational therapists tend to supplement their Bobath-based assessment findings using specific performance component evaluation tools, e.g. of perception and visual–motor integration (Menken et al., 1987; Reid and Drake, 1990; Colarusso and Hammill, 1996; Beery and Buktenica, 1997). The assessment process may be illustrated by case example 4.

Assessment is carried out on an individual basis and of the whole child, because the therapist must be concerned with posture and functional movement throughout the whole body, *not* so much with the ranges of movement in one joint, or with the contraction and relaxation of specific muscle groups, although this is also considered important. Analysis is of the patterns of activity, including the quality and distribution of abnormal postural tone, and the patterns of posture and movement seen and felt. Clinical questions that guide the problem-solving process include: How is the child moving/functioning? What combination of patterns of movement does the child use and why? How do these patterns interfere with movement and function? How does the child compensate and what components are missing? Although needing to be noted, the focus of assessment is *not* on assessing reflexes, unless the presence of retained responses impacts negatively on the child's functional abilities, e.g. the startle response frequently impacts balance and increases tone. The therapist is interested in the quality of tonus/movement and in identifying what is missing in the course of her observation and handling of the child. Assessment always begins with looking at what the child is able to do, and how much help is required and where, followed by what the child is not able to do. It is important to evaluate the child in a variety of positions, including prone, supine, sitting, standing and walking. The outcome of assessment is to identify the child's main impairments/problems and how this impacts on function and development. Answering 'how' and 'why' questions leads to treatment. Critical thinking is vital in Bobath/NDT. Furthermore, systematic reliable thinking tools that would potentially guide assessment and clinical reasoning from the basis of a top-down functional approach, rather than from that of the traditional bottom-up, component/impairment perspective, are being explored (Simmons Carlsson and Recordon, 2000).

During assessment the Bobath-trained therapist will take into account factors such as: the functional task; the child's communicative intent/ expression; his/her level of arousal;his interactions/emotional–social status; any observable expressions that may point to the presence of associated conditions, which may require further in-depth, more specific evaluation, e.g. language; oral–motor functions; visual–perception; and sensory processing. Most importantly, assessment aims to make contact with the child and his/her parent or caregiver and to establish a mutual rapport of trust and open communication. Parents and caregivers, and the child, form a vital part of a collaborative assessment framework and Bobath-trained therapists should always seek to find out and understand the parents' (and the child's if possible) main concerns, including their wishes, hopes and dreams for their child, as well as those of the child's respective caregivers, such as teachers, nannies, etc. This is often carried out during the initial interview phase and may be re-visited during the course of treatment sessions. In addition, the therapist is interested in learning about the child's life story, who he or she is as a person, child, sibling, friend, student, player, and where these life roles and events may occur. The child's likes and preferences for toys, people, sensations, textures and movement experiences, for example, need to be assessed. Parental expectations of therapy and their perceived roles and goals for therapy are also important to identify and discuss during the assessment phase. These may need to be periodically re-visited, re-negotiated and reviewed as treatment progresses. Data-gathering from other team members and agencies involved with the child, including the referring agency and any relevant discipline-specific assessment findings, also form a vital part of assessment.

Case example 4 – Joshua

Joshua is a 4-year-old boy with moderate–severe spastic quadriplegia, right side more than left, and cortical visual impairment. The therapist's assessment begins as she enters Joshua's house. Joshua is lying on his back on the floor with his toys beside him. The therapist immediately observes Joshua's postural patterns in supine, his postural alignment, or rather asymmetry, and his lack of ability to take up the base of support offered by the floor and pillow. She notes that his postural tone and patterns increase slightly as Joshua hears his mother's voice. She also notes that, although Joshua listens, he does not turn his head in response to his mother's voice; however, he stills and smiles when the therapist says hello. The therapist observes that this social response further increases Joshua's hypertonia. As part of the initial interview, the therapist has decided to administer the Pediatric Evaluation of Disability Inventory (PEDI), in order to gain an overall baseline view of Joshua's capabilities in the functional skills domains of self-care, mobility and social functions. The PEDI also allows the therapist to determine the extent of caregiver assistance and modifications that Joshua requires in the course of his daily management. During administration of the PEDI questionnaire, the therapist also seeks more qualitative information and asks Joshua's mother about how she handles Joshua during self-care activities and what his postural/tonus responses are during these activities, e.g. the therapist is interested in learning about how Joshua is positioned for eating and drinking and what happens to his oral–motor coordination when eating/drinking.

The therapist's assessment also includes playing with Joshua and handling him in a variety of positions on her lap and on the floor, after ascertaining that both Joshua and his mother are happy for her to do so. The therapist places Joshua in prone, supine, and supported sitting and standing. In all positions, she ensures that he feels secure and then slowly handles him, assessing and analysing his responses to being handled and moved. She notes his postural patterns and the degree of variability in all positions, as well as the degree of tonus change and the conditions that change tone. During assessment she also experiments with handling to see what TIPs do and/or do not work in terms of reducing tone and achieving alignment and activity. She also experiments to determine Joshua's potential for active participation in reaching out to his environment, as well as in terms of his potential for postural control.

The therapist also takes particular note of Joshua's communicative signals and specifically observes his visual and auditory responses, as well as his responses to touch. Joshua's mother's knowledge of her son's abilities and responses is vital in determining this, including Joshua's likes and dislikes, and play preferences. The therapist talks with Joshua's mother to determine the family's main concerns, hopes and wishes for Joshua. Through her handling, analysis and initial assessment, the therapist collaborates with Joshua's mother to identify his main problems from the perspective of motor control and motor learning, and what these may mean in terms of restriction/limitations on his participation in life. Most importantly, they also identify the main functional goals for Joshua in the short term, with a view to the long term. The therapist also identifies areas for further assessment, such as visual functioning, play, communication, and eating and drinking. In addition, she identifies with the mother those areas of positioning that require immediate follow-up in terms of adaptive equipment. The therapist takes care during the entire assessment process to explain clearly and simply what she is doing, and why, as she handles Joshua, and answers his mother's questions as they arise, as well as explaining to Joshua's mother that the assessment process will be ongoing.

Treatment

The Bobath approach aims to assist the child with CP to learn to move in a more efficient and functional way, so that he may actively participate in activities and tasks that are meaningful to him and his family/caregivers. This requires collaborative problem-solving with the child's family/caregivers to devise management programmes that may be carried over into the child's home/school environment. Treatment involves many factors including: handling of the child by the therapist/parent/caregiver; adapting and orchestrating the environment; and involving the child in meaningful tasks. As mentioned above, handling techniques are but one tool of treatment that must be adapted and modified to suit the individual needs of the child, based on the assessment/analysis data, the child's age, abilities and disabilities, and classification. Treatment tools are used to 'bring about change' (Luebben et al., 1999, p. 27). Treatment does not comprise a set of exercises, nor is it a recipe or a rigid and standardised method of treatment (Bobath and Bobath, 1984). Bobath/NDT treatment tools include skilled observation and analysis, problem-solving, specialised handling techniques, the therapist's conscious use of self, and use of the non-human environment. In treatment, the therapist is conscious of the effects of her handling on the child and the role she plays as 'an agent to effect change within the therapeutic process' (Luebben et al., 1999, p. 28), e.g. how much pressure she applies through her hands; the directional movement cues/feedback she gives the child through handling and verbal guidance; the type of touch she uses, light or firm; how much skin-on-skin/body-to-body contact she has with the child; the tone of her voice; how she relates to the child's parents/caregivers; and even the type of clothing she is wearing which may visually overstimulate some children.

Use of the non-human environment includes the use of adaptive/therapeutic equipment such as wedges, bolsters, plinths, benches and therapy balls, which may be incorporated during handling to provide support, stability and/or movement opportunities. Adaptive equipment for positioning and daily management of the child is also vital to ensure carry-over of treatment aims, e.g. the use of a standing frame may be helpful in ensuring that James (case example 3) is provided with adequate opportunities for aligned weight-bearing in standing while he plays at the kitchen table, or has a daytime snack, while his mother prepares a meal. The standing frame would also be a useful position for James to learn to use his pencil and to access the computer with switch input.

The physical environment in which treatment/management occurs is an important consideration, e.g. consideration is given to the types and range of toys and activities to which the child may be exposed at home/school, and during treatment. The therapist's skill in task analysis and adaptation, and her ability to select, match and build-in the appropriate objects and playful opportunities within the context of therapy is highly desirable. Skills in identifying what is motivating and meaningful to the child is paramount in eliciting active participation. Technology, including low-tech and high-tech options, also plays a role in practice depending on the child's needs, e.g. intervention for James (case example 3) at school may focus on working on sitting on his adapted school chair during story writing, while using switch access on his computer. The therapist handles James to facilitate his postural alignment in sitting, as well as to help him to grade and coordinate the placement of his arm movements during switching, working towards 'hand's-off'. The ergonomic dynamics of the computer in relation to James's position and seating system, as well as the physical aspects of the room such as lighting and noise distraction factors, would also be considered.

Treatment should be tailored to meet each individual child's needs. It is important to elicit the child's own, more normal activity while he is engaged in a goal-oriented task because the best 'inhibition' of abnormal tone often comes from the child's own more normal activity. TIPs allow the therapist to help the child become more active. The therapist may use weight shift and weight bearing as techniques of treatment to counteract hypertonus, as well as to grade the environment, activity and handling accordingly to 'inhibit' and/or facilitate more normal active patterns of movement from the child. During treatment, the therapist aims to take a 'less hands-on' approach to allow the child to control his own activity and his own postural adjustments and movement. The therapist also aims to establish functional carry-over into daily life through collaborating with and educating the child's parents, and/or caregivers. This may include: discussion and teaching handling/management strategies to counteract, or minimise, structural deformity and contracture; education related to the child's capabilities and disabilities; and educating parents/caregivers about how to handle the child during the day, so that it becomes a natural part of family life – not a rigid set of exercises to be carried out once a day. The therapist combines and applies principles of the biomechanical approach in the evaluation and prescription of positional and adaptive equipment. In this way, carry-over into daily life contexts may also be achieved in the absence of regular handling.

Integrating play with handling

Play combined with handling can provide the medium for the therapist to elicit the active participation of the child in meaningful goal-oriented activities, which provide opportunities for practice of movement components and whole sequences of movement. Play activities may be used to achieve treatment goals; however, they should not become the means to the motoric end at the expense of play and playfulness itself (Blanche, 1997). Therapists who use handling techniques are often at risk of 'doing to' rather than 'doing with' the child with CP, when play is part of the treatment context (Blanche, 1997). Play is the recognised medium through which children may naturally learn and explore, have fun, be active and be playful. It is intrinsically motivating, spontaneous and flexible. Play provides the child with a reason to move, interact and engage with the objects and people in the child's real and pretend world. In the treatment context, play can help the therapist to tap the child's intrinsic motivation to become an active participant in tasks that are meaningful to the child (see Blanche, 1997). Children know and respond accordingly when they are not playing. Therein lies the challenge for the Bobath/NDT therapist to reconcile the use of play as a tool to achieve a goal, while at the same time to maintain the meaning of the play activity for the child and, most importantly, to maintain the playful, interactive, fun, spontaneous and intrinsically motivating aspects of the tool. Bobath-trained therapists must learn to 'incorporate play into . . . treatment and into the life of the child with CP . . . as a context for learning as much as an intrinsically rewarding experience' (Blanche, 1997, p. 203). They need to develop competencies not only in how to use play activities playfully as a motivator, or reinforcer, but also in how to use play as a context for the child to learn and develop adaptive skills (motor, cognitive, social). Most importantly, they need to develop competencies in using play as an end in itself (Blanche, 1997).

Carry-over into daily life

Bobath recognised the need for carry-over early in the concept's evolution. Carry-over allows the necessary opportunities for practice and repetition of new learning and skills so that these may be consolidated and integrated into the child's repertoire of function. Carry-over of activities and handling into the child's daily life is an integral part of the Bobath concept, and as such it is essential that the therapist empowers parents and caregivers to learn to handle their child in the most helpful way, so that he or she may participate in the everyday activities that occur in the home and school settings. Without parent/caregiver participation, there can be little to no carry-over of treatment into the child's daily life. Treatment is handling and handling is treatment, and the role of parents and caregivers in treatment cannot be emphasised enough. Training of parents and caregivers takes time, and may take much time to do well. It should be done gradually and take into consideration the child's life story: his/her home background; family circumstances; family supports; his needs, wishes and wants; the family's main concerns/goals; the risks and benefits of intervention; as well as the child's occupational performance status and potential, and even such practical aspects as space. This type of training requires the therapist to work in open and honest partnership with parents/caregivers, to identify collaboratively their main concerns, and to educate and train the key people who come into regular contact with the child.

In the course of intervention, Bobath/NDT therapists provide parents and caregivers with suggestions for home/school activities. These may include: strategies for modifying/adapting play or school activities; suggestions for handling and positioning including prescription of adaptive equipment; and specific activities/positioning to lengthen tight muscles/align and strengthen body parts. Home programmes may be provided in written form, or via visual aids, such as video recording, photographs and pictures. They are discussed, modelled, demonstrated and tried out during treatment before being recommended. Suggestions are individually tailored to meet the child's needs, and those of the parent/caregiver, e.g. how the therapist handles the child when she is carrying him may not work, or 'feel right' for the child's parent, who may be left-, rather than, right-handed, and who may be taller, or shorter, than the therapist, and of a different body build. The therapist must therefore be able to problem-solve with the parent/caregiver to find a way of handling the child that is right for them and to ensure that the parent/caregiver understands the principles of handling, including the nature of the child's condition, and the application of TIPs and KPCs. Therapists may assist parents/caregivers to make the necessary links between the child's motor control/learning potential, the limitations and restrictions on participation, and the different handling techniques and positions. In this way, parents and caregivers may be empowered to analyse and problem-solve how to help/handle the child themselves in a variety of situations when the therapist is not there – which is most of the time! Finally, the therapist must be conscious of the additional demands she may be placing on the family in recommending a home programme, and therefore must ensure that the suggestions are realistic, functional and meaningful for the child and family/caregivers. The ecological context of family life must be taken into account and home programmes should be realistic and helpful, rather than an added burden, and/or a set of prescribed exercises to be carried out daily.

The link with occupational therapy

Weaving occupation into Bobath/NDT-based intervention

Occupational therapists use the Bobath/NDT approach to address the neuromotor problems exhibited by children with CP; however, their primary concern as a profession must be centred around enabling occupation and person–environment interactions (Case-Smith et al., 1996; Townsend et al., 1997). Townsend et al. (1997) define occupation as 'groups of activities and tasks of everyday life, named, organised and given value and meaning by individuals and a culture' (p. 181). In other words, occupation encompasses 'everything people do to occupy themselves' (p. 81). This includes the activities and tasks involved in looking after one's self (self-care), those that are performed in the course of enjoying life (play/leisure), and those activities/tasks that contribute to the social and economic fabric of people's communities (productivity). Occupations are selected because of their meaningfulness to the individual and/or groups of individuals. Occupational therapists apply occupation-focused intervention through use of the medium of occupations to effect change in occupational performance. Occupational performance results from the dynamic, interacting relationship of the person, environment and occupations (Townsend et al., 1997), e.g. in simple terms, the child's play is a result of the dynamic interaction of the child's sensory–perceptual–cognitive and neuromotor capacities, the contexts in which he is playing, such as on the floor, including the sociocultural context; the human and non-human environment; and the play tasks/activities in which he/she is engaging. For instance, catching a small ball in sitting is likely to demand a higher level of sensory–motor organisation and physical skill from the 1-year-old child than a large beach-ball would.

The importance of person–environment–occupation interactions has been recognised by the profession of occupational therapy for some time, and even more so over the last decade. This pivotal theme has increasingly emerged in motor control/learning theories, with postural control being seen as a result of the interaction of the individual, the task and the environment (Shumway-Cook and Wollacott, 1995). Occupational therapists who work with infants/children and young people may conceptualise postural control as one of the performance components that underpin occupational performance. The continuation of case example 1 illustrates this section.

Case example 1 – Jack (continued)

Enabling Jack to gain postural control in sitting would allow him the dynamic stability in sitting to free his arms to reach out with his hands to play. Jack's meaningful occupations encompass the many and varied play activities/tasks and playful experiences of a 13-month-old child, as well as those in which he engages as co-occupations with his mother and caregivers, such as dressing, bathing, mealtimes, communicating and reciprocal play. At his age, Jack's occupational productivity activities and tasks encompass contributing to the social, rather than the economic, fabric of his immediate and extended family group, as well as his group of playmates, plus those groups with whom he may be in contact in his community in the course of his life. Jack's occupational performance is embedded in the dynamic interweaving of Jack, the person/individual, his environment, which not only includes the physical environment, but also includes the adults on whom he depends for nurturing, safety and meeting his basic needs, and his occupations, which include playing, eating, sleeping, socialising. In addition, Jack's life and occupational participation occur within the context of time and space, in that he has daily routines, and his life takes on the flow and pattern of his family group.

As a result of the nature of his movement disorder, Jack's capacity to participate in meaningful occupations is compromised and may be restricted and/or limited by the motor and associated impairments. Helping Jack to do what he needs and wants to do, i.e. to participate and engage in and perform the roles and occupations of childhood and family life, as well as assisting Jack's parents and caregivers to find ways to care for and play with him, for example, are primary goals of occupational therapy intervention. The goal of postural control/motor coordination itself, although vitally important for the efficient execution of occupation, is secondary. The Bobath/NDT approach would provide an intervention tool within occupational therapy practice to support intervention for postural control issues, as part of the occupational therapist's brief in enabling occupation with Jack and his family members.

Posture and movement subserve function

Movement is not an entity on its own and does not occur in a vacuum. Rather, movement subserves all function, whether it be adequate dynamic postural support as a basis for use of eyes when reading a book, or for handwriting, or the weak squeeze of a hand to communicate 'yes'. Occupational therapists who use Bobath/NDT must do so while focusing on meaningful, functional, goal-directed activities. Many disorders of movement can be compensated for through the application of external postural supports and environmental adaptation via application of the biomechanical approach (see Colangelo, 1999); however, when problems of abnormal postural tone and patterns of posture and movement arise as a result of CNS damage, it is not enough only to consider a compensatory approach to treatment, and the Bobath approach becomes a useful tool to address all aspects of daily life.

Children learn movements as they relate to function, so occupational therapists must consider function in relation to movement. The presence of abnormal postural tone and abnormal patterns of movement may bring about movements that can be restricted, or disorganised, and incoordinated. There may be altered, distorted and/or abnormal perception of movement and processing of sensory information, and lack of ability, or inability, on the child's part to be able to achieve the necessary experiences for the development of desirable (more functional) patterns of posture and movement for effective and efficient functional performance. There may be restricted/limited/lack of adequate sensorimotor experiences, which may lead to secondary problems with higher-level functioning. In addition, the child's own intention and effort may further exacerbate the secondary limitations that stem from abnormal postural tone and patterns, in turn further compromising functional ability. Learning may be based only on abnormal sensorimotor input and output, further reinforcing the use of abnormal patterns of movement in function. Thus, in order to address all of the needs of all children with CP fully, occupational therapists must be able to understand the interrelationship between normal and abnormal postural tone, postural control, functional performance and context. In other words they must recognise, understand and integrate the concepts driven by motor control and motor learning theories into occupational therapy practice (Kaplan, 1994; Janeschild,

1996). The Bobath concept provides occupational therapists with one practice model that would enable this.

Occupational therapists aim to develop function through the use of carefully selected activities and occupations, graded to suit age, culture, past experience and client needs. They apply self-care, work/school, play/leisure activities in order to help the child achieve maximum function and enhance development and their quality of life. The occupational therapist's legitimate tools of practice include 'conscious use of self', the non-human environment, purposeful activities and occupation (Kramer and Hinojosa, 1999). Further, they are skilful in task and environmental analysis and adaptation. All therapists, however, whether occupational, physio- or speech and language therapists, need to be concerned with the development of function. Occupational therapists who use Bobath/NDT must do so while focusing on meaningful, functional, goal-directed activities. The Bobath concept can provide the occupational therapist with a framework to help understand the importance of postural control for functional participation. Further, it can enable the occupational therapist to understand, and learn potent skills of observation and analysis in order to see/hear/feel the impact of disorders of movement/abnormal postural tone and patterns of posture and movement have on function. The concept assists occupational therapists to interconnect better the components of sensory and motor function with psychosocial functions, cognitive development and all other aspects of occupational performance. It provides a unique approach which addresses the possibility for the child to achieve a better quality, or rather efficient means of movement for, and during, function, and presents a logical and practical approach to the problems of the child with CP and allied neurological conditions.

The concept enables the occupational therapist systematically, and analytically, to look at 'why' the child has difficulty with movement and function, as well as to determine what is required by the child in order to achieve a better functional level, or rather potential, for occupational participation. As a treatment tool within occupational therapy, Bobath/NDT may be used to support and facilitate more normal movement within the context of purposeful and meaningful activities. Implications for the practice of occupational therapy using the principles of the Bobath concept include reflecting on the following issues. First, how can we facilitate/make possible more efficient functional movement and postural control for enhanced participation in occupations? Second, how can we provide the child with the appropriate experiences, so that he/she may experience 'more normal' motor control and sensory feedback, in order to learn about the environment, thus enhancing sensorimotor, cognitive and psychosocial development? And, last, how do we remain true to the philosophy of occupational therapy, while applying an intervention approach that potentially could place us at risk of becoming component focused, rather than occupation focused?

Review of practice

The astute 'best practice' practitioner of today would be wise to critique the Bobath concept in the light of the paucity of current and respectable studies/publications, and in the light of it primarily being founded on clinical observation, experience and practice; however, as Mayston et al. (1997) point out, it is this very element that has given the concept not only its stability, but also one could say 'face validity' in the practice arena, and this, in part, has ensured that the concept has continued to evolve and that it has stood the test of time. Until recently, formal literature describing the Bobath concept as a practice model has been sparse. Course notes (Bobath Centre, 1997) continue to be updated and published and are available only to those who attend Bobath/NDT postgraduate courses. There have been a few unpublished works (Higgins, 1999), as well as numerous newsletter publications (Bly, 1991; Bryce, 1991; Mayston, 1995; Simmons Carlsson and Savage, 1995; Wilson Howle, 1999a, 1999b; Anderson, 2000; Correll and Dodd, 2000; Romano and Dodd, 2000); however, these Bobath-specific newsletters tend only to reach a limited readership. The literature, in particular that related to adult treatment, depicts the Bobath concept as a traditional approach (Kielhofner, 1997; Shumway-Cook and Wollacott, 1995; Bennett and Karnes, 1998); however, theories of the 1940s to the 1970s, albeit being 'traditional', need to be credited as providing the backdrop against which today's neuromotor treatment programmes have been developed (Bennett and Karnes, 1998). Some of the early approaches, including the Bobath concept, form the foundation for the current understanding of the CNS, and that of abnormal movement observed when damage occurs to the system (Bennett and Karnes, 1998; Mayston, 2001). Many of the techniques of these respective treatment approaches remain evident in practice and are functionally significant when they are integrated with contemporary task-oriented practices (Bennett and Karnes, 1998).

Over the past 10 years, and especially in the last 3 years, there has been a resurgence in published chapters and books related to Bobath/NDT (Mayston, 1992; Freeman, 1995; Blanche et al., 1995; Blanche, 1997, 1998; Bly and Whiteside, 1997; Finnie, 1997; Schleichkorn, 1988; Bly, 1999; Elenko, 1999; Erhardt, 1999; Pruzansky and Farrington, 1999; Schoen and Anderson, 1999; Dunn, 2000; Mayston, 2000a, 2001). Studies to test application in practice (Lilly and Powell, 1990; Law et al., 1997) have been relatively few in the paediatric field, and the need for sound, robust research is high. Results of effectiveness studies to date are mostly cited as not supportive (Dunn, 2000) as a result of poor methodology, difficulties around measurement focus and ethical issues in research design. Romano and Dodd (2000) suggest that the evidence is currently insufficient either to support or to refute the use of Bobath/NDT. Correll and Dodd (2000) found that the quality of research studies was insufficient to allow therapists to accept whether or not NDT is effective. Sasad's (1998) paper provides a useful overview of 10 efficacy studies and suggests that, while clinicians may believe in the effectiveness of Bobath/NDT treatment, practice falls 'short of initiating and designing research studies to prove the effectiveness of the NDT approach . . .' which in turn '. . . makes it difficult to defend . . .' (p. 1) the approach. Others (DeGangi and Royeen, 1994; Law et al., 1998) have explored current practice of Bobath/NDT in a specific population of therapists. The author recommends that, in addition to reading the current literature, therapists who wish to study the Bobath concept and apply the treatment approach in their practice with infants, children, and young persons should pursue the following: (1) include attendance on a basic Bobath/NDT course as part of their professional development plan; and (2) seek dialogue with Bobath/NDT-trained clinicians who have participated in a basic course in the last 5 years.

Conclusion

Current thinking around motor control and motor learning revolves around a dynamic system's viewpoint which focuses on the interaction of the human system with the environment. The emphasis is on the heteroarchical, interactive nature of the CNS and musculoskeletal systems, acknowledging the importance of the active participation of the individual in occupations, including the vital role that the functional task and context play in learning and motor control (Shumway-Cook and Wollacott, 1995; Kielhofner, 1997; Bennett and Karnes, 1998; Mayston, 2000a, 2000b, 2001). Treatment approaches that reflect these concepts are commonly classified as contemporary approaches to motor control (Kielhofner, 1997), or contemporary task-oriented models of practice (Shumway-Cooke and Woollacott, 1995; Bennett and Karnes, 1998). These constructs are explicitly reflected in modern-day Bobath/NDT courses, theory and practice (Mayston, 2000a, 2000b, 2001). There is a strong emphasis on the role of motor learning while acknowledging and emphasising the need to focus on goal-directed, meaningful, functional tasks. The theoretical basis of the Bobath concept of the millennium is explained in terms of the current concepts that relate to motor control and motor learning. Hypotheses are underpinned by new knowledge derived from advances in neurophysiology, neuroplasticity, movement sciences, motor control and learning theory.

The Bobath concept has continued to evolve in keeping with developments in knowledge and clinical experience, and in this sense it is on a par with contemporary treatment approaches. This is not surprising, given that we are dealing with the human nervous system and human occupation within an ecological context. Thus, it is possible that, in the end, all approaches may reach the point whereby 'the boundaries between approaches [should be] less distinct as each approach integrates new concepts related to motor control into its theoretical base' (Shumway-Cook and Woollacott, 1995, p. 106). As a practice model, the Bobath concept continues to be highly relevant and current. It continues to be a useful approach within the practice of occupational therapy with children who have CP, and allied neurological conditions.

Berta Bobath was a living testimony to the value of continual learning through clinical experience and problem-solving. This 'way of being' continues to be embraced by Bobath/NDT practitioners, and Bobath/NDT tutors/instructors alike today (Bly, 2000; Mayston, 2001) as they continue to grapple with, criticise, question, test and challenge the Bobath concept, and in doing so continue to evolve the original work of Berta Bobath and her husband, Dr Karel Bobath. Although the Bobath concept may be criticised for its lack of sound methodological studies and publications over the last decade, it nevertheless remains a valued approach in the treatment of children with CP – an approach that has stood the test of time. It has and will continue to develop and grow with each new clinically tested hypothesis and with the advent of more robust studies, and it will continue to evolve as new theories of motor control and motor learning emerge and as knowledge, and understanding of person–environment interactions and human engagement in meaningful occupation, unfolds over the next 50 years.

Chapter 4
Conductive education

HEATHER LAST AND LINDSAY HARDY

Conductive education or conductive pedagogy is a method of working with individuals presenting with motor disorders created by Andras Petö (1893–1967).

Born in Hungary, Petö completed his education in Budapest before moving to Vienna to study medicine. Alongside his interest in medicine, Petö studied the writings of Steiner and the work of Kodaly, and their schools provided inspiration for the basic elements of Petö's own institution.

Petö studied Ivan Pavlov's work in inborn and learnt reflexes, and the use of speech as a conditional stimulus. He also worked with the relatively new gestalt psychology, and its concept of the whole being more than the sum of its parts. These provide some of the theoretical foundation to his development of conductive pedagogy. Petö's method treated motor disorder with directed movement education. It sits at a junction between health and education philosophies.

What is conductive education?

Conductive Pedagogy is a method that does not treat separate muscles or limbs but turns cortical functions into events

(Petö)

Conductive education is a pedagogy that deals with the neurologically impaired child or adult as a whole human being, not viewing this condition as an illness or disability. It aims to promote the personal development of each individual with motor impairment and helps address their needs as full human beings.

> It recognises that each child (or adult) as a unique and special individual with cognitive, physical, social and emotional needs as well as a range of personal qualities, concerns and difficulties. The emphasis is on the development of the positive abilities and gifts of each person.
>
> McCettrick (1999)

The development of an active 'intending' child is of paramount importance in conductive education. The child's own active participation and initiative are vital in the learning process. It is a 'personality centred education', whereby the child with a motor disorder learns an active problem-solving approach to life, building self-esteem and a functional personality.

> Andras Pető created Conductive Education, the essence of which is to change incorrect ways of working, dysfunction, into correct ones, orthofunction, by means of Conductive Pedagogy. It aims for the children with motor-disorders to become participants in a system of education.
>
> Forrai (1999, p. 9)

Orthofunction is the ability of individuals to adapt to environmental and biological demands made upon them. These demands differ depending on age or society, but are usually achievable by those with an unimpaired central nervous system (CNS). Orthofunction is not the isolated improvements of movement and other functions but the development of the whole personality, which promotes the adoption of an active way of life, realisation and problem-solving capability.

The philosophy, planning and organisational strategies and programmes in conductive education elicit, maintain and develop this active attitude until it becomes an integral part of the personality.

Dysfunction is a lack of orthofunction, a lack of adaptive capacity leading to an inability to adjust to and satisfy all the demands made.

A child with cerebral palsy is going to react in a stereotypical pattern when asked to do something. At the time when Pető developed his system, other approaches recognised this too. Their methods were often based in the theory of sensory feedback and tended to avoid the problem of stereotyped movements by the adult taking more control through handling, initiating and facilitating the child's movements. Pető believed that, if a child was going to learn to do something, he or she must do it actively. He felt that children would not evoke a motor memory purely through the sensation of a movement; they had to be active in the process. They had to initiate, plan and execute the motor activity themselves. The conductors would guide and assist only when necessary. This is a cognitive approach, individuals being shown the plan of action, speaking the action plan to themselves out loud or internally, and then executing the action, inhibiting the unwanted pattern of movement and facilitating a more useful one. With practice, these plans should become more automatic and provide foundations for higher skills.

To carry out the philosophy and practice of conductive education, Petö created a complex system of education in which the many aspects of learning are interlinked. The education curriculum is developed and delivered by trained and qualified people called conductors. They use the tools of the group, the daily schedule, the task series, rhythmical intention and the motivation of the child to achieve these aims of conductive education. To facilitate active learning, these component parts of conductive education are used together in a unified system.

The conductor

Understanding conductive education depends on understanding the central role of the conductor in planning, delivering and monitoring a complex educational system. They ensure that there is continuity and consistency right throughout the day.

Conduction helps and facilitates something that comes from within the individual. The conductor acts as a catalyst. It is the conductor's role to provide:

> Guidance to the person's finding of the new co-ordination way. The person's cognitive learning is the principal means.
>
> > Hari and Akos (1988)

Conductive education stresses the vital role played by interpersonal relationships in enhancing the learning process. The conductor's own positive expectancy and belief in the child's ability to learn is essential in order to motivate the child and support their learning. To facilitate the activity of the child, the daily schedule and the specific tasks within it are all designed to encourage each child's readiness, attentiveness, concentration, imagination, self-control and introspection.

In considering the vital role of conductors within conductive education, it is helpful to recognise a 'hierarchy of learning' which includes learning how to: repeat, learn, do, be and finally learning how to become. Learning how to become requires a concern for motivation and self-belief.

One of the roles of conductive education and, therefore, the conductors is to ensure that:

> Education is not about the acquisition of skills of movement alone. Education has to be concerned with the formation of the person.

The values and ideas
The aspirations and dreams
The service to humanity
The life of the young person as a peace-filled fully human citizen.

McCettrick (1999)

The conductors must have warmth, love and commitment, and be dedicated to the child and his or her family. They also need to be sensitive, flexible, imaginative and creative, and have a sense of humour and fun. Working with children in groups also requires them to have the ability to captivate an audience and, by using their acute observational skills, lead, guide and encourage all the children within the group.

The conductor is able to get to know the child so well and know the child in all situations, so that the child learns to trust the conductor. This enables the conductor to understand how to help the child to attend and to develop intrinsic motivation and concentration, the building blocks to learning.

In essence, the Conductor is a professionally trained mother who directs or conducts the activity of her child. In this process everything we do is included, because it is the mother who teaches the child to sit, walk, talk and live. In Petö's method, it is the Conductor who assumes this role.

Forrai (1999, p. 95)

Conductive assessment, observation and planning

To implement a complex educational system requires the integration of very detailed and skilled assessment, observation and planning. The task of the conductor is to plan, deliver and monitor an educational programme that meets the motor, sensory, cognitive, emotional and social needs of all the children within the group, and enables them to achieve their short- and long-term goals. To do this, the interrelationship of all aspects of learning within every single daily living task must be recognised.

To assess, observe and plan for the children effectively, conductors require a detailed knowledge of all areas of child development and their interrelationships. This includes a need to appreciate the impact of disability on a child and the family. Conductors require keen observational skills. Planning needs to be at both the macro- and the micro-level because they are planning for a group and the individual children throughout the day. Planning needs to encompass daily living activities and curriculum targets.

Assessment includes performance of each child and member of staff, use of the room, balance of the daily timetable, the effectiveness of the programmes, use of resources and time, equipment needs, facilitations, whether effective or otherwise, and interpersonal relationships within the group.

Specific assessments within conductive education are aimed at eliciting specific information about a child's neurological and orthopaedic status at that given point in time. They are used to give an accurate picture of the child in order to determine a baseline, evaluate progress and at times try to identify why a child may be having particular difficulties in specific areas. Assessment can be formative (where you are now and what your future could be) and summative (how things are now). Both subjective and standardised tests can be used within conductive education as in other educational and therapeutic interventions.

The child's own self-assessment is also very important within conductive education. It is encouraged from a very early age. At the end of group sessions the lead conductor will ask children what they feel they did well, what they enjoyed and what they learnt. They will be helped to think about this with the other conductors assisting them in the programme. Even when working/playing with young babies and toddlers, the emphasis is on telling the children what they are achieving, e.g. 'Oh look your arm is straight'. Self-assessment plays a very important role in the development of metacognitive strategies, i.e. the process of becoming aware of one's own learning.

Conductive observation is a means of observing the child and the group. The main focus is not the registration of problems, issues or performance (although this occurs during the process). The emphasis is on the components necessary for each child to achieve the next step in his or her development, determining the necessary conditions for that learning process to occur. Observing in this detail, while actively running or assisting in a group class, requires the conductors to be well focused and perspicacious. They need to know each child in depth, have a detailed knowledge of neurological conditions and their impact on the child, understand task analysis and also have the professional skills to understand and foster the teaching–learning process. They have to be able to use parallel observation (observe a child as an individual and also as part of a group with which he or she is in dynamic contact) and continuous observation (constantly observing while working in order to see/interpret incidental changes and unplanned problems).

> Her observation is continuous because it is directed not at the condition at the time but at bringing the developmental process into being, so it is not just restricted to particular examination periods but is constant, both during occupations and the breaks in between them.
>
> Hari and Akos (1988, p. 183)

> The Conductor observes the behaviour of each individual in the group and makes facilitation instructions in order to enhance the behaviour. Observation is like a snapshot instantly followed by corrective facilitation: then a newer observation is made and preventative facilitation is applied.
>
> Rab (1997)

Conductive observation is an essential part of conductive education. There are three types of observation: operative, comparative and progressive.

Operative observation refers to the ongoing form of observation, which ensures that each child receives the appropriate facilitation that they need throughout the whole programme, so that they can achieve success.

Comparative observation is a dynamic process which ensures that optimum conditions for task solution are present at all times. The conductor observes each individual child within a group learning task and is able to determine when he or she needs to create differentiated conditions, so that each child can complete the task, e.g. with a sit–stand task series, some children will be asked to stand up and then step up and down off a box whereas others will perform the stepping up and down but do so while sitting.

Progressive observation is an integral part of operative observation because it enables the conductor to observe and anticipate the development of the child. The conductor has to be aware of the sequential building of tasks, facilitations and solutions which will enable the child to move towards achieving his or her goals.

Planning is an integral part of conductive education – it is the starting point and the priority is the needs of the whole child. It is the meticulous planning of the weekly, daily timetable and the components of the task series, together with lesson plans within that timetable, that allows for complex learning across the day. Planning incorporates how to meet the long-, medium- and short-term goals for all the children within the group.

When planning, the conductors have to consider a whole range of factors and every minute of the day is accounted for. Factors include:

- The needs, aims and priorities for each child in the group
- The diagnosis, age, sex, race and culture
- The developmental stage of each child
- The personalities of the children
- The requirements of the pre-school or school curriculum
- Daily living skills
- The need for differentiation within the programmes
- Staff resources

- Equipment and teaching materials
- Time constraints, traffic flow (described under daily schedule)
- Opportunities for flexibility and spontaneity.

It is the meticulous planning within conductive education that allows the children to work together in groups, where they benefit tremendously from social interaction with their peers, while their unique individual needs are being met and their aspirations and dreams have the opportunity to be realised.

The group

Within conductive education, children work together in large and/or small groups. The group is seen as an essential part of conductive education. It is the basic teaching unit and it is the main vehicle for interpersonal relationships. When developing his system of conductive education, Petö believed that children learnt best when working and living together with their peers. Almost all of the activities in the child's daily schedule take place within the group, regardless of the child's level of disability.

The children who share common goals and tasks shape the atmosphere of the group. The groups spend the best part of the day together, eating, working and playing together within the same room. The room becomes their second home. For children who are residential, the group rooms are also where they sleep.

This structure enables the group to provide a safe and stable environment for the children. The familiarity of the daily routines, the consistency of the adults and children with whom they are working, and the continuity of the programmes all help to provide the emotional security that Petö felt was the foundation for learning. Although the educational aims may be the same, the children in the group are not necessarily at the same level or may not even have the same diagnosis, so this means that individual solutions to tasks must be developed. To enable this to happen the structure of the group must be well planned and coordinated. The individual child's abilities and needs must be known and considered.

As the uniformity of the group does not depend on the levels of the children's ability, the conductors use the daily schedule to develop consistency. The keeping of the daily schedule principally ensures the organisation and conformity of the group, and the rhythm of the group. Every group effectively has its own favourable rhythm.

The group fosters collective responsibility in the children, because they become concerned for each other's well-being and success.

Age groups at the Petö Institute

The following age groups are identified:

* Parent and child (babies and toddlers)
* Nursery age
* School age

Parent and child group

One of the bases of conductive education is that conscious education needs to be started as early as possible, well before school age, and that mothers or carers must be taught 'healing educational ways' to assist the child's development.

Early intervention within conductive education is delivered through individual parent and child training sessions, as well as parent and child groups. In these groups the parents/carers attend with, and work with, their child during the programme. As well as receiving individual guidance and support from the conductor, the parents/carers develop mutually supportive relationships among themselves.

Petö felt that, when a child was born with a disability, the usual mother–infant bonding was altered. This bonding needed to be rebuilt. It was therefore important that it was the mother who worked with her child during the group sessions and that it was she who was guided by the conductor rather than the conductor handling the child. In this way the child's success was seen to be the parent's success also, which was considered to be an important step in the bonding process.

Nursery and school age

Children of nursery and school age may attend the Institute on a residential or day basis. In both cases they are working in the programmes without a carer or parent with them. The conductive programme for these children incorporates the nursery and school curriculum required within all schools in Hungary. In the UK, most centres delivering conductive education programmes on a full-time basis also integrate the early learning goals (nursery) and core subjects from the National Curriculum (school).

At the Institute in Hungary, both residential and day groups are made up of between 20 and 30 children. It may be that, for lessons, children move to different groups. Also, for a particular task series, such as the walking task series, small groups are formed from children who are at a similar level and require a similar level of facilitation, e.g. one group may need the assistance and stability of chairs between which to walk, whereas others may require only the steadying capacity of rope hand rails.

Follow-up

The Institute also has a follow-up service which enables children who have moved out from the centre into other schooling to return for sessional input on either a regular (weekly) or a periodic basis. Within UK centres, a range of follow-up and outreach schemes is being developed.

Planning the groups

The structure of the group is another factor in developing cohesiveness of the group. The structure does not form spontaneously but is planned and developed by the conductors. There are many factors to consider, e.g. in planning the layout of the room, the children with the greatest mobility difficulties may work and sleep nearest the bathroom area.

Within the daily schedule, during a transfer time when children are moving from one part of the room to another, a child waiting for physical walking assistance is encouraged to take an active part by watching and encouraging another child. This also helps to foster awareness and care of each other among the children, which reinforces the feeling of security.

Children's individual successes are always shared, which gives the child a great sense of achievement. When success is highlighted a huge beam of pride spreads across their faces.

The daily schedule

> Every situation in life can be used as a learning situation. No other time of day is better for learning than any other.
>
> (Petö)

The daily schedule considers every aspect of life and includes the biological and social activities required depending on age, race and religion.

> There is no single event in the day, which does not serve its general educational purposes.
>
> Hari and Akos (1988, p. 108)

Every event of the day is seen as part of an educational programme. Every activity presents many opportunities for developing, and for practising, skills.

> A meal not only provides nourishment but also a whole complex of requirements, giving opportunities for learning.
>
> Hari and Akos (1988, p. 152)

For example, while some children work on mobility skills to get to the breakfast table; others help to lay the tables, pass out the food or develop sitting balance. Thus the daily routine includes age-appropriate activities, but the way these activities are carried out is tailored to the specific educational needs of the children.

To develop a schedule in this way, conductors make use of their knowledge of the whole child and their ability to break down the development of daily living skills into component parts.

The daily schedule is a timetable of activities that reflects an integrated system of learning. The most essential element is the linking and practice of tasks and activities in a way that enables children to find solutions to problems, thus reinforcing other functional habits.

Within the Petö Institute many of the groups are residential. The educational programmes run from 6.30 in the morning to 9.00 at night. The challenge for day programmes in the UK is to cover all the daily life tasks but in a shorter time span.

There is a rhythm and sequential flow to the routine of a conductive day. The programmes are designed to allow learning from one task to lead into the next and learning from one day to be developed further in the next. In this way the children's learning is constantly reinforced, successes built on in a planned way. To enable this to happen, the daily schedules are part of a planned weekly schedule.

In planning the daily schedule, the conductors have to formulate the specific 'task series' as well as give careful consideration to 'traffic planning'; the terminology is used to cover the times in the daily schedule when children are moving from one place to another and may have periods of 'free time'. A conductor's daily plan will, for example, detail how the first arrivals at the lunch table will occupy themselves while other children are still walking from the toilet area.

The continuity of active learning throughout the daily schedule is enhanced because there is continuity of staff working with the children throughout the day. The daily schedule has to fit into a weekly and termly programme and is therefore developed with this in mind.

Within the daily schedule, conductive education believes that it is vital that every child learns to:

- become as self-sufficient as possible;
- define their aims consciously;
- seek out ways to achieve these aims;
- participate in mutually cooperative relationships thereby becoming an active member of the group.

Task series

The task series are a unique aspect of conductive education. They are part of the whole system of education and therefore can be understood completely only when fitted together with the other integral parts of the system. Task series are often seen as an end in themselves and have been practised in countries outside Hungary under the name of conductive education. Essentially, however, to be successful, task series must be delivered within the context of a carefully planned day, which has a rhythmical sequential flow to the activities.

Task series are made up of a sequence of complex tasks that provide the children with the opportunity to learn and practise the motor aspect of their self-expression and behaviour. Task series can take many forms depending on their aims, the particular group of children they are written for and the place they have within the daily routine.

Task series are the means by which the performance of activities, usually learnt spontaneously by children without motor disorders, are taught in a step-by-step fashion so that children with motor difficulties can learn how to move or do activities in a functional, non-stereotyped way. However, although the term refers to a series of intentional activities with a primary focus on learning motor behaviour, they also consider cognitive communication, social and emotional arousal, and motivational needs and goals. They are not a repetitive set of exercises, although this is how they may appear to the uninformed observer.

In order that a child with a motor disorder can eat or write, he or she may first have to learn to achieve a more basic goal of learning to sit independently. To do this, the child may well need to learn the prerequisites of sitting. In constructing a task series, it is necessary to move down the hierarchy of goals until reaching an activity where the child is able to achieve goals and be successful. The task series is created from here, building on a foundation of activities that can be carried out successfully.

The aim is to provide the child with opportunities for problem-solving in a variety of ways. Initially, the task series breaks down the activities into the component steps, thus allowing the child to be better able to motor plan. In this way the child begins to understand what a task will require and persevere in the quest to seek solutions and achieve goals.

The conductor will say what he or she is going to do and demonstrate the movements, the child gaining reinforcement in an auditory and visual way. At the same time, the children can watch their peers, so receiving reinforcement from all directions.

There is a rhythm, flow and sequence to the task series where one task prepares for the next, e.g. children are lying on their backs and the task is learning to rise from lying into long sitting. The children are asked to abduct and extend their legs, turn their head to one side, put their arm down to one side and push up. The work they did first in moving legs apart before sitting up means that when in sitting their legs are in the correct position. The preparation helps to achieve a good position in sitting.

Task series are always goal oriented. An active movement starts with an intention and ends with a goal. Through the guidance of the task series, orthofunctions develop that become the foundation blocks to higher skill development. They should result in the laying down of neuronal models, which become motor memories that facilitate the evolvement of a repertoire of routine activities.

They are always sequential, going from gross to fine and from easy to complex. The aim is to improve the quality of movement. In developing a task series for children with severe problems, there is a trial period, where the conductor tries to find a method that works best for the child.

The sequence of activities within a task series prepares the child for and assists him or her through functional activities in a similar way. A logical sequence of activities provides the preparation as well as the assistance to get the child successfully through the series. In constructing the task series, special emphasis is given to the needs of particular groups of children, e.g. the children with spasticity will benefit from particular emphasis on abduction of hips and dorsiflexion of the ankles in any position or task series.

A task series for lying, sitting, standing, hand grasping, etc. would last anything from 20 to 90 minutes, depending on the needs of the children. To help the children to attend for lengths of time and also in order to achieve educational or occupational goals, the task series will often take place within a theme, e.g. an autumnal theme.

Before the start of the lying task series, the children sit on chairs at the ends of their plinths. They listen to a story about autumn. They sing a song and think about their sitting. They prepare to stand, to pull on to the plinth and begin their lying programme. Using rhythmical intention to facilitate, and the story of animals collecting food for winter to motivate, the children begin their task series. The children move around the plinth in sequences of movements: combining the intention and execution of movements with rhythmical narration of song, looking for pictures of animals, and finding food for them to eat.

For the standing and walking task series that comes next, the children are taken for an imaginary walk through the woods. Ladder back chairs, rope and pole supports and wooden ramps make a walkway through autumn leaves and painted cardboard trees. In the trees are toy squirrels and owls; standing on the ground are cardboard woodland animals. As the children walk along the 'woodland path' they practise standing and walking skills, squatting to feed the animals, stretching up high to feed those in the trees. In this way the children are motivated to attend and concentrate for considerable periods of time.

When designing a task series the conductor must know and consider the following:

- Each child's abilities and difficulties in all aspects of development (motor, cognitive, social, emotional).
- Each child's individual goals in all areas.
- The group goals.
- The way the particular task series will fit into the day and the week.
- How this task series will lead into and prepare the children for their next activity, and how movements and actions practised within the task series will be practised again in different positions/activities.
- The options with the task series for a wide repertoire of movements, positions, postures and transitions.
- The appropriate facilitations for each child – when and where required
- How to use the assistance of the other conductors (second conductors) during the task series.
- The motivational academic communicative components to be built in.

Rhythmical intention

Rhythmical – to give rhythm to movement
Intention – to help activity be a child's own voluntary action

Rhythmical intention is another form of facilitation used within conductive education. The music, singing and rhythm that are synonymous with conductive education are rooted deeply in Hungarian culture. They are very much part of everyday life; it is not so surprising therefore that these support the process of conductive education.

Hari felt that, although it is important to talk about and understand rhythmical intention, it is not the only form of rhythm within conductive education that is important. There is also planned rhythm and flow to the whole day.

'Intention' is the conscious setting of objectives. It involves the anticipation, projection and visualisation of the goal. Intention is usually vocalised and helps to eliminate other thoughts and activities. The child does not actually move until the intention has been expressed by the conductor and the child when possible. This helps the child to anticipate and plan the action.

The rhythmical part of rhythmical intention then assists them to control the quality, timing and speed (temporal) aspects of the action.

I = involves the child as a key person
Lift my arm = action
Up, up, up = key word repeated rhythmically
1 2 3 4 5 = rhythmical counting = time for action to occur.

The rhythm may be:

Unemphasised counting: 1–5
Emphasised counting: 1, 2, 3, 4, 5
Emphatic: 1, 2
Dynamic: Stretch, stretch, stretch

Rhythmical intention is used within specific task series. Alongside this, personal guidance is frequently used by the conductors where necessary. This is where conductors give reminders or additional cues, e.g. within a task series where the children are standing tall, the conductor may remind the children really to straighten their knees by leading with 'I straighten my knees' rather than using rhythmical intention.

The type of rhythm used within the groups varies according to the needs and composition of the group.

Traditionally, within the Petö Institute, children with different diagnoses were grouped separately, e.g. athetoid group. The reason for this was largely to do with the different rhythms required. Groups within the UK are often made up of children with mixed diagnoses, which presents additional challenges.

Aims of rhythmical intention

The aim of rhythmical intention is to facilitate the child to be actively involved in learning the sequences of movements. It encourages the child to initiate his or her movements, to plan and sequence movements. It is the means by which the child forestalls moving in stereotyped patterns. It also assists the child to learn the various language concepts that are routinely used, facilitating the motor aspects of communication, looking, listening and vocalising. It helps to develop body image and an understanding of their bodies in space. It also helps to encourage orientation, attention concentration and perseverance – helping the child to learn when they are successful.

The child does not learn a movement but a solution to problems. Teaching is through rhythm. Self-instruction comes through thought and saying aloud the intention. Speech and conceptual thinking are character-istics of humans; they mean that activity can be anticipated before it is performed. Rhythmical intention is not intended to be drilling or repeti-tive chanting.

If the child wishes to do something other than that which is intended by the conductor, this should be appreciated by the conductor because the primary objective is for the child to *intend*.

Facilitation

Facilitation within conductive education refers to every single strategy and educational tool that can be used to help facilitate/bring about learning.

The aim of facilitation is to provide the conditions necessary for the child with motor dysfunction to learn how to carry out an activity through his or her own efforts. Its purpose is thus to ensure the development of an active intending child.

The conductor must know the stage the child is at to be able to struc-ture the next stage that they need to reach, and assist the child to reach this by providing the scaffolding that they need to do so. To do this, Pető believed the active interaction and active participation of both parties (conductor and child) were essential.

At any given time a variety of facilitations may be used but the purpose of facilitation is to become redundant. Facilitation is appropriate if, with time, it can be slowly faded out and the child's own orthofunctional habits take over.

When considering the range of facilitations used within conductive education (Figure 4.1), it is important not to underestimate the value of motivation of the child. Motivation is a great energiser and can encourage individuals to take even the most challenging step.

Conductive education within the UK

The establishment of conductive education services outside of Hungary has primarily occurred through initiatives led by families and/or other concerned professionals (psychologists, therapists, teachers).

As a result the schemes vary considerably in their practices, and range from families who employ conductors to work privately in their own homes, periodic holiday schemes run by conductors from Hungary, to small 'conductive type' groups being run within existing educational or health services to centres that have been set up to provide full-time conductive programmes. Within these centres there is also considerable variation in the types of staff employed and the services provided. The

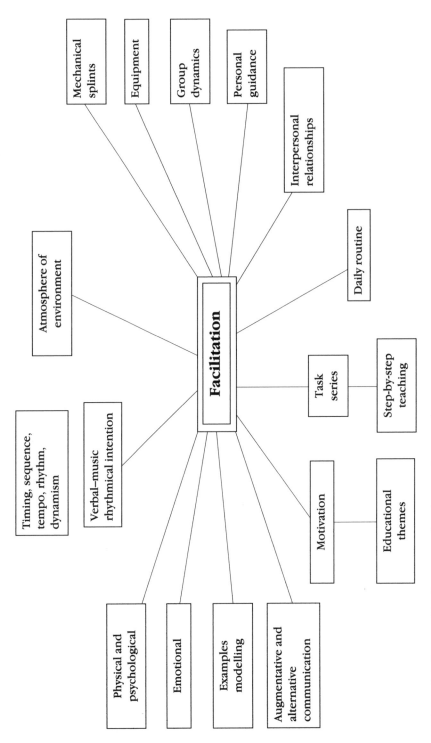

Figure 4.1: Range of facilitation used within conductive education.

Foundation for Conductive Education in Birmingham has developed the National Institute for Conductive Education which provides programmes for children and adults, houses a National Library and has also established the first degree course in conductive education in partnership with Wolverhampton University. The first cohorts from this 4-year degree course qualified in July (2000).

After a physiotherapist's visit to the Institute in Hungary, the charity SCOPE has also shown considerable interest in conductive education. Several schools run by SCOPE have incorporated conductive education programmes into their provision and SCOPE has also been active in establishing a network of small 'school for parents' groups throughout the country.

SCOPE also co-developed a Conductor–Teacher Degree Course with Keele University and the Petö Institute. The first graduates qualified in 2000 and there will be further graduates qualifying in 2001, 2002 and 2003. The course is, however, not being continued and thus, at the time of writing, the only opportunity for training as a conductor in the UK is through the Wolverhampton and Birmingham degree course.

Other centres have been established within the UK specifically to provide conductive education but they have adopted a transdisciplinary staffing policy. This means that, while employing conductors trained in Hungary or in the UK, they also employ a range of other professionals to work alongside them (teachers, therapists, classroom assistants). The largest of these centres include the PACE Centre at Aylesbury and the Craighalbert Centre in Cumbernauld.

It can be argued that to truly deliver conductive education it would be necessary for occupational therapists to work with a skilled conductor, and work within a unit specifically providing a conductive education framework. While respecting this, it is recognised that the former is not always available. The occupational therapists' added value in relation to other therapy approaches is an ability to look at the child from a sensory, social, emotional and motor perspective. The ability to analyse tasks, break them down and then teach the component parts are well-developed occupational therapy skills. These will enable the occupational therapist to incorporate the ethos and knowledge of conductive education into a variety of other situations to the benefit of our clients.

It is almost certain that occupational therapists would benefit from gaining a greater understanding of conductive education and the provision of shorter courses within the UK may be a way forward.

Conclusion

Conductive education is about developing an active intending child. Intention leads to an outlook on life that has wide significance. Children must learn to want to live, to solve problems, to struggle and to fight for something. Conductive education teaches this and it is of much greater significance than just learning movement. Conductive education is about teaching children to live.

Chapter 5
The environmental approach: major and minor adaptations

SUE PRICE

This chapter focuses on the environmental concerns for children with disabilities. The theoretical section considers how the works of Reed and Sanderson (1983) and that of Elisabeth Kubler-Ross' bereavement process (1982) can be applied to considering how the environment can influence children with disabilities. Basic assessment techniques look at points to consider when planning any environmental adaptations. The relationship between the theory and practice of occupational therapy is considered with reference to a case study, and the final section includes a review of current practice.

Theoretical background

In planning adaptations for a child with a disability, it is first important to realise that the whole environment must be taken into consideration. The environment is not just the bricks and mortar of a building, but also the emotional, cultural and psychological environments in which people live. These will all impinge on any adaptations that the therapist may be able to make to the physical environment. The family as a whole must be considered: it is not possible to treat the child in isolation.

One model of occupational therapy that incorporates this view is that of Reed and Sanderson (1983). This model demonstrates very clearly how every aspect of the environment is interlinked, and therefore must be taken into account when planning any work for a child with disability.

A family lives in a home – this may seem an obvious statement, but the point to be made is that it is the home environment rather than the house is that must be adapted. Home is where the child plays, sleeps, has fun, grows up with his or her siblings, and learns – the adaptations and equipment need to fit into the 'home'. The typical comment 'we don't want this

94

place looking like a hospital' is justified, because the design of some equipment is very clinical. However, by adapting the physical environment well, a child's ability to increase his or her self-management skills, leisure activities and 'productivity' can be greatly enhanced.

The biopsychological environment can be influenced by how the family are coming to terms with their child's disability. Families have different ways of coping – this is part of an ongoing grieving process that they go through as part of slowly coming to terms with what is happening to their family. If one looks at the grieving process as described by Kubler-Ross (1982), this can help one to understand some of the dynamics that may be going on within the family setting.

Kubler-Ross (1982) describes the bereavement process in a number of stages. The first stage is denial, moving on to guilt, anger, bargaining, hope and finally acceptance. Although Kubler-Ross sees these as distinct stages, it can be argued that this process is more of a spiral, with people moving between stages and going back to stages at different times. It must also be remembered that different people are going to work through these stages at their own pace. Each will be dealing with his or her own concerns, feelings and emotions, which are part of the bereavement process; each may be at a different stage. This will, therefore, affect the understanding and acceptance of any suggestions that a therapist may make.

The bereavement process can begin at any point; it could be when the diagnosis is given, which may be before the child is born. It could be as the child develops and the full impact of the diagnosis starts to become clear. It could be when a child is older and a progressive degenerative diagnosis has been given. As one mother has described it: 'It is grieving for what might have been, it is knowing that I will not see him running, or walking or playing with the others on the swings, it is not knowing how he might have developed.'

Having an understanding of Kubler-Ross' bereavement cycle can help therapists to understand why some parents react in the way that they do, e.g. the parent who will not allow their teenage child to use the wheelchair within the house, leaving the adolescent to resort to crawling round on his or her hands and knees, may be in denial. For this parent, there is no acceptance that his or her son will not walk, and everything in the house is geared to that child gaining independent mobility without equipment. Therapeutically, it is clear to the professionals involved that, for this child, independent mobility can best be achieved using a wheelchair. It therefore becomes a delicate task to achieve a ground-floor design for an adaptation that will promote the child's independence without alienating the parent.

For some parents, guilt is the overriding emotion: 'This is my fault, I am responsible.' This could be particularly so when a child has an inherited condition such as muscular dystrophy. It can also be evident when one parent has become the main carer: the other parent may find this difficult and wants to compensate in some way. This can take the form of wanting an adaptation, or a piece of equipment immediately, of getting 'everything sorted out now'. Unfortunately, this is rarely practical and can so easily spiral into anger.

Anger can be a very difficult emotion to deal with in any situation. Working with some parents seems to provoke an angry reaction, no matter what the therapist tries to do. This could be because, however gentle, client centred and calm an approach a therapist uses, as soon as an adaptation is mentioned it becomes confrontational: it is making the parent aware that the child's disability is here to stay, and is not going to go away. It is also making a public statement – a concrete ramp is not possible to hide – it shows that someone with a disability lives there. For some this can be too much to bear, and so the therapist becomes the target for their anger.

The bargaining stage, when applied to adaptation work, seems to take the form of the parents accepting that an adaptation is needed and that this is going 'to make everything better' once it is all completed. However, no one can bargain for is the stress levels involved in any building work. Once the adaptation is completed, it may raise many other issues that need to be resolved within the family, e.g. how do the rest of the family cope when the child with a disability has the biggest bedroom and his or her own bathroom? Can the parents cope with the idea of a vulnerable child sleeping on the ground floor while the parents sleep upstairs? There are ways around all of these difficulties, but they need to be considered and discussed.

Hope is so important – it can keep parents going through the stressful times; however, it can work against the therapist's aims if the hopes are based on false expectations. Many parents and children with a disability focus their hopes on the child being able to walk. When working on adaptations with families for whom this is a false hope, it can act against the realistic plans of the therapist for the child.

For many parents, however, they will have worked through these stages and have come through to some form of acceptance of their child's disability. Thus, they are more focused on what is best for the child. This creates a good working partnership with these families – the therapist being able to provide clear information that enables the parents to make an informed decision.

The sociocultural environment of the family will also influence the adaptation, because it will involve their cultural, religious, ethnic and economic status, e.g. in some families the custom will be that everyone sits down together for a meal – so the eating area will need to be large enough to accommodate whatever equipment is needed. For others, there may be religious requirements that have to be considered, such as washing before prayers. The child's main carer may also be an influencing factor.

The economic status of a family will have a direct bearing on the adaptation work that is done. Many families find that they need to have extra heating, increased laundry (especially if a child is incontinent), adaptations to their cars and extra care needs.

Funding of minor adaptations will either be through social services or, if families live in council properties, through the local housing departments. The funding of major adaptations will depend on the type of property and/or local authority practice. The general rule is that council tenants will have their properties adapted via the local authority. People living in owner-occupied, privately rented and some housing association properties will need to apply for a Disabled Facilities Grant, which has a test of resources/means test. This means that the family's income is taken into consideration, but not their outgoings. For many families this can create hardship. Frequently the result of the grant application states that, on paper, the family can make a contribution towards the cost of the work, whereas in reality many families are unable to do this. They are entitled to apply for a top-up grant from their local authorities to meet this contribution, but this can depend on the resources that the local authority has available.

The alternative may be to consider moving – however, the type of property that would suit such families could be a large three- to four-bedroomed bungalow. This is not always easy to find, and often financially impossible.

Sometimes it is possible to get a family re-housed via a local authority or a housing association because of the special needs that the family have: again it will depend on what is available locally and on local policy for people with disabilities. It is often necessary for the occupational therapist to act as an advocate for the family, writing reports detailing the specific needs.

So far, the viewpoint of the parents has been the main focus – but the point of any adaptation work in these circumstances is that it is for the child. The child's viewpoint has to be considered. Sometimes this can be hard to establish, but, wherever possible, the child needs to be consulted, involved in the planning and decision-making. It must also be remembered that these children can be very vulnerable. It has been estimated that a child with a physical disability needing assistance with their personal care, can have as many as 16 different adults involved in 1 day. The child's viewpoint such as the need for privacy, the ability to indicate whom he or she wants to help, and how, is important and must be taken into account when making any plans.

Both parent and child may find it difficult to estimate the best solution for the long term. If possible the adaptation will need to 'grow' with the child. The needs of a 5 year old are very different to those of a young adolescent; in turn, these needs will change by their late teens. These changing needs must be taken into account if the resulting adaptation is to achieve its potential to transform the lives of child and family.

Basic assessment and techniques

This section aims to consider how to apply the occupational therapy process to assessing an adaptation for a child. It considers the need for close liaison with other professionals, how to take a child's possible development into account and the need to ensure that the aims of the adaptation are consistent with other professionals' aims.

The assessment process for planning an adaptation for a family with a child with a disability falls into three sections: assessing the child, assessing the family and care input, and assessing the environment.

Assessing the child

This needs to start with a great deal of background research and liaison. Background information is needed about the diagnosis, the likely prognosis, medical background and the therapeutic aims of other professionals. Part of the assessment process is to consider what a child can do now, what the child hopes to achieve in the future and the potential that other professionals are working to will influence the overall planning. (For example, a child may not be toilet trained yet, but the aim is that they will become so; therefore, the adaptations have to meet current needs and projected needs.)

Assessing the family and respite care

It is worth considering how the family view their situation. This needs to be sensitively handled and may well be best achieved by working with a social worker. The respite arrangements may also need to be assessed, even if all that can be done is to give advice. This will ensure that the aims for the child within the home setting can be carried over to the respite setting as far as possible.

Assessing the environment

The type of house, the ownership and its position within the locality will all influence what is possible to achieve. Once the work has got to the planning stage, it will be essential to work with the local housing and grants officers who will have access to the necessary structural and surveying advice.

The initial task is to find out which other professionals are involved – social worker, health occupational therapist, physiotherapist, school, respite carers. What are their current treatment programmes and what are their aims for the future?

It may be appropriate to arrange a joint visit – social service occupational therapists are often involved only for a specific piece of work, whereas the other professionals concerned may have long-term involvement and know the family. Working together is essential to deliver a seamless service to the family. It is worth seeing the child at home and at school – he or she may function differently in these locations.

From the initial visit, the beginnings of a plan of action can be made. It is essential to involve the child as much as possible. It is good practice to send a copy of the recommendations to the child whenever feasible, with a second copy sent separately to the parents: this helps to establish that this work is focused on the child's needs.

Providing relevant clear information about the processes that are involved, the grant procedures (e.g. the Disabled Facilities Grant) and possible other sources of funding is essential. This will enable informed choices to be made.

The assessment process may be influenced by the local procedures for children with a disability. Some local authorities will have a formalised procedure based on the requirements of the Children Act 1989 – the Level II assessment procedure. This is an excellent opportunity for joint working and can ensure that different professionals do not ask the family the same questions.

The information gathered from the assessment process needs to be recorded: most local authorities will have a standard form that is used, some will have a specific form for children. Figure 5.1 is an example.

The assessment acts as a baseline to gather enough information about the child, the family setting and the existing property. From this a treatment/care plan can be designed, which in these circumstances means adaptation work. It seems appropriate to consider adaptation work for children as treatment – if it is done well, it will enhance independence, allow space for play and create a happier home environment, which will enable the child to thrive.

The aims need to be clearly thought through: are they for independence, for safety, for providing a better caring environment or for a combination of the three?

Once this has been established, then the type of adaptation work that will best meet these aims can be planned. This can range from the simple

Functional occupational therapy assessment form Social Services		Date assessment begun:
Occupational therapist involved:		
Child's name:	Date of birth:	
Home address:	School address:	Respite/care address:
Family at home: Parents: Siblings: (+ ages)	Teacher: Learning support assistant:	Type of care provided: Carers:
Accommodation: Type of property: house/bungalow/flat owner occupied/council/rented/ housing association		Accommodation: Type of property:
Other professionals involved:		
Social worker: Family doctor:	Health occupational therapist: Physiotherapist: Consultant:	Respite coordinator/ contact person:
Diagnosis:		
Medication/medical background:		

Figure 5.1: Example of a standard assessment form.

Presenting physical impairments/behavioural problems:
Upper and lower body:

Sensory impairments:

Cognitive and perceptual impairments:

(contd)

Activities of daily living:

	Home	School	Respite
Mobility equipment **Wheelchair** indoor/outdoor: Walking equipment: Standing frame: Future aims:			
Steps/stairs/access in/out of property: Future aims:			
Transfers:			
Bed (incl. turning): Future aims:			
Chair – type and method of transfer: Future aims:			
Toilet and toileting programme: Future aims:			
Bath/shower: (including special equipment used and method of transfer and use of taps) Future aims:			
Floor/wedges: Future aims:			

(contd)

Car: method of transfer, equipment transported Future aims:			
Daily living skills:			
Eating and drinking: Equipment used: Future aims:			
Washing/cleaning teeth/hair washing (incl. access to sink): Future aims:			
Grooming - self, hair, shaving: Future aims:			
Dressing/undressing (including access to clothes): Future aims:			
Communication skills: Language used: Equipment used: Reading/writing: Future aims:			
Safety issues: Future aims:			

(contd)

Domestic activities of daily living:

Future aims:	Home	School	Respite
Laundry – is access required to washing machine, tumble drier? Cleaning/household tasks: Future aims:			
Cooking: access required to: Microwave: Hob and oven: Sink: Fridge: Work surface appliances: Future aims:			
Leisure activities: Access required to: indoor activities, e.g. TV, CD player Outdoor activities: Future aims:			
Study/educational needs: Access to work area/ computer: Future aims:			
Environmental control systems Future aims:			

(contd)

Accommodation:
Sketch plan of floor layout of current accommodation:

(contd)

Action/care plan for . . . .
Occupational therapist . . . .

Summary of problems	Assessed needs	Action to be taken and by whom

Signed: (Therapist) . . . .   Date: . . . .

(A) I am in agreement with this summary of my identified needs and the subsequent action/provision/recommendations.

(B) Furthermore, I give permission for the Occupational Therapist to contact my Doctor/Consultant/Housing Dept/Grants Officer for further information/if required.*

Yes . . . .   No . . . .

(C) I would like a copy of my care plan: Yes . . . .   No . . . .

Signed: (client/parent/guardian) . . . .   Date: . . . .

*Delete as applicable

grab rail next to the toilet to a complete wheelchair-accessible ground floor extension comprising a bedroom with en-suite shower room.

The following are types of adaptation work to consider.

Minor adaptations

The work includes:

- grab rails
- banister rails
- half-steps

For a child who can walk or transfer from a wheelchair independently, appropriately placed grab rails will give them something to steady themselves and help keep that independence.

Banister rails need to be at the child's height and can assist with walking up/down stairs.

Half-steps for access in or out of a property will assist the child who can walk with a walker or sticks, tripod or walking frame. The steps need to be wide and deep enough to accommodate the walking equipment, the child and the carer.

Major adaptations

Major adaptations take time: the whole process from initial referral to final completion of work can take at least 2 years, if not longer. It needs careful planning, taking time to consider all that is required.

There are other constraints: the Disabled Facilities Grant process operates with funding and design limits – work has to be 'reasonable and practical', 'necessary and appropriate'. The building to be adapted may have design limitations as a result of planning and constructional constraints. There is also the need to ensure that the occupational therapist's recommendations are clearly understood by the family, the surveyor/architect, the builder and anyone else involved. It must also be remembered that any building work is stressful: the social worker involved may need to arrange extra respite care or alternative accommodation.

The work includes the following.

Access

Consideration needs to be given to where ramps will be placed – access is needed into the house and also into the garden for outdoor play. As far as possible the gradient of the ramp should be as gentle as possible – 1 : 20 to make it easier both for the child to self-propel or for a carer to push.

Level access areas throughout the property allowing the child sufficient wheelchair turning spaces, need to be considered.

Door entry systems may be recommended, with consideration given to how the child is going to operate them.

Access to the second floor of a house may be possible using through-floor lifts or stairlifts. However, consideration must be given to how the child is going to transfer on and off a stairlift and to the space requirements for a through-floor lift.

Bathing

Careful consideration needs to be given to whether a bath or shower, or both, are installed. Many children find a shower a distressing experience – for example they may become cold very quickly; or if the spray is not carefully introduced to them, it can cause a startle reflex and the whole experience becomes distressing. For many younger children, bathtime is fun: it is part of the bedtime routine, allowing playtime with other siblings and being immersed in warm water. This allows the child to relax and so sleep can be easier.

For older children, a shower with controls set at a height that they can operate and shower chairs that they can self-propel promote greater independence in personal care.

For very dependent children, a bath and a shower may need to be considered – a shower can be a quick way of assisting a child to get clean, especially if they are wearing pads most of the time, whereas the bath provides a time of relaxation.

How the child is going to transfer in and out of the bath or shower must be considered, and whether or not special supportive seating is needed in the bath or shower. It is also worth considering where the child needs to transfer to dry and get dressed: is a changing bench or area required?

Toilet

The toileting programme for the child will influence the adaptations. A child who will remain in pads will need a toilet for the disposal of waste, storage space for pads, a changing bench for carers to use, with a sink close to the changing bench for good hygiene. It may be possible to have a combined shower and height adjustable changing bench to provide the greatest flexibility.

It may be necessary to consider a special toilet that will wash and dry – again promoting maximum independence, e.g. a toilet that washes and then air dries the individual.

Wash-hand basin

Consider who is going to use it. For the child, it needs to be height adjustable so that it can grow with them, with clear wheelchair access underneath it. A mirror at the correct height for the child above the sink and shaver points need to be included, and consideration given to the type of taps.

If the sink is mainly for the carers to use, then its location needs to be appropriately sited for them.

Bedroom

Careful consideration needs to be given to the location of the bedroom. Although ground floor extensions can provide wheelchair accessibility and so promote independence and a greater degree of privacy, some families feel that this is isolating one of the children from the rest of the household. Access can be made upstairs via a through-floor lift or a stair-lift, but these are not always appropriate or suitable.

The size of the bedroom needs to accommodate mobility equipment being used, with consideration given to the need for a study area and play area, as well as adequate storage for such equipment as standing frames.

Kitchen and laundry facilities

This is particularly important for young adults as part of their independent living skills training. Consideration needs to be given to providing access within the family kitchen to an accessible work surface, a sink, fridge and some method of cooking: will they be using a microwave, or a hob and oven? It is also important to consider access to washing machines and tumble driers.

It may be difficult to provide a fully wheelchair-accessible kitchen under the terms of the Disabled Facilities Grant. In most areas, the criteria demand that the kitchen will be used by the main cook for the family. However, it is important to provide as accessible an area as possible.

Special considerations for adaptations for children with behavioural problems

This will often fall under the discretionary part of the Disabled Facilities Grant, but it is important to pursue as far as possible. For some children with severe behavioural problems, it is essential to provide a safe area – for the child and the family. Careful consideration must be made, together with other professionals involved, about containment issues: there could be legal implications, there may be a behavioural programme in place and any recommendations must be made in line with it.

General points to consider include use of the following:

- Stable-type doors: the top half can be left open so that a parent can see and hear a child, but the child can be safe within a contained area.
- Electrical sockets and light switches: all wiring and sockets can be chased into the wall so that no surfaces are proud; high-level isolating switches can be provided so that power to the sockets is restricted for safety. Light fittings may need to be fixed into the ceilings.
- Flooring and wall coverings: may need to be washable; padded surfaces may be needed.
- Windows: may need to consider the provision of safety glass, window-opening restrictors and window locks.
- Water supplies: thermostatic taps and the provision of isolating stop-cocks may be needed.
- Heating controls and radiators: may need to be at a high level, within a lockable box. 'Cool touch' radiators may be needed. Any radiator provided needs to be robust enough if it is likely to be used to climb on: an alternative method of heating may need to be considered.

Provision of a safe environment where a parent can leave the child with behavioural problems may help to manage the situation within the home.

Other types of adaptations that may be considered via a Disabled Facilities Grant include the following:

- Heating: this can be a difficult area and it will depend on local authority policies – many requests are made for central heating to be installed for medical needs, e.g. cardiac problems, asthma. As these are not part of the functional assessment of occupational therapists, the recommendation will need to be made in consultation with the family doctor or the consultant. For some children, e.g. children with cerebral palsy, their muscle tone and therefore their ability to function independently can be affected by the temperature within their home. It will be essential to maintain an even temperature throughout the areas of the house used by the child.
- Fencing: this comes under the discretionary part of the Disabled Facilities Grant, but it can often be essential for the safety of the child, particularly if they live near a main road. It is worth considering whether or not the child can climb because this will influence the type of fencing recommended, as well as any locks that may be required.

- Adaptations for children with visual impairment: it is possible to get extra lighting, tactile tiles, safety glass and guide rails fitted as part of the Disabled Facilities Grant. This is likely to be considered within the discretionary part of the grant: it is worth working with the specialist visual impairment team to formulate the recommendations.
- Adaptations for children with hearing impairment: it may be necessary to provide special facilities for a child with a hearing impairment. This could include a separate quiet room as a work area, which can accommodate specialist equipment – loop system, computers. These recommendations will need to be considered with advice from the specialist workers involved and are likely to be considered within the discretionary element of the Disabled Facilities Grant.
- Environmental controls: these are funded from a special local health authority budget. It is worth considering what can be provided and incorporating the environmental control system into the overall design. The systems need to be assessed by whoever is responsible for their recommendation within the health authority; however, joint working will mean that any extra sockets, cabling, etc. that may be required will be part of the adaptation rather than an extra piece of work to be done at a later stage.

All adaptations will be unique because they are for a particular individual. It is difficult to give specific detailed recommendations within the context of this chapter; however, there are excellent guidelines produced by Harpin (1999a) for the Muscular Dystrophy Society, looking at the specific needs of children with muscular dystrophy. Often the adaptation ends up being a compromise for what a family will accept, what is possible to do within building and grant restraints, and what is recommended as essential and necessary by the occupational therapist.

Case study: Susan

Susan was referred to the department by her district nurse for an assessment for equipment to help her turn in bed. Susan was 14, living with her parents and younger sister in their own three bedroomed bungalow. Susan has spinal muscular atrophy type II, is totally wheelchair dependent and, at the time of the initial assessment, is reliant on her parents for all her personal care. This involved lifting Susan in or out of bed, on or off the toilet, in or out of the bath and in or out of her electric wheelchair. From the baseline assessment, it quickly emerged that turning in bed was not the main problem (this was resolved by referring back to the district nurse for a pressure care mattress), but was much more about looking to promote more independence for Susan and looking at the moving and handling issues.

The key to planning this piece of work was to start with Susan and her thoughts about her needs. She recognised that she wanted more privacy and she needed access to her own bathroom because the one currently used was the family one. The time she took to get ready meant that this caused problems for the rest of the family. The occupational therapist's main concern was the amount of moving and handling carried out by Susan's parents, both of whom were complaining of severe back pain. Susan was also keen to have better access in the kitchen to a work surface and a sink.

The Disabled Facilities Grant process was initiated, with the recommendation to provide Susan with her own bathroom with, if possible, direct access from her bedroom. The recommendation also included provision of a bath, a Clos-o-mat toilet, a wheelchair-accessible sink, a body drier and a height-adjustable changing bench. The work would need to ensure that overhead tracking could be installed. Kitchen adaptations to include a height-adjustable sink unit and wheelchair-accessible work surface were included, along with a request for a wheelchair store accessible from the kitchen.

There were design constraints on this adaptation as a result of the existing layout of the bungalow. Building regulations meant that the building could not be extended on the ground floor; an existing workshop attached to the house could not be converted because of its concrete construction. There was some loft space available and the final proposal was to convert the existing family bathroom into Susan's en-suite bathroom, turn the younger sister's bedroom into the family bathroom, and provide the younger sister with a bedroom via a loft conversion.

Susan's bedroom had full ceiling-height doors leading into her bathroom installed – this meant that the overhead tracking can run from over her bed, through the doors, over the toilet, the changing bench and the bath, and then round to the body drier. Susan devised the route for the tracking: planning the tasks and sequence that she felt would work for her. She decided that the Clos-o-mat was not necessary; it did not suit her posture which meant that for her the cleansing and drying mechanisms would not be effective.

The kitchen adaptations became a compromise as a result of financial constraints – a full grant had been awarded as well as a discretionary grant to complete the loft conversion. This meant that the budget was tight, but a wheelchair-accessible work surface was fitted, enabling Susan to use the microwave more easily. A wheelchair store was created adjoining the kitchen.

This case was interesting because it was so client led. Susan knew what she needed and it was very important to take her viewpoint into consideration. She now has her own carers – this enables her to have her own privacy, and frees the family from her care.

Review of practice

The evidence found by Mountain (2000) in her review of the current literature points to the need for specialist paediatric services that enable housing adaptations to meet the long-term needs of the child and the family. Mountain's literature review also finds evidence for the need for specialist workers and for integrated or joint working between health and social services occupational therapy departments.

This is also reflected in the Social Services Inspectorate report *Removing Barriers for Disabled Children* (1998). This advocates the need for a clear, coordinated approach between all the agencies working with children – social workers, occupational therapists in health and social services, education, respite care and housing, as well as the child concerned and the families or carers. The report recommends the use of a key worker system to help coordinate the many people involved, to ensure that the focus is client led. Practical suggestions are made for good working practice.

One of the studies considered is the research carried out by Oldman and Beresford (1998) who surveyed 230 people living in northern regions and Yorkshire. This gives a good insight into the problems encountered by children and their families in trying to get their homes adapted. Some of the difficulty is caused by families not being aware of help that they could get with adaptation work, as well as cases where the adaptations are service rather than client led, with families having to fit in to what the local authorities are prepared to do.

The work carried out by Medhust and Ryan (1996), considering the clinical reasoning involved in planning an adaptation for a child with a degenerative condition, emphasises the specialist nature of planning adaptations for children with disabilities – it is working with a family to provide a solution that they can accept and that will meet the needs of the child.

The work by Payne (1999) and Andrews (1995) considers the positive and negative aspects for recommendations for a bath versus a shower, and different toileting equipment. The evidence clearly shows that the consequences of the recommendations need to be thought through with the families and children, e.g. although a shower may allow a child to wash him- or herself, will he or she remain warm enough?

Stewart and Neyerlin-Beale's (2000) work looks at outcome measures for adaptations for children. Their study has demonstrated that there is an increase in independence levels for the children. However, it would appear that there is little reduction to the levels of carer input. This study highlights the importance of using effective outcome measures within a social service setting, which can make a valuable contribution to 'best value' and highlight the need for effective occupational therapy intervention.

Useful addresses

Centre for Accessible Environments
Nutmeg House
60 Gainsford Street
London SE1 2NY

Family Fund Trust
PO Box 50
York YO1 9ZX

Muscular Dystrophy Group of Great Britain and Northern Ireland
7–11 Prescott Place
London SW4 6BS

National Care and Repair Agency
3rd Floor, Bridgeford House
Pavilion Road
West Bridgeford
Nottingham NG2 5GJ

Chapter 6
Play therapy

CAITLIN GOGGIN, CHIA SWEE HONG AND LYNNE HOWARD

Play therapy is an emerging field within occupational therapy. This chapter consists largely of a review of practice from the literature.

According to Jeffrey (1990), play serves many functions. It is used to establish a therapeutic relationship with a child. The child, through different play activities, can regress and use play symbolically to release tension and aggression. His or her needs, both unconscious and conscious, and his or her fears and fantasies can be acted out through toys and play materials. By interpreting all these activities, the therapist assists the child to gain insight, develop new skills and use his or her creativity, sublimating basic needs in a socially acceptable manner.

Play and its relationship with occupational therapy

The importance of play for children has been recognised since the late 1800s when views towards play emerged and it began to be considered as meaningful behaviour. Until then it had been perceived as merely an expression of surplus energy (Breathnach, 1996). Researchers have all tackled the definition of play quite differently, sometimes arriving at apparently conflicting answers, from Winnicott's view that it is 'the gateway to the unconscious', to Piaget's assertion that play 'is primarily mere functional . . . assimilation' (Bracegirdle, 1992a). Millar (1968, cited in Bracegirdle, 1992a) suggests that this confusion arises because play is not a uniform activity.

Clancy and Clark (1990) suggest there is common agreement running through the diverse theoretical propositions. Opie and Opie (1969, cited in Clancy and Clark 1990), assert that play enables children to realise who they are and gives them an opportunity both to experience many of life's emotions and to view their position in life in relation to the rest of the world.

115

A commonly expressed idea is that play is vital in the development process of children, an important means of communication and a mechanism by which children prepare themselves for future roles and responsibilities as adults. Winnicott (1971, p. 41) suggests that 'children develop through their own play; by enriching themselves, they gradually enlarge their capacity to see the richness of the externally real world'. He also suggests that play serves as a function of self-revelation. Jennings (1993) argues that it is important to emphasise the preventive values of play. As children are able to play, they are also able to help themselves, to develop their own repair systems as a self-regulator of experience. She suggests that 'the child who is able to play will have more resources to draw on, both in childhood and in the future' (Jennings, 1993, p. 3).

The literature suggests that play is central to both physical and mental development of children.

Occupational therapy literature has made several statements about play, especially in more recent years, e.g. Mosey (1986, cited in Read, 1996) described play as 'the work of children' and Michealman (1971, cited in Read, 1996) considered play as 'the most vital activity of childhood'. Wood (1996) suggests that play constitutes a major category of human occupation and that the predominant occupational behaviour of childhood is play, so play is a major concern of occupational therapy (Pratt, 1989).

Reilly (1974) appeared to have a significant impact on play in occupational therapy when she formulated a theoretical explanation of play and proposed a theory of occupational behaviour. She presented occupation as 'a meaningful need in life' (Kramer and Hinojosa, 1993). Pratt et al. (1989) believe that Reilly's major focus was to formulate a theoretical explanation of play, which gives substance to clinical impressions that play has an organising effect on human behaviour and is a critical base for adult competence. The central issue raised was how play enables meaning to be attributed to events of everyday life. Read (1996) suggests a developmental continuum between work and play, which was also a concept proposed by Reilly, where emphasis was placed on play and its effects in later life. According to Cronin (1989, p. 520), Reilly suggests that we use the work–play continuum because 'the play of childhood . . . contains a critical ability to transmit the adaptive skills necessary for complex work . . . and urban living today'. However, Cronin (1989) points out that it is important to remember that Reilly's focus is different from psychoanalytically oriented play therapy, which uses play as a modality to promote external expression.

Approaches in play therapy

Play therapy emerged in the early 1900s and has since developed new approaches and built on existing ideas. Cattanach (1994) suggests that play is a symbolic process through which the child can experiment with imaginary choices appropriately distanced from the consequences of those choices in real life. It is children's natural means of self-expression. Play has also been considered to be a form of self-therapy for children, through which anxieties and conflicts are often resolved. It serves as a language for children, a symbolism that substitutes for words (Oaklander, 1988). Play can help children resolve problems arising from stressful situations by means of connecting the safety of their dream world with the harsher realities of their life predicament (Lonie, 1974, cited in Doverty, 1992).

Play therapy can be directive, where the therapist may assume responsibility for guidance and interpretation (Axline, 1947), or non-directive, where the child directs his or her own activities and the therapist is seen as a facilitator of therapy (Wilson et al., 1992). Clancy and Clark (1990) argue that the varied examples of models of play serve to emphasise the complexity of the play phenomenon. No one model provides a wholly satisfying general explanation of the range of activities labelled 'play'. Jeffrey (1982) suggests that, from the earliest days of helping disturbed children, child psychoanalysts and psychiatrists in their search to find effective treatment techniques have appreciated and used the therapeutic potential use of play. The study of the history of play therapy gives the opportunity to consider different play therapy techniques used by child psychoanalysts and psychiatrists over time, and how these influence play therapy today. Wilson et al. (1992) break different play therapy approaches up into subcategories.

Modalities of play therapy

Psychoanalytical play therapy

Clancy and Clark (1990) suggest that pioneers in the study of childhood play were mainly psychoanalysts, so it is not surprising that early studies were linked to understanding psychodynamic processes associated with disturbed behaviour. Although the psychoanalytical approach to therapy is currently used infrequently with children, it is historically significant in that the work of Freud, Klein and Anna Freud provides a stimulus to developments elsewhere in the therapeutic use of play (Wilson et al., 1992). According to Gunn (1975), the psychoanalytical theory assumes that play has the need to repeat unpleasant experiences in a playful way, thereby reducing their seriousness and allowing for acceptance. Freud (1940; cited in Clancy and Clark, 1990) argued that a motivation for play is to attempt to resolve conflicts in the absence of a realistic opportunity to do so (Clancy and Clark, 1990), and suggested that children create worlds of their own and arrange and order things of that world in a new way which pleases them better. He argues that children take play very seriously and expend significant emotion on it (Wilson et al., 1992).

Clancy and Clark (1990) suggest that Klein and Anna Freud developed and refined Freud's ideas of the creation of model play situations for the acquisition of skill mastery by a child, and applied psychoanalytical ideas to treatment of disturbed children through play (Bracegirdle, 1992b). Both believed that child mental health disorders were a result of unconscious conflicts and felt that these would be resolved by bringing the unconscious elements to consciousness through the interpretation of child's play by the therapist. They considered insight to be an essential part of resolution (Wilson et al., 1992) and the task of the analyst was to understand and interpret the symbolic content of the child's play.

There were differences between Klein and Anna Freud concerning the nature of the relationship between the therapist and child, and the extent of interpretation of the child's verbal and non-verbal communications (Wilson et al., 1992). Klein especially equipped the therapy room with a wide range of toys designed to stimulate imaginary play. She saw spontaneous play of the child as substitution for free association of adults. Cattanach (1992) suggests that she emphasised the immediate use of interpretation to the child without delaying to establish rapport. Anna Freud, on the other hand, felt that it was important to wait to interpret the child's play until rapport had been established.

Although child psychoanalysis is very specialised and time-consuming, many working with children have drawn on their methods, and this approach has largely given way to what Woolf (1973) terms 'psychoanalytically oriented psychotherapy', i.e. approaches that draw on the same principles and techniques, but that are more focused, briefer and with more circumscribed aims (Wilson et al., 1992). In development of this concept, Winnicott has been significant.

Object relations therapy

It is believed that a child's natural form of communication is through play. Winnicott (1971) believed that 'to stop playing was to stop thinking'. He felt that play is a way in which rapport is established and, given a trusting relationship in an environment that facilitates communication, the therapist invests in the child's ability to express his or her inner world through play. Jennings (1993) suggests that, although Klein introduced the technique of play through which interpretations can be made about a child's unconscious world, it was Winnicott who recognised the importance of the creative and playful relationship between mother and child, therapist and client. Winnicott's theories are embedded in a classic

Freudian framework and draw attention to the series of relationships that the child forms. Play in Winnicott's view was 'the means whereby the child manages the transition between the inner world of the psyche and outer reality' (Winnicott, 1998, cited in Wilson et al., 1992, p. 6). Winnicott (1976, cited in Bracegirdle, 1992b) claims that children play in order to master anxiety and the ideas and impulses that lead to it. According to Cattanach (1992), Winnicott suggested that through play in therapy the child can dare to reach back for what he or she has lost or was never given or for what was too painful to be absorbed. His approach has been described as directive, in that the therapist sometimes selects the form of play as a means of communicating and interpretation (Wilson et al., 1992). It is, however, at times similar to non-directive play therapy. It is perhaps pertinent to note that his methods sometimes seem elusive and difficult to follow, because, for example, the methods tend to rely heavily on the therapists' personal creativity.

Release therapy

According to Wilson et al. (1992), this form of play therapy is directed towards helping a child who has experienced some sort of traumatic event, to work through and gain control over feelings related to this. It is based on the psychoanalytical idea of re-enacting or experiencing a particular event, so that blocked-off feelings are released and eventually extinguished. Although this approach was developed by an American, Levy (1938, cited in Wilson et al., 1992), it is similar to the world technique introduced by Lowenfeld in London in the 1920s, which is currently used by many occupational therapists using play therapy. In this technique, children are encouraged to construct a series of miniature worlds in a sand tray, choosing from a large collection of miniature figures, ranging from people, to animals, houses, cars and trees. When it is finished, the child is asked to explain it to the therapist whose role is to encourage, but not interpret. Lowenfeld felt that this was more useful than making interpretations, which she did only sparingly (McMahon, 1992). She considered it important for specialists to be properly trained. Lowenfeld also developed a mosaic test which gives the child a large number of pieces of different geometrical designs, sizes and colours, with which they can construct anything they like on a standard size tray (Lowenfeld, 1951). This seems to be less commonly used, but can provide a clear idea of how children go about things in their life. The advantage of the Lowenfeld techniques is that it appears to teach about observation and allows the child to make his or her own interpretations of play.

Structured play therapy or focused techniques

This has principally been developed by Oaklander (1988) working in a gestalt framework (Wilson et al., 1992). Oaklander (1988) believes that, whatever activity she engages in with a child, the basic purpose of a session is always, 'to help the child become aware of herself or her existence in the world' (cited in Jennings, 1993, p. 133). She suggests many guided fantasy and projective techniques, often through the use of art or drawing as a starting point, e.g. she may ask a child to identify with people or objects in their drawing and say 'You be that flower. What does it say?' (Oaklander, 1988). McMahon (1992) suggests that in this approach the therapist does not interpret the child's play, but the child may be asked to do so and in this way is helped to 'own' his or her feelings and projection. If it feels right, the therapist can direct the child's awareness to the content or process of the play. An advantage of these techniques is that multi-media can be used and it gives the child some choice, but allows the therapist to direct at the same time.

Drama-based techniques

Jennings (1993) has a background in drama and drama therapy and has always taken the significance of play as implicit in the development of drama. She saw the play of children as the basis of both drama and the capacity for human beings to create and recreate. Jennings (1990) developed a model of three evolving developmental stages from early infant sensation (embodiment play), when the child evaluates the immediate environment using the senses, through projective play with toys and objects, to the dramatic, social role-play of children. These stages can be worked through in play therapy to help the child progress emotionally. The advantage of this approach appears to be that it enables children whose emotional needs have been inadequately met in the past to regress to re-experience earlier stages of emotional growth, before they can mature and move on (Bell et al., 1989).

This is sometimes used in conjunction with Landy's model (Landy, 1992) involving role-playing appropriate to the developmental level of the child. Landy (1992, cited in Cattanach, 1994) suggests that role-taking gives form and meaning to our behaviour. He described a model of 'aesthetic distancing'. Emunah (1995) suggests that Landy's (1985, cited in Emunah, 1995) theory about distance in therapy involves the human capacity for working through matters of concern to the individual, by creating a distance from the issue in question. At an aesthetic distance, the individual is capable of feeling, without fear of being overwhelmed by the emotions and thinking (Landy, 1992). Although this approach allows the child to talk indirectly about the problem, it seems to have received little use or support in practice.

Non-directive play therapy

Jeffrey (1981, cited in McMahon, 1992) suggests that 80 per cent of play therapy undertaken by occupational therapists is non-directive. Axline (1947, p. 8) described non-directive play therapy as being based on the fact that 'play is the child's natural medium of self-expression. It is an opportunity that is given to that child to "play out" his feelings and problems just as, in certain types of adult therapy, an individual "talks out" his difficulties'.

Non-directive play therapy is seen as a client-centred humanistic approach, based on the principles of the non-directive counselling techniques developed by Rogers in client-centred therapy for adults. Axline (1947) applied these principles to child therapy. Wood (1996) argues that play, which by its very nature cannot be produced on demand, must be controlled by the player. Jennings (1993) suggests that non-directive play therapy emphasises that play in itself is a healing process, with which Jeffrey (1982) agrees, suggesting that the child plays out feelings rather than repressing them; the child then relaxes emotionally, realises how he can direct his own life and matures. Axline (1947) asserts that non-directive therapy allows the individual to be himself. It accepts that self completely, without evaluation or pressure to change, and recognises and clarifies the expressed emotions by a reflection of what the client has expressed. Axline (1964) describes the treatment of a little boy, Dibs, and offers an account of the therapeutic relationship, which illustrates the way individuals, through play, can achieve the resolution of, and mastery over, inner conflicts. This text appears to have inspired many of those using play therapy today.

Axline (1947) developed eight principles of practice for non-directive play therapy. In this model, the play therapist reflects the child's actions and feelings back to them, participating in the play if so requested. In the early stages the play therapist does not structure the sessions, but having tried to help the child feel secure, waits to see what emerges (West, 1992). The emergence of this form of play therapy in the 1950s seems to suggest that children have the ability to solve their own problems in their own time, given the space and freedom to do so, in the presence of non-judgemental therapists.

In a study by Goggin (1997), she found that the number of different approaches the occupational therapists used seemed to overlap. All the occupational therapists in the study adopted an eclectic approach. In some instances, it was unclear as to why these approaches specifically had been selected from the many available. What stood out was that most of the occupational therapists adopted the Lowenfeld (1993) and parts of the Axline (1947) approaches.

The fact that Axline's (1964) text prompted some therapists' initial interest in play therapy makes it understandable that they use this approach. Axline's (1947) approach also teaches a lot about being non-judgemental in approaches to play therapy, which was a reason why some of the therapists adopted this approach. It is described by the therapists as very child centred – the child takes the lead, directing the path of play. Yet, the Lowenfeld technique was the most commonly used among the therapists in the study. Perhaps it is popular among the therapists because it is one of the only forms of specialist training in a specific play therapy technique in the UK and also because the course is run near to most occupational therapists in the study, which could also explain its popularity.

Review of practice – non-directive play therapy

Trafford (1997) described how she used play therapy with a child, Noonie, a victim of emotional and physical abuse and rejected by her parents. Noonie was assessed in three sessions. The team made some recommendations including: to separate mother and child for a limited period with the aim of preventing further child deprivation and abuse; and to encourage Noonie to participate in play therapy three times a week. After an initial period of investigating the toys in the playroom, Noonie settled into symbolic social play. She spent many sessions making tea or preparing food for the occupational therapist and the interpreter. She consistently tried to appease and gain attention and recognition from them. Once she felt accepted, Noonie felt free to express her suppressed feelings. She became aggressive and attacked the toys, the occupational therapist and the interpreter. The occupational therapist reflected on the feelings expressed by the child. The occupational therapist also spent time counselling and supporting Noonie's foster mother. Noonie continued to feel angry but gradually stopped the violence and used toys to play out angry scenes. Unfortunately, the play therapy had to stop as Noonie went to live with her grandmother. Had the play therapy been able to continue, Noonie would have been given space to regress and experience the integration that she had missed with her mother.

Within the secure, supportive, therapeutic environment advocated by Axline, emotional health can develop. Kaplan and Telford (1998) have used the chronological development of a case study called 'Amber' to explain and illustrate the theoretical and practical application of non-directive play therapy. Amber is a composite of a number of children who were victims of sexual abuse. Ainscough and Telford (1995) feel that Axline's non-directive play therapy provides a framework for occupational therapists to interact with the child in therapy. They suggest adopting a second but compatible theoretical framework, i.e. psychodynamic theory, to gain an understanding of the child's interaction and response in therapy. Besides a trusting relationship, the occupational therapist needs to establish good rapport within the child. A child's natural means of communication is through play. Play gave Amber some insight into her inner world. To help Amber further, the occupational therapist had to be responsive to the feelings that the child was expressing and reflect them back so that some insight into her behaviour was achieved. Similarly, the therapist had to be alert to identify emotions from Amber's non-verbal communication and reflect them back to her as to how she might be feeling. This was an attempt to establish communication and gain an understanding of Amber, who made use of this link to make sense of the internal and external world. Readers are urged to read the publication in order to understand further how emotional and behavioural problems may be worked out through play therapy.

Conclusion

Many children with disabilities may need only one or two application models to address their specific needs. At times, this is sufficient, with improved sensory processing or learning strategies to compensate for deficits. Children then begin to participate in everyday activities without difficulty. Others may remain with poor self-esteem and are withdrawn, resistant or immature (Olson, 1999). In addition to being supportive and empathetic, it may be helpful for the occupational therapist to assess and intervene with these children using a psychosocial frame of reference such as play therapy. There are different modalities of play therapy; the application therefore needs to be tailored to a specific situation or problem with which a child presents. Such selection needs to be intuitive and may involve aspects from different modalities used appropriately, in view of the skill and experience of the occupational therapist and the requirements of individual children, rather than rigidly adhering to one treatment modality.

Chapter 7
Sensory integrative therapy

SIDNEY CHU

Some children have exceptional difficulties in motor organisation, perceptual functions, academic learning, behavioural organisation and psychosocial development, despite having normal intellectual capacity and supportive parents. These children are not generally delayed, and have no classic hard neurological signs.

Many of these children are referred to occupational therapy and found to have significant incidence of sensory integrative dysfunctions (Chu, 1996). Therefore, it is essential for occupational therapists to have a better understanding of the theory of sensory integration (SI), and the concepts and principles guiding the processes of assessment and intervention. This chapter will provide an introduction to sensory integrative therapy (SIT) within the practice of paediatric occupational therapy.

Theoretical background

The theory of sensory integration was developed by the late Dr A. Jean Ayres, PhD, OTR, between the 1960s and the 1980s. She studied the relationship between sensory processing functions and dysfunctions in the brain, and the presenting perceptual, motor, behavioural and learning problems of children with specific developmental disorders (Ayres, 1965, 1968, 1972a, 1979, 1989). The theory is validated by three decades of scientific research. The sensory integration model of practice is the most extensively researched and developed area in occupational therapy (Kielhofner, 1992).

Table 7.1 summarises the milestones in the development of the theory and practice in sensory integrative therapy by Ayres. Ayres died in 1988. Her theory of sensory integration is continually being developed and researched by other occupational therapists worldwide.

The development of sensory integrative concepts was based on the foundation of clinical questions, review of literature and research studies

Table 7.1: The development of the theory and practice of sensory integrative therapy by Ayres

Years	Events
1972	Ayres published her classical book *Sensory Integration and Learning Disorders* (Ayres, 1972a)
1972	Ayres developed the Southern California Sensory Integration Tests (Ayres, 1972b)
1972	The Centre for the Study of Sensory Integrative Dysfunction (CSSID) was established
1974	Henderson et al. (1974) edited the book *The Development of Sensory Integrative Theory and Practice: a collection of works of A. Jean Ayres*
1975	Ayres published the Southern California Postrotary Nystagmus Test (Ayres, 1975)
1977	Ayres opened the Ayres Clinic in Torrance, California. It provided an avenue for her to further research the theory of sensory integration
1979	Ayres published the book Sensory Integration and the Child
Early 1980s	Ayres expanded her work to children with autism (Ayres and Tickle, 1980; Ayres and Mailloux, 1983)
1984	The CSSID was changed to Sensory Integration International (SII)
1985	She also began to look at the concept of praxis and dyspraxia in much greater detail (Ayres, 1985)
1986–1989	In 1986, the Occupational Therapy Department of the Rush University of Chicago initiated the process to revise the SCSIT. The Sensory Integration and Praxis Tests (SIPT) was published in 1989
1988	Ayres passed away in 1988

to develop standardised evaluation tools and therapeutic methods. The concepts are then further defined and validated by research studies on the efficacy of interventions, i.e. 'research-then-theory' and 'theory-then-research' (Kinnealey and Miller, 1993; Blanche et al., 1995).

The knowledge base of sensory integration is complex and advanced. Therapists need to have a good grounding in neuroscience and to attend different stages of postgraduate training to learn the theory, evaluation and intervention procedures.

What is sensory integration?

Within the literature of neuroscience, sensory integration is used as a term to describe a neurological process related to an intricate synaptic connection within different levels of the central nervous system (CNS). Ayres did not use the term solely as a neural process, but as a neurobehavioural concept in relating it to functional behaviour (Parham and Mailloux,

1996). For the practice of paediatric therapy, sensory integration is a theory and remediation approach that addresses problems presented by many children with specific developmental disorders (Ayres, 1980).

Ayres (1972a) first defined sensory integration as the ability to organise sensory information for use. She stressed that the brain must organise all sensory information if a person is to learn and behave normally. She equated dysfunction in sensory integrative processes to a rush-hour traffic jam, i.e. when the flow of sensation is disorganised, the brain cannot use these sensations to form perceptions, behaviour and learning (Ayres, 1979). She further defined sensory integration as:

> ... the neurological process that organises sensation from one's own body and from the environment and makes it possible to use the body effectively within the environment. The spatial and temporal aspects of inputs from different sensory modalities are interpreted, associated, and unified. Sensory integration is information processing.
>
> Ayres (1989, p. 11)

The process of sensory integration is believed to begin in the womb and continue to be refined through adulthood. It is the process by which the CNS develops and matures by organising sensory information to produce an adaptive response. Ayres (1979) defined adaptive response as a purposeful, goal-directed response to a sensory experience. In normal development, adaptive responses are powerful forces in making the child an active learner. It enables the brain to attain a more organised state and increases its capacity for more complex integrative processes related to learning. Thus, sensory integration leads to adaptive responses, which, in turn, result in more efficient sensory organisation (Parham and Mailloux, 1996).

Sensory integrative processes are different from other information processing functions in that they occur on an unconscious level and in an automatic manner. Ayres (1972a, 1979) hypothesised that the development of basic sensory systems and the integration of their information in the lower part of the brain (i.e. brain stem, thalamus and other subcortical neural substrates) is necessary before higher cortical functions will appear and develop normally. It forms the building blocks for emotional development, cognitive growth and behavioural organisation (Quirk and DiMatties, 1990).

The original theory adopted a hierarchical view of the CNS functions, i.e. bottom-to-top approach. It is different from other educational and neuropsychological approaches which emphasise cortical-based functions and dysfunctions. Ayres (1979, p. 9) stated that:

> Educators often call reading, writing and arithmetic the 'basics', but actually these are extremely complex processes that can develop only upon a strong foundation of sensory integration. A sensory integrative problem that is 'minor' in early childhood may become a major handicap when the child enters school.

The processes of sensory integration

The terms 'sensory integration' and 'sensory processing' have been used interchangeably. Ayres (1979) described three aspects of sensory processing function as (1) the registration of sensory information, (2) the modulation of the registered sensory inputs and (3) the ability to organise and discriminate different sensory inputs in order to produce an adaptive response. Although these three processes are described as separate aspects, it is important to note that they are actually interlinked and somehow happen sequentially and simultaneously. To illustrate the process of sensory integration, a linear model is presented in Figure 7.1.

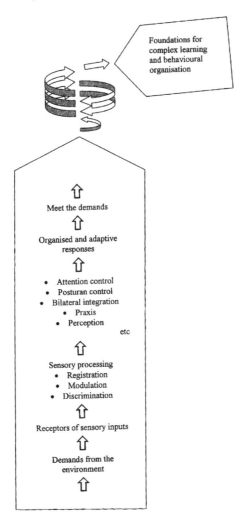

Figure 7.1: Processes of sensory integration.

The reader should refer to the 'spiral process of self-actualisation' used by Fisher and Murray (1991, pp. 18–22) to depict an open-system circular process of sensory integration. Recently, Spitzer (1999) attempted to apply the dynamic systems theory to analyse the theory of sensory integration. It incorporates current views on normal development into the theory of sensory integration.

Sensory registration

It is the reception of sensory stimulus at a conscious or unconscious level that affects alertness and capacity to orient, respond and habituate to stimuli (DeGangi and Porges, 1991). It is also the perception of the intensity of the signal and the orientation to the signal, i.e. orienting response (Royeen, 1997). Orienting response is the mechanism for detection of novel stimuli and orientation of the sensory receptors to the source of the stimulus, i.e. the 'What is it?' reflex. Through a process of match and mismatch, the individual is aroused for sustained and selective attention (DeGangi and Porges, 1991).

Sensory modulation

This is the process of facilitating some registered neural message to maximise a response, or inhibiting other messages to reduce irrelevant activity (Sensory Integration International, 1991). It is the self-regulatory mechanism of the CNS, i.e. it is a 'process of increasing or reducing a neural activity to keep that activity in harmony with all other functions of the nervous system' (Ayres, 1979, p. 70). Thus, sensory modulation refers to process of sensory signals before they are organised for use, i.e. sensory discrimination (Royeen, 1997).

It is important to note that the concept of sensory modulation used by occupational therapists does not refer to a phenomenon at the receptor level, i.e. neuromodulation at cellular level communication through different synaptic activities. Rather, it refers more to an observable behavioural response, from which the therapist makes inferences about how a sensory signal is being processed by an individual. It is artificial to describe sensory registration and sensory modulation as two separate processes because the latter refers to inferences that the therapist makes about how an individual is modulating the sensory input, i.e. they are really two sides of the same coin (Royeen, 1997).

Royeen (1989) suggested that the process of sensory registration undergoes normal variation throughout time. It is expressed on a continuum of sensory registration and modulation. A problem is indicated when an individual spends excessive time at one extreme end of the continuum, or shifts between the two ends. When an individual overreacts, underreacts or fluctuates in response to sensory input in an out-of-proportion manner, we describe this person as having a sensory modulation disorder. The developing theory of sensory modulation disorder hypothesises that the limbic system acts as a modulation centre for sensory input (Royeen and Lane, 1991). It is not surprising to know that individuals with sensory modulation disorder will always have problems in arousal level, attention control and self-regulation of activity level. Table 7.2 illustrates the continuum of sensory registration and modulation, and the effect of the sensory modulation disorder on the state of the CNS and possible observable behavioural responses.

Sensory discrimination

This refers to the process of refined organisation and interpretation of sensory stimuli (Parham and Mailloux, 1996). It is related to the central processing of sensory information through a single system or interaction between different systems. The discrimination of different sensory information contributes to the development of different sensory integrative processes and end-product behaviours and abilities (see 'Sensory integrative development').

The sensory systems

Our brain can process and perceive seven different kinds of sensory information through the tactile, proprioceptive, vestibular, visual, auditory, gustatory and olfactory sensory systems. In the theory of sensory integration, the processing functions of the tactile, proprioceptive and vestibular systems are particularly emphasised because they mature earlier in life. These three sensory information systems are mostly unconscious in nature and processed at the subcortical level. They all have a survival and discriminatory role, and serve as a foundation for the development of higher cognitive function, social and emotional functions, and behavioural organisation.

Knowledge of the development, functions and dysfunctions of these three sensory systems and their interaction with each other and other parts of the brain, may assist the therapist in identifying a child's underlying dysfunctions and devising a therapeutic programme to regulate/modulate and enhance the child's sensory discriminative functions.

Vestibular system (sense of movement)

The receptor of the vestibular senses is the vestibular apparatus, which is located in the inner ear and next to the cochlea. It consists of three semicircular canals arranged at right angles to each other, with utricle and

Table 7.2: The continuum of sensory registration and modulation

Continuum	SENSORY REGISTRATION AND MODULATION		
SENSORY REGISTRATION	FAILURE IN ORIENTATION i.e. poor registration	NORMAL REGISTRATION AND ORIENTATION	OVER-ORIENTATION i.e. too much registration
MODULATION-inferred from behaviour observed	HYPORESPONSIVITY/ UNDER-REACTIVITY	NORMAL SENSORY RESPONSIVITY/REACTIVITY	HYPERRESPONSIVITY/OVER-REACTIVITY
STATE OF CENTRAL NERVOUS SYSTEM (CNS) FUNCTIONS	SENSORY DORMANCY i.e. 'a syndrome or collection of behaviours indicative of atypical perceptual processing of sensory input so that all or selective sensory stimuli are damped down or "tuned out", and the organism does not orient to or perceive the stimulus. It may be associated with extreme parasympathetic responses' (Royeen, 1997, p. 12)	NORMAL STATE OF FUNCTIONS i.e. sensory filtering and habituation	SENSORY DEFENSIVENESS i.e. 'a syndrome or collection of behaviours suggesting atypical perceptual processing of sensory input so that non-noxious sensory stimuli are perceived as irritable and threatening; it emotionally biases the organism toward survival-oriented (versus discriminatory) responses. It may be associated with extreme sympathetic responses' (Royeen, 1997, p. 12)
BEHAVIOURAL RESPONSES	• HIGH THRESHOLD TO SENSORY INPUT i.e. need stronger stimulation to elicit a response • SENSORY SEEKING BEHAVIOURS • AROUSAL LEVELS: a. primarily under-aroused, i.e. lethargic or passive state of the CNS, but may become b. over-aroused-sensory seeking state, active seeking behaviour	NORMAL RANGE OF BEHAVIOURS	• LOW THRESHOLD TO SENSORY INPUT i.e. small amount of stimulation will produce a response which is out of proportion • SENSORY AVOIDANCE BEHAVIOURS • AROUSAL LEVELS: a. primarily over-aroused – 'fight and flight' state, avoid sensory input, but may become b. under-aroused – intermittent shut-down state, over-exhausted

© Sidney Chu MSc, SROT, OTR, May 1999. Based on Royeen (1997); Royeen and Lane (1991); Kimball (1993).

saccule connecting to the base of the semicircular canals. There are hair cells gathered at the base of the semicircular canals, with endolymph flowing through the structure. It is responsible for detecting angular acceleration and deceleration of the body and head movement, and resulting in phasic postural tone for dynamic body movement. The utricle and saccule are responsible for detecting linear movement, vertical motion and vibration, and result in tonic postural tone for maintaining static posture.

The primary functions of the vestibular system are to:

- maintain static and dynamic muscle tone for postural stability and body balance
- help to maintain upright posture against gravity
- coordinate the movement of eyes, hands and body automatically, i.e. enable the eyes to move in order to compensate for movement of the head
- coordinate two sides of the body, i.e. bilateral integration
- provide information about where the body is in space, and whether the body or the surroundings are moving
- inform the position of one's body and the speed and the angle of the movement.

Proprioceptive system (sense of body position and movement)

Proprioception is the unconscious awareness of the position of body parts, their relationship to each other, and their movement in space. The receptors of the proprioceptive senses are located in the muscles, tendons, joint capsules, ligaments and mechanoreceptors of the skin.

The primary functions of the proprioceptive system are to:

- give feedback to the brain about the positions of different body parts and whether or not they are moving or keeping still
- guide the movement of body parts without having to rely on vision
- interact closely with the vestibular system in maintaining static and dynamic muscle tone for postural stability and body balance
- help to grade muscle contraction and control smooth movements
- allow the performance of certain gross and fine motor skills at automatic level.

The interaction of the vestibular and proprioceptive system provides a reference point for relating one's body position in space, and regulating postural control in relation to the gravitational pull. As the two systems are closely linked, they are always placed together and referred to as vestibular–proprioceptive system.

Tactile system (sense of touch)

The receptors of the tactile senses are located at different layers in the skin structure. Some are responsible for detecting light touch, temperature and pain sensation; others discriminate different textures, shapes and contour of surfaces.

The following are the primary functions of the tactile system, to:

- regulate emotional and social development, e.g. bonding between parents and baby.
- contribute to the development of body scheme which was first postulated by Ayres (1961). It is related to the sensorimotor awareness of different anatomical elements of the body (Ayres, 1972a) and is referred to as an internal model of the body in action (Cermak, 1991). Ayres (1972a, p. 168) suggested that 'sensory input from the skin and joints, but especially from the skin, helps develop in the brain the model or internal scheme of the body's design as a motor instrument'.
- serve as a basis for the development of praxis through the establishment of body scheme, i.e. the ability to formulate the idea of what to do, plan and execute the sequence of actions for a task.
- contribute to the development of fine motor skills.
- form the foundation for perceptual and cognitive development.

Vestibular–proprioceptive–tactile information is classified as 'near senses', whereas visual and auditory information is classified as 'distant senses'. The former is processed unconsciously and mostly at the subcortical level, whereas the latter is processed more consciously and at the cortical level. Both levels of information-processing function are important for learning and behavioural organisation.

Sensory integrative development

The integration of different sensory information allows the child to develop different sensorimotor and perceptual functions for performance in different daily life, school activities, play and leisure activities (Figure 7.2). Sensory integrative development progresses in a natural manner in the first 8 years and continues to be refined throughout adulthood. Ayres (1972a, p. 12) stated that 'cognitive function has its tap root in the spinal cord, most of the rest of its roots in the brain stem and other subcortical structures, and the cortex assumes a mediating role over all'.

The three stages of sensory processing functions described (i.e. registration, modulation and discrimination) contribute to different aspects of development. Any deficits in the process of sensory registration and

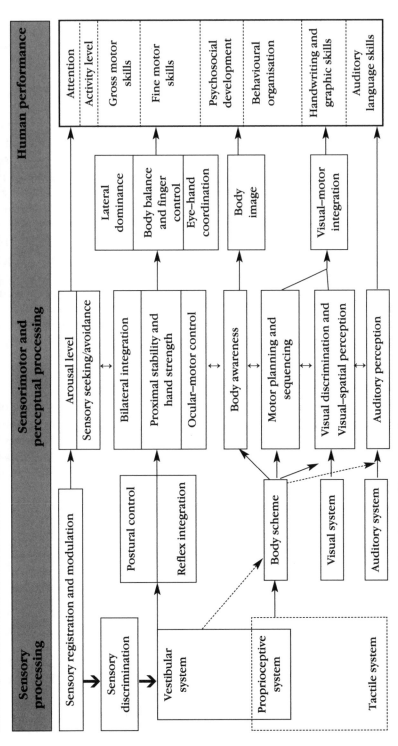

Figure 7.2: Sensory integrative foundation of human performance.

modulation will affect a child's arousal level and attention control. A child may be overreactive, underreactive or fluctuated in response to sensory inputs. As a result, the child may exhibit a spectrum of sensory-seeking or sensory-avoidance behaviours (see Table 7.2). Ayres (1964) described the link between tactile dysfunction and hyperactive behaviour as early as 1964, and later identified the pattern of tactile defensiveness (Ayres, 1972a).

The discrimination of different sensory information and interaction of different sensory processing functions form the 'building blocks' for more complex and more mature development. First, the child develops the senses that tell him or her about his or her own body and its relationship to the gravitational field of the earth, i.e. body scheme. The formulation of a map of the body enables the child to develop different perceptual functions, e.g. the visual perception involved in reading is the end-product of many building blocks that form during sensorimotor activities (Ayres, 1979). Cabay and King (1989) described the contribution of sensory integrative processes in the development of perceptual functions that serve as a foundation for conceptual development. Praxis is also another end-product of sensory integration. Through different factor analyses, Ayres (1989) identified a consistent link between praxis and somatosensory processing function, i.e. the discrimination of tactile and kinaesthetic information.

Sensory integrative evaluation

Evaluation is the planned process of gathering and interpreting objective/subjective data necessary for making a diagnosis, selecting appropriate treatment methods, and planning treatment programmes with stated goals and objectives. The therapist needs to adopt a multi-faceted assessment approach in order to determine whether or not a sensory integrative dysfunction is present, and how it affects the child's development and performance in different areas of function.

Basic assessment procedures

The process of gathering information in a sensory integrative evaluation could include the following procedures:

- Clinical observations (CO) on the evaluation of sensory processing functions.
- Sensory Integration and Praxis Tests (SIPT).
- Parents' questionnaire on developmental history and specific behavioural patterns suggesting different sensory processing functions and dysfunctions.

- Teacher's questionnaire on school behaviour and academic performance.
- Other standardised tests, scales and checklists.
- Observations at home, school and during interaction with peers.
- Interview/discussion with key individuals, e.g. parents, teachers, etc.
- Information from other professionals, e.g. psychologists.
- Review of the child's medical file.

Clinical observations

The CO is a set of non-standardised procedures designed to measure a child's neurobehavioural and neuromuscular functions, e.g. reflex integration and postural control, etc. (Ayres 1972a, 1976). The items are selected to supplement the information gathered through other standardised tests, e.g. the SIPT. As the administrative procedures and scoring criteria of the CO items have not been standardised, therapists need to rely on their skills and experience, especially the ability to relate the child's responses to sensory processing theory and functions.

The CO items are closely related to tests of cerebellar–vestibular functions or soft neurological signs described by Touwen (1979). Wilson et al. (1994) published the Clinical Observation of Motor and Postural Skills (COMPS) which provides more objective measures on six items: slow movements, rapid forearm rotation, finger–nose touching, prone extension posture, asymmetrical tonic neck reflex and supine–flexion posture.

Sensory Integration and Praxis Tests

The SIPT was published by the Western Psychological Services in the USA (Ayres, 1989). It was developed from the Southern California Sensory Integration Tests, with input from the Rush University of Chicago, Sensory Integration International, and a group of occupational therapists and physical therapists who helped to gather normative data throughout USA and Canada. It is standardised on a normative sample of 1997 boys and girls, with different ethnic backgrounds and from different rural and urban areas throughout North America.

The SIPT is 'designed to assess several different practic abilities, various aspects of the sensory processing status of the vestibular, proprioceptive, kinesthetic, tactile, and visual system, and the major behavioural manifestation of deficits in integration of sensory inputs from these systems' (Ayres, 1989, p. 1). It identifies discrete dysfunctions. It is a battery of 17 standardised performance tests for children aged 4 years to 8 years 11 months. The 17 subtests are grouped into four types of tests:

1. Motor-Free Visual Perception Tests
   - Space Visualisation
   - Figure–ground Perception
2. Somatosensory Tests
   - Manual Form Perception
   - Kinaesthesia
   - Finger Identification
   - Graphaesthesia
   - Localisation of Tactile Stimuli
3. Praxis Tests
   - Praxis on Verbal Command
   - Design Copying
   - Constructional Praxis
   - Postural Praxis
   - Oral Praxis
   - Sequencing Praxis
4. Sensorimotor Tests
   - Bilateral Motor Coordination
   - Standing and Walking Balance
   - Motor Accuracy
   - Postrotatory Nystagmus.

The whole battery could be administered in one or two sessions, totalling 1.5–2 hours plus an additional 30–45 minutes for completing the scoring on computerised protocol sheets. The protocol sheets are computer scored by the publisher, or by using a Microcomputer Disk for SIPT scoring, published by the Western Psychological Services. A written report will be generated by the computer, with detailed description on the child's performance in individual tests and a ChromaGraph to compare the child's pattern of performance with an identified cluster group. Interpretation of the ChromaGraph with other additional information enables the therapists to differentiate whether or not the child has a sensory integrative dysfunction.

As a result of the complexity of the tests and the levels of knowledge required to interpret the results, therapists are advised to go through postgraduate training in order to acquire an appropriate level of competency in using the test for clinical practice. Further details on the content of the SIPT and its psychometric properties can be found in the articles by Mailloux (1990), Ayres and Marr (1991) and the SIPT Manual (Ayres, 1989).

The use of questionnaires

Structured questionnaires will be useful to gather information from parents and the child's teacher. Larson (1982) developed a sensory history to assess developmentally delayed children with and without tactile defensiveness. There have also been different versions of the questionnaires developed and constructed by different therapists throughout the years, e.g. Knickerbocker (1980), Carrasco and Lee (1993) and LaCroix et al. (1997). Recently, Dunn (1994, 1997, 1999) developed a sensory profile which proved to be a useful tool for sensory integrative evaluation, especially in the aspects of sensory modulation. A series of studies has been carried out to establish the psychometric properties of the sensory profile (Dunn and Brown, 1997; Dunn and Westman, 1997; Kientz and Dunn, 1997; Ermer and Dunn, 1998).

Observations

Observations of the child's behaviour within a natural environment (e.g. classroom, playground and home) and during an initial treatment session will be useful to support and confirm the interpretation of data gathered through formal and objective assessment procedures. The therapist may concentrate on the following aspects of observation:

- Response to sensory input, i.e. registration, habituation, modulation, and discrimination of tactile, proprioceptive, vestibular, and visual and auditory information.
- Arousal level, attention control and activity level.
- Emotional/behavioural responses to certain sensory inputs.
- Postural–motor control and responses, e.g. tonic and phasic postural control, proximal and central stability, extension and flexion posture, rotation and postural adjustment, etc.
- Bilateral integrative functions, e.g. symmetrical and asymmetrical patterns, bilateral holding and release, etc.
- Static and dynamic body balance and general body control in different coordinated movements.
- Ocular responses, i.e. fixation, tracking, vestibular-mediated eye movements.
- Praxis, i.e. ideation, motor planning, timing, sequencing, spatial organisation, etc.
- Organisation of behaviour, e.g. level of self-control, interactive behaviour, use of language, etc.
- Levels of adaptive responses when engaging in activities with different levels of complexity.

- Other observations, e.g. presence of associated reactions, associated movements, body asymmetry, etc.
- Functional performance, e.g. level of self-care skills, handwriting skills, social interaction with peers, etc.

Interpretation of assessment results

As there is no direct mean to measure the actual sensory integrative processes in the subcortical level, assessment procedures tend to focus on those behaviours that are greatly subserved by sensory processing functions, particularly those related to the tactile, proprioceptive and vestibular systems. Thus, the interpretation of the assessment results is based on an assumption that an underlying sensory integrative dysfunction is the basis of the observed deviation in behaviour and performance.

First, the therapist needs to analyse the information gathered in relation to different domains of functions and dysfunctions in the sensory integrative processes. Table 7.3 illustrates a format of analysis on the domains of function. After this analysis, a hypothesis could be generated as to whether or not the child has a sensory integrative dysfunction. With

Table 7.3: Analysis of the domains of function

VESTIBULAR PROPRIOCEPTIVE SYSTEMS

Registration of vestibular proprioceptive inputs

Hypo-responsive	Hyper-responsive	Discrimination	Cerebellar integrity
Movement seeking Physically active High arousal level	Intolerance to movement Gravitational security Postural insecurity (?)	Slow movements Finger to nose Diadochokinesia Supine lying Kinaesthesia	Slow movement Diadochokinesia (arm) Diadochokinesia (tongue) Supine lying

Integration of primitive reflexes and development of automatic reactions

Reflex integration		Automatic reactions	
Rolling Supine flexion Prone extension	ATNR Anti-ATNR STNR Postural change in arm (SAE)	PER Equilibrium reaction Standing balance (eyes closed)	Trunk rotation (also in SAE head resistance and discomfort, resist trunk rotation)

Table 7.3: (contd)

Postural–ocular motor control

	Postural	Ocular	Others
Muscle tone Body posture Co-contraction Prone extension Supine flexion Postural stability	Shoulder stability Anti-ATNR Trunk rotation PER Equilibrium reaction Standing balance	Vestibular–ocular reflex, i.e. eyes fixate when body moves Hypo-PRN Hyper-PRN	Postural background movements Patterns of movements Associated movements Associated reactions

Bilateral integration and sequencing (BIS)

Laterality	BIS		Other BIS functions
Eye Ear Hand Foot	Eyes cross midline Arms cross midline Slow movements Diadochokinesia Mirror movements	Thumb/finger touching Bilateral motor coordination Jumping (feet together) Sequence of movement	Tying shoe-laces Using knife and fork Cutting with a pair of scissors Sequencing of week days, months and alphabet Sequencing of time

TACTILE SYSTEM

Hypo-responsive	Hyper-responsive	Discrimination
High threshold to tactile input Needs stronger stimulation in order to elicit a response Seeking out tactile inputs, very touchy Usually passive and inactive Under-sensitive to physical hurt Low arousal level	Features of tactile defensiveness, e.g. Does not like to be touched from behind Does not like clothes made of certain material Does not like to have hair washed, finger nails cut, etc. Needs to have obvious emotional reaction to tactile input	Tactile items from the clinical observation of somatosensory perception, i.e. Finger identification One- or two-point touch Graphaesthesia Stereognosis Double-touch discrimination

VISUAL SYSTEM

Form and space		Visual construction		Visual–motor coordination
Results of: TVPS MVPT	Two-dimensional orientation Visual reversal	Results of: TVMS VMI	Three-dimensional orientation Written reversal	The ability to do tracing tasks

Table 7.3: (contd)

PRAXIS		MOTOR FUNCTIONS	
Central processes	**Others**	**Fundamental motor skills**	**Fine motor skills**
Ideation Motor planning Execution **Performance:-** Supine flexion Tongue–lip movements Eye movements Bilateral motor coordination	Sequencing Spatial organisation Follow verbal instructions Imitation of posture Visual–motor integration Constructional praxis Poor organisation of materials Forgetful Shows hesitation of doing new tasks, etc.	Hopping Jumping Skipping **Balance** Standing balance Heel–toe walking **Ball skills** Throwing Catching Kicking Bouncing	Hand grasp Thumb-finger touching Pencil control Scissor skills Two-hand coordination, e.g. threading beads In-hand manipulation **Ocular–motor control** Eye pursuits Eye convergence Quick localisations Visual scanning

HEMISPHERIC FUNCTIONS

Right hemisphere	**Left hemisphere**
Independent eye closure – cannot close right eye Visuopraxis Spatial processes	Independent eye closure – cannot close left eye Praxis on verbal command Sequential processes
IRREGULAR NEUROLOGICAL FUNCTIONING	DISTRIBUTION
Choreoathetoid movements (SAE) Body asymmetry Overt associated reactions Tight TAs, hamstrings and hip abductors	Poor arousal level and attention control Physically active and impulsive Poor figure–ground and short-term memory Poor self-control

ATNR – asymmetrical tonic neck reflexes; STNR – symmetrical tonic neck reflex; PER – protective extension reaction; PRN – Postrotary Nystagmus; SAE – Schilder Arm Extension Test; TVPS – Test of Visual Perceptual Skills; MVPT – Motor-Free Visual Perception Test; TVMS – Test of Visual–Motor Skills; VMI – Developmental Test of Visual–Motor Integration.

further interpretation, based on the knowledge of established dysfunctional patterns, a specific type of sensory integrative dysfunction could be delineated.

Second, it is important to relate the conclusions of interpretation to the reasons of referral and the child's presenting problems (Fisher and Bundy, 1991). The therapist should make appropriate recommendations in terms of the type, intensity and duration of therapy input, and also state the possible outcomes of intervention by setting specific goals and objectives, together with the parents, teachers and other professionals involved.

Sensory integrative dysfunctions

Sensory integrative dysfunction is a heterogeneous group of dysfunctional patterns that are devised from different factor and cluster analytical studies. Different patterns of dysfunctions have been conceptualised into a 'meaningful cluster' when a group of test scores and observations are correlated, and also supported by the neurobiological and behavioural literature (Fisher and Murray, 1991). These clusters of dysfunctional patterns may be identified through clinical observations, the SIPT, and other formal and informal assessment procedures.

Types of sensory integrative dysfunctions

The conceptualisation of different sensory integrative dysfunctions has changed and been refined throughout the past 30 years. There is no single system for classifying the range of dysfunctions. Table 7.4 illustrates the types of sensory integrative dysfunctions as described by Fisher et al. (1991), Kimball (1993), Parham and Mailloux (1996) and the Sensory Integration International Theory and Treatment Workshop Syllabi. The most common sensory processing and integrative dysfunctions are the child's inefficiency in registering, modulating and discriminating different sensory inputs.

Sensory registration and modulation disorders

If a child cannot register information correctly, he or she will pay little attention to most things. It is usually identified among children with severe developmental problems.

When an individual overresponds, underresponds or fluctuates in response to sensory input in a manner disproportional to that input, we say that the individual has a sensory modulation disorder. Disorders of sensory modulation occur in both the vestibular–proprioceptive and the tactile systems, and link with the limbic system.

Sensory discriminative disorders

It is defined as decreased abilities to discriminate touch, movement or body position. It is related to poor central processing of sensory information. Unlike sensory modulation disorders, in which the symptoms often fluctuate from day to day or even hour to hour, disorders of sensory discrimination remain relatively stable over time.

End-product dysfunctions resulting from poor sensory processing functions

There are many different end-product dysfunctions subserved by an underlying sensory integrative dysfunction, e.g. perceptual dysfunctions and poor practic functions. Different patterns of dyspraxia have been identified through the cluster analysis of the SIPT (Ayres, 1989).

Effect of sensory integrative dysfunctions on the development of learning and behaviour

If there are gaps and irregularities in any of the integrative steps before the child goes to school, there will be gaps and irregularities in his or her school work or in life as a whole. Sometimes the deficits in sensory processing may be mild, moderate or severe; sometimes they will be expressed in one way, sometimes in another. A child with an underlying sensory integrative dysfunction may present more than one of the following signs (Sensory Integration International, 1991):

- Overly reactive and sensitive to touch, movement, sights and sounds, with obvious emotional responses as well.
- Underreactive or no response to touch, movement, sights and sound.
- Poor attention control and easily distracted.
- Poor arousal level; activity level that is unusually high or unusually low.
- Physical clumsiness or apparent carelessness in sport and other physical activities.
- Impulsive, lacking in self-control, tends to rush through things.
- Poor adaptation, with difficulty making transitions from one situation to another.
- Inability to unwind or calm self, with outbursts of overt behaviours.
- Delays in speech, language or motor skills.
- Poor self-concept and confidence.

Table 7.4: Types of sensory integrative dysfunctions

Processes	Dysfunctional patterns
Sensory registration and modulation	Sensory modulation disorders 1. Sensory dormancy (hyporeactivity) (a) poor sensory registration (b) sensory seeking behaviour 2. Sensory defensiveness (hyperreactivity) (a) too much registration (b) sensory avoidance behaviour Types: tactile defensiveness intolerance or aversive response to movement gravitational insecurity auditory defensiveness visual defensiveness, etc. 3. Simultaneous disorders of sensory dormancy and sensory defensiveness
Sensory discrimination	Sensory discriminative disorders 1. Poor discrimination of vestibular–proprioceptive information (a) postural–ocular motor disorders (b) bilateral integrative and sequencing deficits (vestibular–proprioceptive based) 2. Tactile discriminative dysfunction
Modulation and discrimination	Simultaneous disorders of sensory modulation and sensory discrimination
End-product	Sensory-integrative based dyspraxia 1. Somatodyspraxia 2. Bilateral integration and sequencing deficits (tactile based) Cortical-based dyspraxia (could be sequel of SI-based dyspraxia) 1. Dyspraxia on verbal command 2. Visuodyspraxia

- Delays in academic achievement, especially those requiring perceptual analysis, motor planning and sequencing functions.
- May develop secondary social and/or emotional problems.

The application of sensory integrative theory in the practice of paediatric occupational therapy

Sensory integrative therapy employs procedures for controlled sensory input and elicited adaptive responses involving total body movement activities. The basis of SI procedures is an assumed developmental sequence of a neurophysiological mechanism that is positively influenced by this intervention. Sensory integrative therapy works to effect progressive organisation of the child's brain in the direction of that of a developmentally normal child (Ayres, 1972a).

Goals of therapy

Occupational therapists have applied sensory integrative therapy to different diagnostic groups and with different efficacy results (Ottenbacher, 1982a). The primary goal of the therapy is to improve the way that the brain processes and organises sensation, and not to teach specific perceptual–motor and academic skills. The following are the expected outcomes of the therapy:

- Regulation of arousal level and attention control.
- Development of body scheme.
- Development of postural–motor and bilateral integrative function, which serve as the basis for efficient and automatic motor coordination.
- Development of praxis for organisation of behaviour.
- Improvement of gross and fine motor skills, including handwriting skills.
- Development of visual–auditory processing involved in learning and daily activities.
- Acquisition of receptive and expressive language.
- Development of psychosocial functions, e.g. self-confidence and self-esteem.
- Independence in daily activities.

Treatment principles

Classic sensory integrative therapy has a unique set of characteristics and tends to be applied on an individual basis. The therapist does not follow a 'cookbook' approach because the handling techniques and interaction with the child need to be adjusted based on the child's sensory needs and responses to sensory inputs (Parham and Mailloux, 1996). The following treatment principles guide the therapist in using different sensorimotor activities, reflecting the postulates or assumption of SI therapy (Ayres, 1972a, 1979; Merril, 1990; Koomar and Bundy, 1991; Kielhofner, 1992; Kimball, 1993; Parham and Mailloux, 1996).

Creation of a therapeutic environment to provide 'just-right' challenges

Basic to all development is the dynamic interaction between the child and the environment. The therapist needs to create an environment that provides multiple opportunities for interaction and just-right challenges for the purpose of organising the sensory information, in order to produce an adaptive response.

To learn how to learn – implied or stated goal of improving neural processing and organisation of sensation

Training of specific skills is not usually the focus of sensory integrative therapy. The child probably will not be drilled on tasks such as walking on a balance beam and using a pencil. Rather, a variety of activities will be used to develop the underlying abilities that enable a child to learn such skills efficiently. Therefore, treatment should aim at tackling the under-lying deficits in sensory processing rather than training in specific skills or behaviour.

See movement, think sensory – the use of planned and controlled sensory inputs

Movement activity is valuable because it provides the sensory input that helps to organise the learning process – just as the body movements of early animals led to the evolution of a brain that could think and read. Therapy will involve activities that provide vestibular, proprioceptive and tactile stimulation, and are designed to meet the child's specific needs for development. It is important to note that the emphasis is on integration not sensory inputs (Kimball, 1988).

Place emphasis on the elicited adaptive responses from simple to complex levels

Adaptive response is an appropriate action in which the child responds successfully to the environmental demand (Ayres, 1979). In therapy the child will be guided through activities that challenge his or her ability to respond appropriately to sensory input by making a successful, organised response. Therapeutic activities will also be designed gradually to increase the demands on the child to make an organised, more mature response, i.e. from simple to complex levels.

Child-centred approach – encourage active participation

The therapist considers the individual sensory needs of the child so that appropriate intervention and therapeutic rapport can be established to nurture the child's growth and development. The child is encouraged to be an active participant in activities. Seldom is the child simply a passive recipient of stimulation, because it is active involvement and exploration that enable the child to become a more mature, efficient organiser of sensory information.

The use of non-directive purposeful activities – balance of facilitation and inhibition

Emphasis is placed on automatic sensory processes in the course of a goal-directed activity, rather than drilling or instructing the child on how to respond. The therapist should use artful vigilance to regulate the child's arousal level by using different facilitatory and inhibitory activities.

Capitalise on the child's inner drive and self-direction – therapy must be fun

Motivation of the child plays a crucial role in the selection of activities, i.e. self-direction. This is an important cue to the therapist because most children tend to seek out those activities that provide sensory experiences that are most beneficial to them at that point of development. Therapy is almost always fun for the child. It may look like play to the adult observer as well. Creating a playful atmosphere during therapy is not done just for fun. It is advantageous because the child is more likely to benefit from time spent in therapy than a child who is disinterested or disengaged.

Clinical application of sensory integrative theory

Sensory integrative theory is intended to explain problems in learning and behaviour in children, especially those problems associated with motor incoordination and poor sensory processing which cannot be attributed to frank CNS damage or abnormalities (Fisher et al., 1991). The theory is not intended to explain the learning difficulties and neuromotor deficits associated with such problems as cerebral palsy (e.g. abnormal muscle tone), Down's syndrome (e.g. low intellectual functions) or strokes (e.g.

decreased tactile discrimination in the affected side), because they are caused by cortical CNS dysfunctions. When applying the theory into practice, occupational therapists may use the knowledge in the following ways:

- To analyse the child's behaviour and presenting problems based on the knowledge in different sensory systems and its related processing dysfunctions.
- To apply the principles of sensory integrative therapy in direct or indirect treatment modes.
- To promote the child's development based on the normal sequence of sensory integrative development.

Treatment guidelines

Providing intervention based on the principles of sensory integrative theory is both a complex and an exciting process. It requires the therapist involved to be able to combine a working knowledge of the theory with an intuitive ability to engender a child's trust and create 'just-right' challenges. The ultimate goal of intervention is to facilitate a child's development, self-actualisation and occupational performance (Fisher et al., 1991). The treatment of sensory integrative dysfunctions should be multi-faceted, individualised and child centred. It generally falls into three categories:

1. Promote the awareness and understanding of the child's underlying sensory integrative dysfunctions and its effect on the child's development and behaviour.
2. Integrate planned and scheduled activity programme into the child's natural environment in order to meet his or her specific sensory needs, e.g. home and school programmes.
3. Implement direct hands-on treatment programme either individually or in a small group.

Therapists also need to consider the following factors in developing and implementing a treatment programme:

- Set treatment goals and objectives that are measurable, observable and achievable in conjunction with other key individuals, e.g. parents, teacher.
- Adopt specific treatment principles of sensory integrative therapy, e.g. use of controlled and planned sensory inputs, provide 'just-right'

challenges, elicit adaptive response, non-directive approach, capitalise on the child's inner drive and self-direction, etc.

- Select appropriate service provision approaches, i.e. remedial, functional, compensatory, adaptive, management and maintenance (Mosey, 1993).
- Implement the treatment programme by using different modes of intervention, e.g. direct therapy, monitoring and consultation (Dunn and Campbell, 1991).
- Communicate regularly with other professionals involved, so that inter-professional collaboration could be established with common goals of intervention.
- Monitor the child's progress and response to the therapy input.
- Integrate different treatment methods in order to address the child's needs in different areas of development.

Review of practice

Sensory integration is described as the most researched conceptual model of practice in occupational therapy (Kielhofner, 1992; Miller and Kinnealey, 1993). In the last three decades, a huge number of research studies and treatment study articles have been published by occupational therapists in different scientific journals. Generally, the studies could be classified into the following categories:

- studies aimed at validating the theory
- studies aimed at standardising assessment tools and other assessment procedures
- studies aimed at identifying the nature of sensory integrative dysfunctions, e.g. patterns and incidence
- studies aimed at developing treatment protocols, methods and techniques
- studies aimed at evaluating the efficacy of treatment.

Ayres (1972c) first identified that the combination of sensory integrative therapy with special education is an effective method for improving academic scores of children with specific learning disabilities. Ottenbacher (1982a) selected eight studies to carry out a meta-analysis on the effectiveness of sensory integrative treatment. Although he noted limitations in the research methodology of certain studies, he concluded that there is empirical support for treatment effectiveness.

In a comprehensive review of paediatric occupational therapy effectiveness, Clark and Pierce (1986) concluded that both single subject and group design studies tend to show positive treatment effect using sensory integrative procedures. However, the results are not consistent across all studies. Ottenbacher (1988) states that, although there are design flaws in existing studies, most sensory integration efficacy studies reveal that sensory integrative treatment is effective. The American Occupational Therapy Association (1988) published a brief summary of research data which supports the efficacy of sensory integrative procedures. It is also important to note that the lack of conclusive scientific evidence does not mean that the construct of sensory integration lacks validity (Kinnealey and Miller, 1993).

Cermak and Henderson (1989) highlighted that considerable attention must be given to the development of clinical evaluation measures that can be reliably used to demonstrate change with therapy. They proposed use of the measures of organisation, learning rate, attention, affect, exploratory behaviour, biological rhythm (sleep–wake cycle), sensory responsivity, play skills, self-esteem, peer interaction and family adjustment to document progress and demonstrate change with therapy. They also pointed out the need to develop models to examine the immediate effect of sensory integrative procedures, as well as a model of examining change over time (Cermak and Henderson, 1989). Cohn and Cermak (1998) proposed the inclusion of the family perspective in sensory integration outcome research.

Ottenbacher (1991) stressed the importance of developing a consensual science that supports and documents the effective elements of sensory integration. He states that:

> Sensory integration is a multi-faceted intervention approach that is difficult to reduce to component parts. To ensure the integrity of sensory integration as an independent variable requires special training. The description of the treatment, the training of individual responsible for implementing the intervention, and the development of procedures to monitor delivery of treatment are vital to any successful investigation.
>
> Ottenbacher (1991, p. 390)

Miller and Kinnealey (1993) pointed out that questions about the effectiveness of sensory integrative treatment may not be answered in an isolated study. They suggested that research studies must be conducted over time, with a large variety of well-defined samples, by numerous researchers, representing a large number of programmes.

In a recent meta-analysis of sensory integration efficacy research studies carried out by Vargas and Camilli (1999), 16 studies were used to compare sensory integration effect with no treatment, and 16 were used to compare sensory integration effect with alternative treatment. Three central conclusions were drawn:

1. In the SI/NT comparison, a significant effect was replicated for sensory integration treatment effects in earlier studies but not in more recent studies.
2. Larger effect size was found in psychoeducational and motor categories.
3. Sensory integration treatment methods were found to be as effective as various alternative treatment methods.

There is strong evidence in the literature that sensory integrative therapy may be effective; however, research evidence is not conclusive. As a result of a variety of methodological problems, many of the studies are open to criticism. Therapists who carry out sensory integration research should be aware of, or familiar with, the papers of critiques by Bochner (1980), Schaffer (1984), Carte (1984), Arendt et al. (1988), Densem (1989), Cummins (1991), Law et al. (1991), Polatajko et al. (1992), Wilson et al. (1992), Kaplan (1993) and Hoehn and Baumeister (1994).

Conclusion

This chapter provides a brief introduction to the theory and practice of sensory integrative therapy. Therapists who are interested to apply it to paediatric occupational therapy practice should attend recognised postgraduate training courses. It is also important to integrate the knowledge into a defined conceptual model of practice in occupational therapy.

It is recognised that on-going research is essential for further validation of the theory and to build up evidence of treatment efficacy. Therapists should employ clinical reasoning in applying the theory to children with appropriate conditions, and recognise the need for other intervention approaches that address certain children's problems with different needs.

Collaboration with parents, teachers and other professionals involved is important to develop an integrated intervention programme. The treatment provided should be multi-faceted, child centred and family centred. The therapist involved needs to consider the integration of treatment activities into the child's natural environment. Contributions to the writing of the child's individual educational plan is essential to establish occupational therapy as an integral part of the child's education.

Finally, therapists need to be aware of the criticisms from other professionals and also from within the profession. We should see sensory integrative therapy as an evolving practice within occupational therapy.

Part III
Examination of the Needs
of Children

Chapter 8
Occupational therapy in the neonatal intensive care unit

BETTY HUTCHON

Introduction to neonatal intervention

Occupational therapy in the neonatal intensive care unit (NICU) is a relatively new area of practice in Britain, although in North America occupational therapists have been working in this area for several decades (Gorga, 1994). It was in the 1970s that the spotlight turned to the NICU as recognition of the developmental needs of pre-term infants grew. Occupational therapists who were equipped with knowledge of infant development and intervention began to apply infant treatment approaches in the NICU.

Early developmental intervention, beginning in the NICU, has been shown to be effective in improving the developmental outcome of pre-term infants (Resnick et al., 1987; Blanchard, 1991). As advances in medical technology and care continue to save smaller and sicker infants, concerns about the developmental implications and sequelae of the NICU have emerged (Collin et al., 1991). As many as 50 per cent of the extremely low-birthweight (ELBW) infants may have behavioural and learning problems, and motor or language delays (Escobar et al., 1991; Allen, 1993; Hack et al., 1995a, 1995b).

Research and literature support the concept of developmentally supportive care in the NICU as desirable and beneficial (Als et al., 1986; VandenBerg, 1990; Becker et al., 1991; Lefrak-Okikawa and Lund, 1993). Awareness and interest in this area has grown, particularly in the latter part of the 1990s; training courses specifically for occupational therapists have now been developed in the UK. In addition to better opportunities for training, the literature is also expanding rapidly.

Training and competencies for the neonatal therapist

Working in neonatology is an advanced area of practice and requires knowledge that is well beyond that of those who are new to paediatrics. Inappropriate intervention could have life-threatening consequences.

A background in the Bobath approach to treatment (neurodevelopmental therapy or NDT) and sensory integration (SI), as well as experience of working with families who have young children with disabilities or developmental problems, are essential in order to begin to understand the complexities of these tiny patients, and to look at the neonate in a holistic way. This viewpoint is confirmed by the American Occupational Therapy Association's official document on *Knowledge and Skills for Occupational Therapy Practice in the NICU* (AOTA, 1993.) It specifies that occupational therapists working in the NICU should have experience in general paediatrics, as well as the willingness, and resources, to develop specific strategies to generate specialised skills and knowledge necessary for safe practice in the NICU (e.g. relationship with a mentor, study group, advanced certificate in assessment) (Anzalone, 1994). Risks to medically fragile infants are profoundly increased when therapists have insufficient experience and training (Sweeney and Chandler, 1990). Therapists should evaluate their own competence and measure it against the standard for best practice outlined in the AOTA's official document.

The AOTA also state that:

> . . . the specialised knowledge required for practice in the NICU includes familiarity with relevant medical conditions, procedures, and equipment, an understanding of the unique developmental abilities and vulnerabilities of the infant, an understanding of theories of neonatal behavioural organisation, family systems, NICU ecology, and the manner in which these factors interact to influence behaviour.

Anzalone (1994) expresses the view that:

> . . . although the neonatal occupational therapist has the same domains of concern as other occupational therapists (i.e. performance of developmentally appropriate goals or occupation and the performance components underlying function), . . . in neonates the occupations or functional areas are not work, play and self-care; they are responding to the environment, maintaining homeostasis, beginning social interactions with parents, and taking in nourishment.

Also of concern to the occupational therapist working in the NICU are the occupations of the parents. As occupational therapists, we are able to provide a unique and invaluable perspective on the treatment of neonates and their families in the NICU.

Occupational therapy in all areas of practice is concerned with providing a holistic approach, but this can be achieved on the neonatal unit only by a knowledgeable therapist who understands the needs of the infants, families and environments found there.

NICU environment

Over the last few decades, advances in technology and improved understanding of the pathology of neonatal problems have reduced mortality and the incidence of major neurological sequelae (Brezman and Kimberlin, 1993; Hack et al., 1995b; Paneth, 1995).

Accompanying these advances have been concerns about the impact of the NICU environment on the pre-term infant.

It is widely accepted that the NICU is a harsh environment which contrasts sharply with the warm, dim, supportive and soothing confines of the uterus. The effect of this environment in the neonatal period is increasingly being recognised as a major contributing factor in long-term development (Graven et al., 1992). It is felt by many specialists that infants receiving care in most NICUs are exposed to bright lights, loud noises, painful or uncomfortable procedures, relatively hard surfaces and lack of a supportive, confining microenvironment.

According to Als (1986), the extrauterine 'fetal neonate' is in a mismatch situation by virtue of having irreversibly left the intrauterine environment, with all that that entails (oxygenation, nutrition, waste clearance, protection against infection, sensory control), yet his or her nervous system is geared to many more weeks of the intrauterine environment's specific inputs.

The intensive care environment is dominated by life support equipment (Figure 8.1) and, in the midst of all the technology, developmental assessment and developmental care of the sick newborn are often ignored or forgotten.

Developmental care

In the last 15 years, however, more attention has been focused on the intensive care environment and the outcome for high-risk infants. Many researchers have repeatedly demonstrated the need for an appropriate environment in which to care for the developing pre-term infant. Several studies proposed intervention approaches that would change the environment to reduce the infants' stress, a factor that may interfere with recovery (Cole, 1985; Goffried and Gaiter, 1985; Wolke, 1987). It has been shown

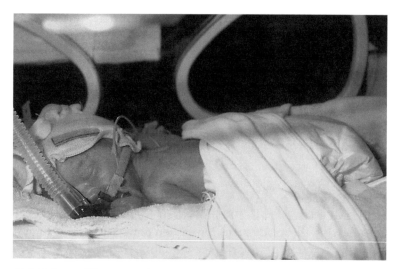

Figure 8.1: Baby on life support in intensive care.

that these infants have markedly improved outcomes when the stress of over-stimulation is reduced in their environment through a reduction of noxious stimuli (light, sound, traffic) and the promotion of proper positioning and handling. One of the most influential authors on the developmental care of pre-term infants is Heidleise Als whose work on the development and application of synactive theory is discussed later. Als' Synactive Theory of Development and the Neonatal Individualised Developmental Care and Assessment Programme (NIDCAP) has led to a greater emphasis on developmental care for high-risk infants and their families to enhance neurodevelopmental outcomes. Als et al. (1986) found that assessing the individual infant's ability to cope with excessive stimulation provided the caregiver with information to modify each infant's environment and treatment strategies.

Developmental care has been investigated in many studies and significant outcome improvements cited include (Grunwald and Becker, 1990; Becker et al., 1991, 1993; Mouradian and Als, 1994; Stevens et al., 1996; Westrup et al., 1997; Als, 1998):

- Fewer days on the ventilator
- Earlier feeding success
- Shorter hospital stay/earlier discharge
- Marked reduction in the number of complications
- Improved motor and state control at term age
- Improved neurodevelopmental outcomes during the first 18 months of life

- Lower nursing care costs
- Reduced incidence of intraventricular haemorrhage
- Reduced severity of chronic lung disease.

Optimal developmental care for the pre-term infant can be provided by minimising stress, increasing the ability to self-organise and interpreting the infant's non-verbal cues to influence care-giving. Modifying the environment through the development of care-giving protocols can be accomplished without compromising medical treatment.

The synactive theory of development

The work of Als and colleagues has provided a theoretical basis for understanding behaviours of pre-term infants, including the infant's efforts to cope with the stresses of the extrauterine environment and to maintain homoeostasis in the NICU (Als, 1982, 1986).

The theory focuses on planning and implementing care that is individualised and appropriate for the infant's current developmental goals, and promotes a strong family-centred approach.

Not only has Als' work facilitated the move of occupational therapy into individualised developmental care (Gorga, 1994), it has also emerged as the state-of-the-art transdisciplinary approach to recognising and meeting developmental needs of each infant and family in the NICU (Als, 1982; Creger and Browne, 1989; Blackburn and VandenBerg, 1993).

In the past, newborn babies were considered to be unaware of their environment and unable to participate in meaningful interaction. There was a general belief that they were unable to see, hear or experience pain, and that they were passive and helpless beings.

This is no longer felt to be the case. Newborn infants can respond, although obviously not at a cortical level, to visual and auditory stimulation, smell and taste. They can also respond to different types of touch and are able to move away from painful stimuli when necessary (Brazelton, 1979; Lott, 1989).

In Als' model, it is proposed that newborn infants interact with the environment through five separate but interdependent behavioural subsystems:

1. Autonomic
2. Motor
3. State
4. Attention–interaction
5. Self-regulation.

She states that, in the mature, well-organised, full-term healthy infant, these subsystems:

* support and enhance one another
* function smoothly.

But in the pre-term infant these subsystems:

* generally do not develop simultaneously
* are often characterised by disorganised behaviour and signs of stress.

Als' theory is called 'synactive' because during every stage of development the subsystems are developing independently, yet they are continuously interacting with one another and the environment (Als, 1982). The developmental process is described as a series of concentric circles, with each subsystem continually providing feedback to the others.

It is through the occurrence of recognisable approach and avoidance behaviours in these subsystems that infants continually communicate their level of stress and stability in relation to what is happening to, and around, them.

Als states that the autonomic system is the first to become functional and is believed to form the foundation or the core for the stability of the entire system. Channels of communication within this subsystem include colour, breathing patterns and visceral signs (e.g. bowel movements, gagging and hiccoughing). There may also be motor behavioural signs (e.g. twitches of the face, extremities or body).

The motor system is characterised by posture, muscle tone, movements and activity. State organisation is observable in the infant's ability to achieve a range of states of consciousness, from deep sleep to crying. Ease of transition between states is also considered.

Attention and interaction are observed by the infant's ability to maintain attention and engage in interactions with caregivers and the environment. The self-regulation subsystem gives infants the ability to control and modulate other subsystems and, as a result, be able to calm themselves even when exposed to potentially stressful situations. These behaviours are frequently protective mechanisms – allowing the infant to 'shut-down' or avoid interaction.

Self-regulatory balance is reflected in regular respiration, good colour, stable visceral functioning, smooth movements, modulated tone, softly flexed posture, and steady sleep and awake states (Als, 1998). Extension and diffuse behaviours generally reflect stress, whilst flexion and robust behaviours generally reflect self-regulatory effort and competence.

One of the most important tasks of the neonatal occupational therapist is to develop competency in learning to recognise these behaviours and their implications for care-giving and programme planning.

The ability of healthy full-term infants to interact with the environment in an organised, smooth, balanced and relatively stress-free way results from the maturity and integration of this behavioural system complex. Als and her colleagues call this process neurobehavioural organisation. When an infant who lacks stability and control in a subsystem is required to elicit a response within that subsystem, signs of instability in other subsystems are likely to appear. Infants give clear signals of stress when stability of the subsystems is being affected (Table 8.1).

Table 8.1: Synactive theory of development: neurobehavioural subsystems, signs of stress and stability

Subsystem	Signs of stress	Signs of stability
Autonomic	Colour changes Changes in vital signs (heart rate, respiratory rate, etc.) Visceral responses (gagging, hiccoughs, etc.) Yawning not in isolation Sneezing not in isolation	Physiological stability Regular respiratory rate Stable colour
Motor	Generalised hypotonia Hyperextension of extremities Finger splaying Frantic, flailing movements	Smooth well-regulated movements Hand clasping Balanced flexion and extension postures
State	Diffuse sleep states Glassy eyed Staring Gaze aversion Hyperalert, panicked look Irritability	Clear states Smooth transition between states Focused clear alertness Good self-quieting and consolability
Attention/ interaction	Effort needed to attend and interact to specific stimulus elicits stress signals of other subsystems	Focused, alertness

Instability increases when the stressful stimulus is not removed and, although an infant may initially be showing interactional or attentional stress reactions, these may progress to state, motor and eventually autonomic stress reactions. As stress increases, the infant's self-regulation power decreases, unless appropriate care-giving intervention is given to restabilise the system. In some instances, care-giving intervention in the form of a 'break' from the stimulation may allow the system to become reorganised.

Self-regulatory behaviours include the infants' ability to achieve and maintain self-organisation in each subsystem as required. Examples of self-regulatory behaviours are (Als, 1986):

• postural change
• hand to mouth
• grasping
• sucking
• hand clasp

Behaviours that are interpreted as stress reactions in Als' approach are very common in the behavioural repertoire of pre-term and high-risk infants, because of their lack of ability to inhibit or protect themselves from stressful stimulation. There is much current knowledge to support the view that stress prevention is very important in the management programme of fragile infants.

The occupational therapist working in the NICU needs to learn to recognise and effectively respond to infant cues. NIDCAP focuses on developing observational skills to individualise the intervention with high-risk newborns, based on behavioural organisation and response to stress (Figures 8.2 and 8.3). Many neonatal therapists are now becoming NIDCAP trained. Details of training are given in the section on Assessments p. 173.

Classification of age and birthweight for pre-term infants

Age

Newborn infants are classified according to their gestational age (GA):
37–42 weeks: full term
28–36 weeks: pre-term
< 28: extremely pre-term

Once pre-term babies reach term or pass their due date, they have both a chronological age and a corrected age. Chronological age is calculated from the actual date of birth. Corrected age is calculated from the due date or EDD (expected date of delivery). Corrected age is used until 2 years of age in developmental assessments, after which time the infant's chronological age is used.

Weight

> 2500 g: average birthweight
1500–2500 g: low birthweight
1000–< 1500 g: very low birthweight
< 1000 g: extremely low birthweight

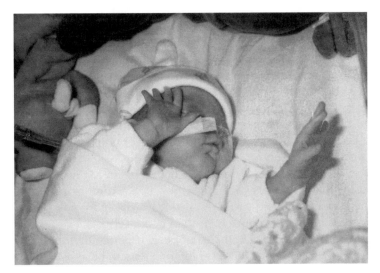

Figure 8.2: Infant showing signs of stress in the motor system.

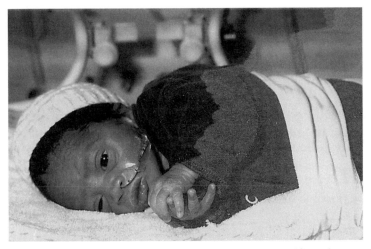

Figure 8.3: Infant in hyperalert state but showing attempts to self-regulate.

Newborn infants are also classified according to their birthweight in relation to their gestational age:

AGA: appropriate for gestational age (between 10th and 90th percentile)
SGA: small for gestational age (below 10th percentile)
LGA: large for gestational age (above 90th percentile)

Neuromotor development of the pre-term infant

The postures of pre-term infants vary considerably from the typical postures adopted by healthy full-term infants. As pre-term babies lack the physiological flexor tone observed in full-term infants, they tend to adopt extended postures. Although their muscle tone is low, pre-term infants should not be described as hypotonic because their muscle tone is normal for their gestational age, and immaturity is not the same as a pathological condition.

The development of postures and movements in the pre-term infant follows a predictable sequence of maturation.

From 28–40 weeks' gestational age, infants begin to develop flexor tone in a caudocephalic progression. Therefore, flexor tone is usually observed first in the lower limbs and progresses to the arms and trunk. The development of active and passive muscle tone in extremely sick pre-term infants is often delayed but, once it begins to appear, it generally follows the same caudocephalic progression. Pre-term infants need to be assisted to maintain more flexed postures, but even at term these infants often do not display the same degree of physiological flexion as the full-term infant.

According to Amiel-Tison and Grenier (1986), after term age, as extensor tone begins to appear, infants begin to experience a decrease in flexor tone which follows a cephalocaudal progression. This is true for both passive and active muscle tone where head control develops first, followed by trunk control and finally lower limb control.

Reflex development

Most normal infants manifest all of the primitive reflexes at birth because the development of reflex activity begins *in utero*. However, pre-term infants often initially exhibit an absence of a number of the primitive reflexes. Most of the reflexes begin to appear around 28 weeks' gestational age and gradually improve until around 37 weeks. At term age in the normal infant, it should be possible to see or elicit most of the primitive reflexes.

Motor activity

The pre-term infant at 40 weeks' gestation has accomplished major developmental progress. He will have developed flexor tone against gravity, resistance to full extension of the knees, hips and shoulders, and his active movements will have become more fluent and smooth. However, it is important to remember that neonatal motor behaviour can be affected by many factors, including autonomic instability, stress, environmental temperature, infection, electrolyte disturbances, jaundice, respiratory distress and medications.

A summary of pre-term neuromotor development is provided in Table 8.2.

Table 8.2: Pre-term neuromotor development

The pre-term infant at 27–28 weeks
Resting posture
Low muscle tone appropriate to gestational age
Response to handling
• Full passive range of movement without resistance is demonstrated by the heel-to-ear manoeuvre in the infant at 27–28 weeks
• When both arms of the infant at 27–28 weeks are extended parallel to his body and then released, he makes no attempt to recoil his arms into a flexed position
• The infant at 27–28 weeks shows no attempt to align head and body when pulled to sit
• When pressure is placed on the ball of the foot, the infant at 27–28 weeks makes no attempt to grasp with his toes
• The placing response is absent in the infant at 27–28 weeks

The pre-term infant at 30 weeks
Resting posture
Flexion beginning in lower extremities
Response to handling
• Arm recoil is seen in the infant at 30 weeks. Grasp now involves some flexion of the arm. The combination of grasp and traction may begin to lift the infant's body from the supporting surface
• Although head lag remains extreme, once in the sitting position, the infant at 30 weeks succeeds in righting the head both anteriorly and posteriorly. He is able to maintain his head in this position only momentarily
• The infant at 30 weeks makes no attempt to bear any weight on his legs in a supported stand, but does exhibit some resistance to the supporting surface with his feet. There is still little attempt to assume an upright posture

The pre-term infant at 32 weeks
Resting posture
The infant at 32 weeks flexes his thighs and begins to show development of hip flexion. This is evidence of the development of tone in the lower extremities before development of tone in the upper extremities
Response to handling
• There is a decreased range of passive movement of the legs of the infant at 32 weeks
• The elbows now go only to the body's midline when testing for the scarf sign
• When pulled to sit, the infant at 32 weeks rights his head consistently and more smoothly when compared with the younger infant
• While in a sitting position, the infant at 32 weeks shows more ability to maintain his head in alignment with his body
• When held in a supported stand, the infant at 32 weeks places some weight on his feet. His head begins to right and there is extension of the knee with some effort to extend the trunk
• The Moro reflex shows complete extension and abduction of the arms with extension of the fingers. The flexion and adduction component is not yet evident

(contd)

Table 8.2: (contd)

The pre-term infant at 34 weeks
Resting posture
Displays development of hip flexion by assuming frog-like resting posture
Response to handling
- The infant at 34 weeks is able to grasp and maintain traction with the upper extremities
- Traction continues to be demonstrated in the lower extremities
- The infant at 34 weeks resists passive knee extension
- The infant at 34 weeks attempts to right his head when in a supported sit
- The placing response is now demonstrated
- The infant at 34 weeks attempts to extend the hips and knees in a supported stand
- When held in ventral suspension, the infant at 34 weeks maintains some flexion in the elbows and knees, and makes an effort to lift his head
- The infant at 34 weeks extends and abducts the arms, followed by partial flexion and adduction when exhibiting the Moro reflex

The pre-term infant at 36 weeks
Resting posture
Wide variety of resting postures; flexor tone dominates in trunk and extremities
Response to handling
- All newborn primary reflexes can be elicited in the infant at 36 weeks
- The Moro reflex remains incomplete
- Resistance to extension of the knees and adduction of the hips is noted
- Leg recoil is brisk
- Attempts to maintain head in alignment with body when pulled to sit
- When placed in the prone position, the infant will pull into flexion using trunk and legs
- Stepping and placing responses are demonstrated

The pre-term infant at 40 weeks
Resting posture
- All four extremities are held in a flexed position
- The flexor tone of the pre-term infant who has reached the equivalent of full term is never as great as that of the infant born at term
Response to handling
- By 40 weeks' gestation, the pre-term infant resists full extension of knee, hip and shoulder
- At 40 weeks, the pre-term infant recoils his arms within 2–3 seconds after release by the examiner, flexing them at the elbow at an angle of less than 100°
- The pre-term infant aged 40 weeks lacks the shoulder muscle tone of the infant born at term. As a result, he may not be able to maintain his head in alignment with his body when pulled to sit
- In a supported stand, the pre-term infant at 40 weeks can usually bear weight easily on his legs, but may not yet be able to reciprocally step like the infant born at term

Adapted from Creger and Browne (1989)

General movements from pre-term to term age

Prechtl et al. (1997) have described the spontaneous general movements (GMs) in pre-term, term and post-term infants. Normal GMs are described as:

> . . . gross movements, involving the whole body. They may last from a few seconds to several minutes or longer. What is particular about them is the variable sequence of arm, leg, neck and trunk movements. They wax and wane in intensity, force and speed, and they have a gradual beginning and end. The majority of sequences of extension and flexion movements of arms and legs is complex, with superimposed rotations and often slight changes in direction of the movement. These added components make the movements fluent and elegant and create the impression of complexity and variability.
>
> GM Trust – course handout

Around term age, normal general movements take on a writhing quality which are characterised by small-to-moderate amplitude and slow-to-moderate speed. Fast and large extensor movements may occasionally break through, particularly in the arms. Typically, such movements are elliptical in form; this component creates the impression of a writhing quality of movement.

The quality of GMs can be observed even when the infant is still in an incubator, so long as he or she is awake and not crying.

Medical management of the high-risk neonate

A sound medical foundation is essential to address an infant's developmental needs safely. Occupational therapists must therefore ensure that they are knowledgeable about intensive care equipment, the prevailing medical problems of newborn infants, their medical management and the ways in which a medical problem may affect intervention. It is essential to be familiar with medical equipment including the different types of incubators, and the range of ventilation tools available.

Apnoeas and bradycardias (As and Bs)

Pre-term infants tend to have a higher and more irregular heart rate than full-term infants and have a higher incidence of apnoeas. Apnoeas are respiratory pauses that last over 15 seconds. Apnoeic spells are frequently accompanied by bradycardia (heart rate below 100 beats/min) because the heart rate tends to drop when there is a respiratory pause. Most infants recover spontaneously, but sometimes oxygen administration is required. Babies usually grow out of apnoea of prematurity.

Nutritional support

Nutritional support to the pre-term infant aims to achieve a postnatal growth rate that is similar to normal intrauterine growth. For the average infant, this corresponds to a weight gain of 15 g/kg per day (Adcock and Consolvo, 1993). Pre-term infants may receive parenteral nutrition or enteral nutrition. Parenteral nutrition such as intravenous dextrose solution or total parenteral nutrition (TPN) is administered outside the digestive system. Enteral nutrition, given through an orogastric or nasogastric feeding tube or nipple feeding, is administered directly into the digestive system. Selection of the appropriate method combination is based on the infant's gestational age, medical condition and environment (Hunter et al., 1994). The generally accepted criteria for using TPN include any condition that requires delaying enteral nutrition. TPN provides the infant with water, protein, minerals, carbohydrates, vitamins and fat. Infusion pumps provide controlled infusion of parenteral fluids into peripheral veins, arterial lines or central venous catheters over a prescribed period of time.

Thermoregulation

Lack of temperature regulation is one of the most serious problems of prematurity and such babies have to be protected against excessive heat loss. Extended postures, thin skin, pulmonary dysfunction and frequent care-giving interventions, and a lack of brown fat, allow heat to transfer from the body to the air. The special 'brown fat' used by neonates to metabolise heat is not produced until the third trimester. The infant may lose heat by convection, conduction, radiation and evaporation.

Convection refers to heat loss from the infant's body to the cooler surrounding air. Conduction refers to heat transfer that occurs when the infant's body is in direct contact with a cooler object. Radiation refers to heat loss from the infant's body to a cooler solid surface not in direct contact with the infant. Evaporation refers to heat loss that occurs when liquid from the infant's respiratory tract and permeable skin is converted into a vapour.

Medical disorders in the neonate

Most medical problems experienced by pre-term infants result from immaturity of the vital systems. However, sick full-term infants may also exhibit similar conditions. Another cause of medical problems in newborn infants involves often unavoidable complications resulting from medical management of certain serious conditions, particularly respiratory conditions. Neonatal infections are also a common cause of serious medical problems in fragile infants.

A thorough knowledge of the following conditions is vital and should be read in the appropriate literature before undertaking work with the neonates:

- Respiratory distress syndrome (RDS)
- Bronchopulmonary dysplasia (BPD)
- Gastro-oesophageal reflux
- Intraventricular haemorrhage (IVH), periventricular leukomalacia (PVL) and hydrocephalus
- Perinatal asphyxia (birth asphyxia)
- Hypoxic ischemic encephalopathy (HIE)
- Infection
- Sepsis
- Retinopathy of prematurity (ROP)
- Gastrointestinal: necrotising enterocolitis (NEC)
- Persistent pulmonary hypertension (PPHN)
- Patent ductus arteriosus (PDA).

Practical considerations for developing occupational therapy in the NICU

Before the establishment of a plan for occupational therapy involvement in the NICU, the need for developmental intervention should be discussed with the consultant neonatologist. An extensive review of the literature is necessary prior to this meeting, as is contact with other therapists in similar units, which allows a comparison of approaches and roles.

The following are the points to consider before attempting to provide occupational therapy intervention in the NICU:

1. Familiarise yourself with the four levels of neonatal care. Not all neonatal units are able to provide the highly specialised care of the NICU. Is your unit a regional unit or a local unit? What level of care does it provide?
   Level 1: intensive care (maximal intensive care)
   Level 2: intensive care (high-dependency intensive care)
   Special care
   Normal care
   The status of infants will vary according to the type of unit, as will the need for occupational therapy services.
2. Assess the needs of the nursery. This will vary depending on the personnel already available and their skills. For some units, it will be the first time that they have had a therapist on the unit, whereas other

units may already have physiotherapy and/or speech and language therapy involvement. Nursing staff will normally be very interested in the practical input that therapists can provide, e.g. information on special feeding techniques and positioning techniques to minimise future developmental problems will be appreciated, if this is not already being provided.

3. Establish a close working relationship with the nursing staff. Although the doctors are ultimately responsible for the infant's health, it is the nursing staff who will be better informed about the infant's routines, behaviours, responses and individuality. In addition, the nurses will be able to provide up-to-date valuable information about the infant's medical status and family. This is particularly useful for therapists when several days or sometimes even a week may have elapsed since last seeing the infant.

4. Familiarise yourself with the many medical conditions and surgical procedures relevant to pre-term and high-risk neonates. Be aware of the implications for future developmental status and contraindications for treatment. Reassess monitors constantly when providing intervention to unstable infants. Be able to recognise signs of increasing stress and physiological instability. Do not treat those infants whom you feel you cannot adequately assess.

5. Attend training courses in the assessment and treatment of high-risk infants. Visit other centres, network with other therapists, and read all the available literature and self-study manuals. A strong background in paediatric neurology, neurodevelopmental therapy and sensory integration, and maternal–infant bonding is essential to the development of the role of developmental specialist.

6. Familiarise yourself with community agencies so that you can provide information to parents on other services available locally. This is essential if you are planning to run a follow-up programme after discharge.

7. Realise that not everyone is suited to work in the NICU. The therapist will be exposed to infant deaths as well as severe illness and deformity. You will need to be able to deal with parents' depression, fear, anger and frustration. This is difficult if you cannot deal with your own emotions. Not all occupational therapists will have the professional and personal characteristics necessary for this practice area.

8. Start slowly. Attending one of the weekly ward rounds consistently is a very good way of becoming familiar with the unit and its practices. Restrict your involvement to only one or two infants and their families to begin with. Introduce yourself to new and unfamiliar staff so that they learn to recognise you.

9. Offer to run short teaching sessions for new staff and students on your role and your approach to intervention. Nursing staff are extremely interested in developmental care and the synactive theory of development (Als, 1986). Handouts explaining your role are useful for both parents and staff.
10. Introduce yourself to the parents as soon as possible after receiving a referral for an infant. Establishing collaborative relationships with parents is a primary focus of family-centred care and occupational therapy practice in the NICU.

What does the neonatal therapist do?

Positioning

Positioning is extremely important in terms of both neurodevelopmental outcome and preventing stress and promoting sleep in the pre-term infant. The occupational therapist's role is to educate and advise staff about the general principles of positioning, and to carry out individual assessments on specific infants and make recommendations about appropriate positioning. If there is a neonatal physiotherapist, this may be a shared area.

Stimulation

Parents in particular welcome information on the level of stimulation that their baby should receive. There are general guiding principles that should be followed for good practice to prevent babies being 'overloaded' with sensory stimulation. In addition, each baby's tolerance for stimulation should be assessed individually. What one baby may be able to cope with at 35 weeks' gestation, another baby may find stressful.

Parents need to know where to position soft toys and photographs in the baby's cot, and how and when to use visual and musical toys. Background noise and lighting in the unit also need monitoring and appropriate suggestions made to staff about possible improvements, particularly in relation to developmental care principles.

Infant's skills

Therapists need to be able to demonstrate to parents the fascinating behaviour repertoire of their infant and how to interpret these behaviours. The therapist should be able to describe to the parents the baby's competencies, as well as any difficulties the baby may be experiencing at a particular point in time.

Feeding

Therapists provide help with infants who have feeding problems, including positioning for feeding. If there is a neonatal speech and language therapist, the occupational therapist should work jointly with him or her on this area.

Parental support

The occupational therapist's role in the NICU is to offer practical advice in terms of the infant's developmental needs, and to support the parents. Hunter (1996) states that 'the primary roles of the occupational therapist are to support families throughout hospitalisation, to promote attachment between infant and family and to facilitate effective parenting within the NICU and after hospital discharge'.

Transition to home and follow-up

If follow-up is planned it is important to explain clearly to parents what your follow-up will be.

What skills does the therapist need?

* To be able to observe and interpret baby behaviours
* To be able to recognise behavioural states and stress responses (including those that are characteristic of pre-term babies)
* To understand bereavement and the psychological impact that the child's pre-term delivery and fight for survival will have on the rest of the family
* To overcome fear of handling very tiny babies attached to tubes and wires
* Knowledge of pre-term development of movement and sensory skills
* Understanding principles of positioning and feeding small sick infants
* Familiarity with neuromotor assessment of pre-term and term infants.

Criteria for referral to occupational therapy

* Marked prematurity < 28 weeks' gestation
* Developmental concerns
* Questionable or abnormal tone or posturing, i.e. poor head and trunk control, asymmetries, hyper- or hypotonicity
* Prolonged hospitalisation – particularly post-term age
* Feeding or sucking–swallowing difficulties
* Congenital malformations
* Sensory impairments
* Disorganised behaviour, i.e. irritability, inability to self-quiet, jitteriness, excessive startle or hyperexcitability
* Parental anxiety.

Referral criteria based on diagnosis should include the following:

- Grade IV haemorrhage
- PVL (periventricular leukomalacia)
- Asphyxia with:
  - seizure activity
  - abnormal neurological examination
- Neuromuscular disorders
- Chromosomal abnormalities compatible with survival (i.e. Down's syndrome)
- Prolonged hospitalisation (more than 2 months) with associated chronic medical complications such as bronchopulmonary dysplasia
- Brachial plexus injuries.

Overview of assessment

A comprehensive assessment facilitates appropriate intervention. However, neonatal assessment is highly specialised and requires additional training and knowledge and, in many cases, certification. Many aspects of the baby's behaviour and development needs to be included in the assessment, but much of the essential data can be obtained through structured observation, thereby causing as little disruption as possible to the infant. Lengthy hands-on assessments are to be avoided and are both potentially harmful to the fragile infant and unnecessary. There are now many reliable methods of assessment that require minimal handling, some of which are described in this text.

Important considerations for assessment

The infant's response to a stimulus or the behaviour he exhibits during an assessment is affected by many factors, including:

- The infant's gestational age at the time of testing
- The degree of any disorder (visual, auditory, motor, etc.)
- The level of medical support he requires and medical complications such as BPD
- The medications he is being given, e.g. theophylline or caffeine citrate, which are used to control apnoea of prematurity, can result in jitteriness or increased muscle tone (Creger and Browne, 1989)
- Timing of the assessment in relation to his feeding schedule
- His own biological clock.

Assessment tools

- Prechtl's Method of Qualitative Assessment of General Movements (Prechtl et al., 1997)
- Naturalistic Observations of Newborn Behaviour (NONB) (Als, 1984)

- Assessment of Preterm Infant Behaviour (APIB) (Als, 1982)
- The Neurological Assessment of the Preterm and Fullterm Newborn Infant (NAPFI) (Dubowitz and Dubowitz, 1981)
- Brazelton Neonatal Behavioural Assessment Scale (NBAS) (Brazelton and Nugent, 1995).

All the above assessments apart from the NAPFI require training and certification.

Prechtl's Qualitative Assessment of General Movements (Prechtl et al., 1997)

This was developed to assess the quality of GMs as a diagnostic tool for early detection of brain dysfunction (Prechtl, 1990). This technique is suitable for infants from extremely pre-term to 20 weeks' post-term. It is non-invasive and has high reliability and validity. Video recordings are made of the baby's spontaneous movements when awake and lying on his back on a bed or other suitable surface. Normal GMs are gross movements involving the whole body, which may last from a few seconds to several minutes or longer. Around term age and up until 6–8 weeks post-term, GMs are commonly referred to as writhing movements. GMs from the pre-term age up to around 8 weeks post-term can be classified as normal or abnormal and abnormal GMs are further classified as:

- poor repertoire
- cramped sychronised or
- chaotic

At 6–9 weeks post-term, the form and character of GMs of normal infants change from the writhing type to a fidgety pattern. Fidgety movements are continual in the awake infant except during focused attention. They may be concurrent with other gross movements such as kicking and swiping of the arms. Fidgety movements are most commonly seen between 9 and 15 weeks post-term. Fidgety movements are judged as:

- normal
- abnormal or
- absent

Recent research has shown that abnormal or absent fidgety movements are a strong indicator of cerebral palsy. Training and certification are essential in order to use this approach. For further information contact: Professor Christa Einspieler, Department of Physiology, University of Graz, Harrachgasse 21, Graz, Austria.

Naturalistic Observations of Newborn Behaviour (Als, 1984)

The Naturalistic Observations of Newborn Behaviour (NONB) is level 1 of the Neonatal Individualised Developmental Care and Assessment Programme (NIDCAP). It is based on Al's Synactive Theory of Development and is for use with pre-term and term infants who are too fragile for handling.

To carry out this assessment the baby is observed for at least 20 min before an intervention, then during the intervention or care-giving episode, and again after the intervention. Each observation requires a minimum of 50 min. During this time structured observations of specific behaviours are recorded at 2-min intervals as are measures of physiological function (heart rate, respiratory rate, oxygen saturation). By observing the infant's behavioural responses over time to environmental and care-giving interventions, it is possible to assess the maturation and adaptation of the infant's neurobehavioural subsystems (autonomic, motor, state, attention, and interaction and self-regulation).

As a result of these observations, information about the infant's threshold of instability and self-regulatory efforts provides the basis for the recommendations, which are then made in the infant's developmental care plan. In order that the infant's developmental care plan can be updated, periodic reassessment using the NONB is recommended.

The certification process requires formal training and assessment of rater reliability. Further information on training is available from: Heidelise Als, PhD, Enders Pediatric Research Laboratories, 320 Longwood Avenue, Boston, MA 02115, USA.

Brazelton Neonatal Behavioural Assessment Scale (Brazelton and Nugent, 1995)

The Brazelton Neonatal Behavioural Assessment Scale was developed by Dr T. Berry Brazelton and first published in 1973. At that time, many still thought of babies as passive recipients of environmental stimuli and assessment was confined to Apgar scores, paediatric examinations and neurological evaluations.

Brazelton sought to encourage a positive model of child development and parenting, and the aim of the scale is not to focus on or test for pathology but to demonstrate the baby's strengths. The goal of the NBAS is to identify and describe individual differences in neonatal behaviour. The main feature of the NBAS is that it is interactive and the examiner's role is to facilitate the baby's best performance. The NBAS is the most comprehensive examination available of neonatal behaviour and is one of the most commonly used measures of the newborn infant's socially inter-active responses. It can be used with infants from 38 weeks' to 48 weeks' gestation. It is used widely in research and clinically and also as an intervention with parents.

Using the NBAS as an intervention with parents

When using the scale as an intervention with parents, its purpose is to sensitise parents to their baby's uniqueness and to promote a positive parent–infant relationship.

The examiner's role is to draw out and demonstrate to the parents their baby's wide range of skills and capacities. However, the goal is not to dismiss any problems that may arise, but to share them with the parents and support them in dealing with them. Therefore 'difficult' behaviour as well as 'positive' behaviour should be described and discussed.

Parents are also given the opportunity to discuss any concerns that they may have about their baby's development. Examiners using the scale need to be very familiar with and knowledgeable about normal development, so that they can provide developmental information about the range of variability in neonatal responses that fall within the normal range. Parents will often want to know if other babies cry or sleep as much as their own baby, and the examiner needs to be able to answer these types of questions.

Using the NBAS to test neurological function

To measure neurological function, the test includes 18 items which assess reflexes and other relevant responses:

- Plantar grasp
- Hand grasp
- Ankle clonus
- Babinski's reflex
- Standing
- Automatic walking
- Placing
- Incurvation/gallant reflex of newborn
- Crawling
- Glabella
- Tonic deviation of head
- Tonic deviation of eyes
- Nystagmus
- Tonic neck reflex
- Moro's reflex
- Rooting
- Sucking
- Passive movement of arms and legs.

Important factors when administering the NBAS

The infant's state of consciousness or arousal, most frequently classified into six categories (Als, 1982), is monitored throughout the session:

State 1: deep sleep
State 2: light sleep
State 3: transitional state of dozing or drowsiness
State 4: quiet alert
State 5: active, alert and maybe fussing
State 6: crying.

Scoring

Clusters of items are scored:
* Habituation
* Orientation
* Motor performance
* Range of state
* Regulation of state
* Autonomic regulation
* Reflexes.

For further information on the Brazelton Scale contact: Joanna Hawthorne, PhD, Coordinator, Brazelton Centre in Great Britain, Box 226, NICU, Addenbrookes NHS Trust, Hills Road, Cambridge CB2 2QQ.

Neurological Assessment of the Preterm and Full Term Newborn Infant (NAPFI) (Dubowitz and Dubowitz, 1999)

This is widely used by paediatric neurologists as an assessment tool for pre-term and term infants who can tolerate handling. It is designed to record the functional status of the infant's nervous system.

Assessment of Preterm Infant Behaviour (APIB) (Als et al., 1982)

The APIB is based on Als' Synactive Theory of Development. It is intended for use with stable pre-term and term infants. It is a complex assessment designed to provide an integrated subsystem profile of the infant, identifying current levels of function in the face of varying environmental demands. The subsystems, as outlined in the Synactive Theory of Development, are referenced throughout the assessment. The therapist handles the infant as a systematic sequence of increasingly demanding environmental inputs, termed 'packages', is administered. The infant's responses are closely monitored to assess neurological behavioural organisation and methods of attaining self-regulations, as well as the amount of support needed for the infant to achieve and maintain organised behaviour. The examiner identifies tasks that the infant handles well, can handle given environmental supports and are beyond the infant's capabilities (Als, 1986). The examiner is able to assess the infant's threshold from organisation to disorganisation (Als and Duffy, 1989). An infant must have physiological stability to tolerate most of the test manoeuvres.

The APIB is used more as a research tool than for everyday clinical purposes. Training in the APIB is lengthy and rigorous and is not yet available in the UK. For further information contact: Heidelis Als, PhD, Enders Pediatric Research Laboratories, 320 Longwood Avenue, Boston, MA 02115, USA.

Neonatal positioning

Creger and Browne (1989) state that:

> A goal in the care of all high risk infants, premature or full term, is to provide them with developmentally supportive positioning and therapeutic handling to promote more normal motor development and minimize their chances of developing abnormal movement patterns.

Sick and pre-term infants often present with a number of positioning problems which, if not managed appropriately, may lead to the development of a variety of postural and movement problems. For example, pre-term infants often lack the ability to assume the typical neonatal posture of flexion, shoulder protraction and posterior pelvic tilt. It is common for these babies in supine to adopt a 'W' arm position (shoulder abduction and external rotation with elbow flexion). This position, if not corrected, may affect the baby's ability to bring hands to midline. A subsequent delay may be noticed in fine motor control and midline hand play.

Not only can supportive positioning make an infant more comfortable but, by focusing on flexion and midline orientation, positioning may reduce stress and enhance physiological stability. This, in turn, will promote sleep which is critical for growth and weight gain.

The specific positioning needs of each infant must be determined on an individual basis. The infant's physiological, motor and behavioural responses to any one position must be constantly observed and monitored.

The main criteria for selecting a position are the infant's presenting problems:

- Low muscle tone
- Persistent extended postures
- Disorganised movements, irritability, unsettled sleep states
- Gastro-oesophageal reflux.

General goals of developmentally supportive positioning (Creger and Browne, 1989)

- Promote flexion
- Facilitate midline orientation (hand-to-mouth activity) and symmetrical positioning
- Enhance self-quieting skills and behavioural organisation
- Encourage relaxation and improve digestion
- Prevent bony deformities and skin breakdown
- Increase awareness of body in space
- Facilitate visual and auditory skill development
- Facilitate development of head control.

Therapeutic positioning should therefore:

- prevent postural abnormalities
- optimise the infant's developmental potential and functional abilities
- promote a balance between flexion and extension
- minimise energy expenditure
- not interfere with medical interventions or life-support equipment
- make the baby more comfortable by providing a sense of containment and security.

Positioning techniques

A variety of positioning options is available. The medical and developmental advantages and disadvantages of each position need to be considered in relation to the individual baby's needs. The beneficial effects of various positions must always be assessed and monitored in relation to the baby's physiological and behavioural responses.

Prone position

Advantages

- Facilitates flexion (Connally and Montgomery, 1987)
- Facilitates the development of head control (Bobath and Bobath, 1972)
- Facilitates hand-to-mouth activity for self-calming
- Infants sleep more (Hashimoto et al., 1983; Masterson et al., 1987; Baird et al., 1992)
- Conserves energy (Masterson et al., 1987)
- Improves arterial oxygen pressure (Martin et al., 1979)
- Lowers intracranial pressure (Emery and Peabody, 1983)

- Has lower respiratory rate (than in supine)
- Improved oxygenation and ventilation in infants with and without ventilatory support (Alistair et al., 1979; Wagaman et al., 1979; Martin et al., 1979; Fox and Molesky, 1990; Mendoza et al., 1991)
- Significantly reduces the severity of gastro-oesophageal reflux (Ewer et al., 1999).

In addition it has been noticed that infants positioned in prone tend to be calmer and more organised than infants in other positions.

There is also some evidence which supports the view that the head elevated prone position of 15° is more beneficial than the horizontal prone position in terms of reducing hypoxaemic events (Jenni et al., 1997).

Disadvantages

- Access for medical care is more difficult
- Infant may self-extubate
- Some infants, particularly those with severe irritability, cannot tolerate prone – may exhibit trunk hyperextension in this position.

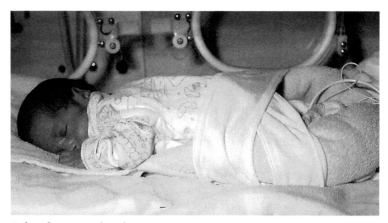

Figure 8.4: Infant nested in the prone position.

Principles

The mattress should be tilted to 15° so that the infant's head is elevated. The infant's hips and knees should be flexed. The arms should be flexed near the head. The head should be turned to one side and the hand on the face side should be near the infant's mouth.

Suggestions

Hip flexion may be facilitated and hip abduction minimised by a small roll placed under the lower pelvis so as to elevate it slightly. Weight bearing should be through the anterior knee and hips should not be flexed more than 90°. Boundaries may be provided by using a blanket nest, a 'Bendy-Bumper' or a 'Cosy Wrap' (Figure 8.4).

Supine position

Advantages

- Easier access to infant for medical care
- Infants who do not tolerate the prone position often respond to supine 'nesting'
- Easier visual exploration by infant.

Disadvantages

- Promotes extensor patterns (Fiorentino, 1965; Anderson and Anderson, 1986)
- Increases energy expenditure (Masterson et al., 1987)
- Increases intracranial pressure (Emery and Peabody, 1983)
- Constantly exposes infant's eyes to bright overhead lights
- More reflux than in prone (Meyers and Herbst, 1982; Orenstein et al., 1983; Ewer et al., 1999)
- Greater risk of aspiration than in prone (Hewitt, 1976)
- Infants sleep less and cry more in supine than in prone (Brackbill et al., 1973; Bottos and Stafani, 1982).

Despite the many disadvantages sick infants often have to be maintained in supine for medical reasons.

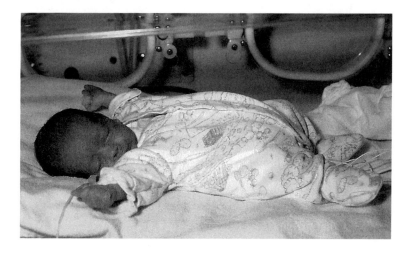

Figure 8.5: Unsupported supine position.

Principles

Infant's knees and hips should be partially flexed up towards the abdomen. Feet should be inside surrounding boundary. The arms should be tucked in by the body with the elbows flexed and off the bed surface. Head should be in midline or comfortably to one side.

Suggestions

A sheet or blanket can be rolled into a tube and positioned in a 'horse-shoe' around the baby. The infant may be swaddled to promote flexion and help maintain hands in midline. Nests can be formed out of blanket rolls to promote flexion, adduction and shoulder protraction. Nesting will also promote symmetry and midline orientation. Nesting with lateral head support will help reduce head flattening.

Side-lying position

Advantages

- Facilitates midline orientation of the head and extremities
- Encourages hand-to-hand and hand-to-mouth activities
- May be used to encourage flexion and adduction; counteracts external rotation of limbs
- Left lateral positions significantly reduces the severity of gastro-oesophageal reflux (Ewer et al., 1999).

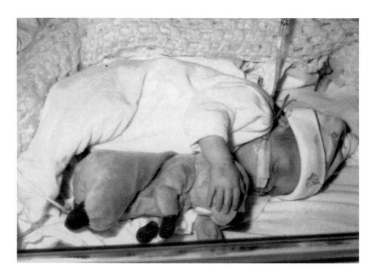

Figure 8.6: Supported side-lying position.

Disadvantages

- Can be difficult to maintain some irritable or hypertonic babies in correct side-lying position
- May be difficult to avoid neck and trunk hyperextension, shoulder retraction and asymmetrical posture.

Principles

The infant's hips and knees should be flexed, with the top hip being securely positioned forward of the weight-bearing hip. Arms should be forward and comfortably flexed. The head should be positioned as close to midline as possible and with slight neck flexion. The infant's back should be well supported to maintain a flexed symmetrical side-lying posture.

Suggestions

A Bendy-Bumper is very useful for providing boundaries and support in side-lying. A roll or soft toy tucked in close to the infant's abdomen and chest will facilitate trunk flexion. Larger babies may require support under the head to maintain alignment with the body. Blanket rolls may be used firmly behind the baby, loosely between the legs and up along the baby's front to maintain the correct position.

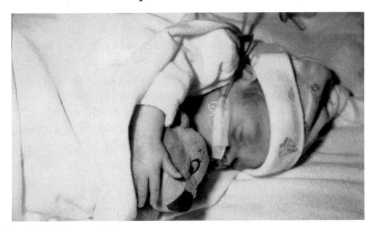

Figure 8.7: Side-lying position.

Seated position

Advantages

- Alternative position which may be more appropriate for older babies when they are awake

- Encourages visual exploration
- Encourages social interaction
- More alerting position.

Disadvantages

- May be difficult to position baby properly without slumping in the seat.
- More upright position increases heart rate and mean arterial pressure in pre-term infants (Smith and Turner, 1990)
- Semi-reclined position may decrease oxygen saturation in some pre-term infants (Willett, 1986).

Principles

Infant should be positioned symmetrically with hips and knees flexed, shoulders forward and head in line with the body or slightly flexed.

Suggestions

A blanket may be rolled into a tube and positioned in a 'horseshoe' around the infant to keep the shoulders forward and the head in midline.

Positioning to prevent head flattening

Doliocephaly refers to progressive head flattening which can result in a narrow and elongated shaped head. Pre-term infants, because of their inability to maintain the head in midline, tend to keep their head turned to one side. The weight of the head causes pressure on the lateral aspect of the skull. This, combined with the infant's soft cartilaginous skull, causes the typical head flattening so often seen in pre-term infants.

Providing lateral support in supine is one method commonly used to prevent head flattening. Water beds, gel pillows and changing head position as and when appropriate will all also help.

Feeding

Newborn infants are anatomically and neurologically predisposed to feeding and normally are able to initiate feeding shortly after birth. Pre-term birth, however, is the most prevalent cause of feeding disorders in newborn infants (Morris and Klein, 1987). Although most of the oral–motor reflexes are functional by 32–34 weeks' gestation, other factors such as lack of flexor or oral–motor tone, small and weak sucking pads, decreased strength, immature respiratory control, and unreliable coordination of sucking and swallowing all contribute to poor or inefficient feeding in the preterm infant.

Difficulties with feeding can be:

- the first sign of neurological damage (Ingram, 1962; Volpe and Hill, 1981) and/or
- a sensitive indicator of CNS integrity (Brazelton, 1970).

Feeding and swallowing difficulties are highly sensitive to the integrity of the CNS and to neurological dysfunction. Pre-term babies are at increased risk for neurological problems and it is well documented that a high percentage of children with neurological damage exhibit either:

- slower sucking rates (Braun and Palmer, 1985) or
- atypical respiratory–swallow patterns (Casas et al., 1994).

Development of sucking

Neither sucking nor swallowing is an entirely new experience for healthy full-term newborn infants because fetal sucking and swallowing has been noted *in utero* as early as 13 weeks' gestational age. Thumb sucking has been seen at 16–20 weeks' gestational age (Dubignon et al., 1969).

More integrated sucking and swallowing is generally thought to appear at 32–34 weeks' gestation, but is not consistently well coordinated with breathing until 37 weeks' gestation. By this time *in utero*, the baby is almost fully grown, developing flexor tone and becoming more flexed, allowing hand–mouth exploration and the opportunity for experiencing sucking of fingers/thumbs.

Some breast-fed pre-term infants may be able to coordinate sucking, swallowing and breathing at 32–34 weeks' gestation.

Sucking is a flexor activity and the predominant flexor tone that results from intrauterine crowding and neurological maturity further enhances the infant's ability to suck (Morris and Klein, 1987). Sucking activity depends on reflex development as well as on muscle strength and coordination of the oral–motor mechanism (Jain et al., 1987). Fatty cheek pads called 'sucking pads' provide stability in the term baby to enhance their sucking efforts. Sucking activity is further supported by a relatively large tongue in a relatively small mouth which provides a mechanical advantage for the full-term baby.

Natural protection of the airway also develops with flexion, and the position of the larynx becomes more anterior and superior as flexion increases. At the same time, the epiglottis approximates the soft palate, again increasing natural airway protection during swallowing.

In contrast, pre-term babies have very little flexor tone – the smaller they are, the less they have. They are born with a predominance of extensor activity, not lending itself to such a highly integrated skill as sucking.

Inadequate proximal stability affects the development of oral stability which is compounded by immature oral musculature, such as:

- small oral cavity
- retracted jaw
- relative small size of the tongue
- decreased cheek stability.

All of this leads to poor oral stability.

Development of coordinated sucking, swallowing and breathing is a highly integrated process (VandenBerg, 1990), and dysfunction in any of these three individual functions or in their coordination can lead to feeding problems, and complications such as aspiration. Often pre-term infants may be able to cope with NNS (non-nutritive sucking), but have difficulties when fluid is introduced, not being able to adjust to the demands of the situation, such as the size and type of teat, viscosity of liquid, etc. The rhythm of the suck/swallow/breathe pattern is very important, and maintenance and regulation of rhythm are often affected. These problems are intensified by the low energy levels of the infant who is often weak and tires very easily.

Neurobehavioural control during feeding affects the infant's autonomic, motor and state systems, and again difficulties are indicated often in either very subtle changes of respiration, heart rate, skin colour/temperature or very obvious signs such as disorganisation of motor patterns, hyperextensive postures and changes in alertness.

Oral motor reflexes, such as rooting and sucking, are fairly well established by 28 weeks' gestation but responses may be slow and imperfect. The rooting reflex is particularly affected in special care babies as a result of decreased/altered oral sensation from overuse of tubes and tapes around the oral/facial area. These babies will often open their mouths only to show that they are aware of the stimulus and those under 34 weeks' gestation may not have sufficient head control actually to turn towards it. The very protective cough reflex is thought to appear between 32 and 34 weeks and is of utmost importance if oral feeding is being considered. The gag reflex is not present until 32 weeks' gestation and, although this is not a protective reflex as such, it gives the feeder some indication as to the baby's intraoral sensory status.

Feeding programmes are usually based on weight rather than gestational age. Most infants under 1000 g are usually fed outside the digestive system and are given parenteral (intravenous) feeding during the first weeks of life. Enteral alimentation is given via the digestive system and is usually started before the infant is ready to nipple feed. Enteral feedings are usually given via a nasogastric (NG) tube or less commonly an orogastric (OG) tube. The infant is fed every 2–3 hours directly into the stomach through the tube. Nipple feedings are initiated when the infant (Vergara, 1993):

- has sufficient intraoral suction to suck the feed into the intraoral cavity
- has achieved adequate suck/swallow/breathing coordination
- is able to tolerate tube feeding without aspirating
- has the necessary endurance and energy levels to feed.

A common practice to increase the infant's endurance is to begin nipple feeding until the infant becomes tired and finish the feed through the tube.

Infants who are fed via an NG or OG tube or who experience prolonged intubation are often predisposed to developing changes in sensation both intraorally and extraorally. This is often thought to be a result of the aversion to the insertion and movement of the tube. Offering NNS during tube feeding is felt to decrease oral hypersensitivity.

Feeding assessment

Feeding assessments are indicated for a number of feeding problems too numerous to mention in this chapter. The occupational therapist should consult with the speech and language therapist about feeding assessment. Medical and physiological readiness for feeding must always be established before beginning a feeding assessment. Heart rate, respiration rate, colour and oxygen saturation changes during the assessment process must be closely monitored. Postponement of feeding training should be considered if the infant develops physiological instability during the feeding evaluation (Vergara, 1993).

Assessment instructions

Very few assessments and checklists are available for use with neonates. The most commonly used feeding assessment is the Neonatal Oral Motor Assessment Scale (NOMAS), which is a diagnostic tool developed by an American speech pathologist, Marjorie Meyer Palmer. The NOMAS evaluates oral–motor components such as sucking rhythm and rate, sucking pressure and lip closure, jaw excursion, tongue configuration and movements, and movement of liquid into the pharynx (Braun and Palmer, 1985).

However, many therapists have developed their own assessments or checklists to evaluate feeding. To do this the therapist needs a good understanding of the basic feeding components and knowledge of other problems such as gastro-oesophageal reflux which may interfere with feeding.

Glass and Wolf have stated that a 'global assessment would determine the infant's feeding function in the key areas of state and behavior, tactile responses, motoric control, oral motor function, physiologic control, and coordination of sucking, swallowing and breathing'. They further state that 'information is obtained through skilled clinical observation as well as from technological monitors or medical tests and procedures'.

Prerequisites for safe and efficient feeding include (Comrie and Helm, 1997):

- intact anatomy and physiology
- intact sensory and tactile systems
- adequate muscle tone and postural support of the oral, pharyngeal and respiratory systems
- stable autonomic nervous system
- adequate state regulation
- enough energy to support the entire process.

Management

There are usually two main groups that babies with feeding difficulties can be divided into.

Disorganised feeders

- Babies with chronic lung disease (BPD) and cardiac babies, where the primary concern is maintenance of the airway.
- Babies who are exposed to harmful drugs during pregnancy and who, consequently, have poor adaptability and difficulties with self-organisation.

Dysfunctional feeders

- Those who have had some neurological damage and do not have the right 'wiring' to coordinate sucking physically.
- Those with anatomical defects such as cleft lip and palate, oesophageal anomalies, etc.

With both these groups, preparation is an essential part of treatment and before feeding it is helpful to do the following:

- Encourage 'soft' flexion by swaddling and helping the baby to organise himself, possibly enabling some hand-to-mouth experience.
- Consider the external environment with regard to grading auditory, visual and tactile stimuli, so that it is easier for the baby to cope with the stimuli while being fed. Elevated levels of environmental stimuli may overload the sensory system of the pre-term infant and cause increased apnoea and bradycardia.
- Encourage the baby to wake spontaneously for a feed, rather than feeding him when half-asleep. Increased alertness enhances the full-term infant's ability to suck.
- Use NNS before feeding, again to help the baby organise himself and begin to develop some sort of rhythm or pace for sucking.

There have been a number of studies carried out to investigate the benefits of NNS, both before oral and tube feeding and during tube feedings. The list of benefits cited include:

- Improved gastric functioning by facilitating oesophageal peristalsis (rhythmic passage of food through the oesophagus and into the gut), increased absorption of calories and minerals, hence enhancing weight gain, growth and neurological maturation (Bernbaum et al., 1982).
- Improved respiratory functioning by reducing energy expenditure and behavioural stress during feeding, thereby facilitating better organisation and calming, particularly after the feed.
- Increased success of earlier oral feedings through consistent use and experience of achieving and maintaining coordination between respiration and swallowing.
- Increased association between sucking and feeling full.

However, every infant must be evaluated individually and on a continual basis, because NNS may not be beneficial to every infant. Parents' preferences must also be discussed because some parents have quite deep-rooted negative feelings towards the use of a pacifier.

NNS characteristics do not necessarily reflect those of nutritive sucking, i.e. some babies who can seemingly cope with NNS have difficulties when fluid is introduced (Bu'Lock et al., 1990).

The disorganised feeders are generally 'hands-off' babies, once the environment and their autonomic, motor and state systems are under control. They are greatly helped with external pacing, to encourage more rhythm and consistency during the feed. This can be done by careful manipulation of the teat intraorally or using other methods such as firm tapping or even having gentle classical music in the background.

Both disorganised and dysfunctional feeders can be affected by the size and shape of the teat, e.g. if the hole in the teat is too big the liquid may flow too fast and not give the baby enough time to deal with it. If the liquid is thickened slightly this will give the baby a little more time to deal with the fluid, and also give him increased sensory feedback as to where the fluid is in his mouth. Care must be taken when thickening fluid because it will make it more difficult to suck the milk through a small-holed teat and should not be used for those with a weak suck or those who tire easily. If sucking is very difficult and energy consuming, a small cup must be considered.

The dysfunctional feeder is more 'hands on' and will need more help with improving the actual function and coordination of his orofacial musculature. This is achieved by facilitating more normal postural tone and patterns of movement – giving adequate proximal stability and better alignment to allow:

- better oral stability, particularly of the jaw and cheeks
- inhibition of retraction of the jaw and tongue
- facilitation of better oral seal – both anteriorly (lips) and posteriorly (tongue/palate).

From here, more normal patterns of sucking and swallowing should develop.

Feeding follow-up clinic

After discharge from hospital, it is very important to provide follow-up advice for parents of babies with feeding difficulties. This advice should be coordinated by the multidisciplinary team, involving the paediatrician, the speech and language therapist and the dietitian. The occupational therapist's role would be to advise on suitable seating or positioning for feeding.

Developmental follow-up

After discharge from the NICU, many developmental therapists will be involved in a follow-up programme. Follow-up provides the opportunity to give reassurance for families and to teach them about their child's development, and to monitor the progress.

Purpose of follow-up

- To identify potential developmental problems as early as the problems arise or become detectable, in order to initiate preventive and remedial intervention that will optimise the infant's developmental potential.
- To provide education and support to enhance the family's care-giving skills and their ability to maximise the infant's developmental potential.

Therapists can also link families to community-based services when necessary.

Frequency of follow-up

The frequency of follow-up depends very much on the family's need and the infant's potential risk for developmental problems.

Children who are at high risk for developmental problems should ideally be offered appointments at the following intervals:

- 6 weeks
- 3, 8 and 12 months (corrected age)
- 18 months (corrected age)
- 26 months (chronological age)
- 36 months (chronological age).

However, not all children need to be seen this frequently. Where there are no concerns the following frequency would be appropriate:

- 3 months (corrected age)
- 9 months (corrected age)
- 18 months (corrected age)
- 2.5 years (chronological age).

Assessments used in follow-up

- The Bayley Scales of Infant Development (BSID II) (Bayley, 1991)
- Movement Assessment of Infants (MAI) (Chandler et al., 1980): this assessment is for use by physiotherapists and is generally not used by occupational therapists
- Prechtl's Qualitative Assessment of General Movements (Prechtl et al., 1997)
- Test of Sensory Functions in Infants (DeGangi and Greenspan, 1989).

The Bayley II

This is the most comprehensive assessment available for use by occupational therapists with this population and is a valuable tool when used in the detailed assessment of these children in the follow-up clinic. The Bayley Scales will help identify those children who have difficulties or delays in the areas of:

- gross and fine motor development
- cognitive development
- speech and language development
- attention and concentration

Prechtl's Assessment of General Movements

This is also strongly recommended for use at 3 months' post-term age when abnormal general movements may be a strong predictor of cerebral palsy.

Once an area of concern has been identified, the child may need to be referred on to a specialist for further evaluation and assessment.

Case study: Nazia

'Nazia' was born at 30 weeks' gestation with a complicated medical history. She was referred to occupational therapy for assessment while she was in the hospital's Special Care Baby Unit. Throughout the perinatal period, she presented as irritable, cried often for long periods and was difficult to console. She slept poorly, mostly in light sleep and only for short periods of time, and had problems sustaining relaxed tone and posture. Difficult to feed, despite a good suck reflex, she seemed quickly to lose interest once her initial hunger was satisfied. It was clear that her parents found her behaviour deeply disturbing and did not understand how they were going to handle her.

At 43 weeks' gestational age, the Brazelton Neonatal Behavioural Assessment Scale (NBAS) was administered. It was astounding to watch her reactions to the habituation items – here was a baby who was unable to switch off the environment. Every time the bell or light was presented, she responded in a highly irritated way.

As suspected, the examination showed that Nazia was a sensitive and poorly organised infant who, in light sleep, could not habituate to visual or auditory stimuli. She reacted to every presentation of stimuli with constant squirming, fidgeting and increased respiratory effort, followed by waking and crying. Such a description is not unusual in high-risk infants who commonly do not have the behavioural or neurological competence or energy to habituate. She displayed none of the self-regulatory behaviours that babies use to calm themselves, such as hand-to-mouth gestures, postural changes or pulling into flexion. She was, in short, very much at the mercy of her environment. Nazia's inability to block out noise and light prevented her from getting into deep sleep. This, in turn, made her irritable, upset and unable to self-console. Staff and family members, all of whom had tried everything they could think of to soothe her, felt frustrated and helpless.

Following the Brazelton assessment, several recommendations were made:

- Pay constant attention to Nazia's behavioural cues
- Provide support for whatever efforts she made to self-regulate, and
- Offer consistent advice in helping her parents understand the reasons for Nazia's hypersensitivity.

Most important were the recommendations that Nazia's environment be modulated and stimuli reduced. Slower, gentler handling and swaddling were recommended, and Nazia was to be allowed as much undisturbed sleep as possible with protection from light and sound.

Nazia was moved to a quiet corner of the NICU where lights were dimmed and staff were told to stand well away from her cot when talking. After these changes were made to her environment and in her individualised care, she became calmer, happier and less irritable. Her eating and sleeping patterns improved, and her parents began to understand their daughter's behaviours and needs better, all the while becoming much happier and more positive about her.

Nazia continued to need an individualised care plan, as a result of complexities related to feeding and sensory modulation. She began smiling appropriately, visually tracking people and objects, babbling and developing good postural tone in supported sitting. Her gross and fine motor skills developed normally as she approached her corrected age of just over 3 months.

Chapter 9
Children with learning disabilities

CHIA SWEE HONG

This chapter introduces the condition of learning disability and its impact on the child's activities, and considers some of the assessments and application models that underlie the practice of occupational therapy with children who have learning disabilities. It uses a case study to illustrate the therapeutic strategies undertaken to maximise the development of a child who has profound multiple learning disabilities at school and at home.

Individuals with learning disabilities

Learning disabilities are usually detected when a child demonstrates an overall delay in achieving developmental skills appropriate for his or her age. According to the *Diagnostic and Statistical Manual of Mental Disorders*, 4th edition (DSM-IV; American Psychiatric Association or APA, 1994), the fundamental characteristic of 'mental retardation is significantly sub average general intellectual functioning' (p. 39). Individuals will also have severe limitations in adaptive functioning in at least two of the following abilities: communication, self-care, home living, social/interpersonal skills, use of community facilities, self-direction, functional academic skills, work, leisure, health and safety. The onset must occur before the age of 18 years. IQs have been widely used by psychologists since the inception of psychometric testing. The current view is that there are limitations in the use of intelligence tests, e.g. their validity in the assessment of cognitive performance. Gates (1997) maintained that, if intelligence tests are used appropriately, they can provide an objective measure of cognitive ability which, if used together with other criteria such as social ability, can be extremely useful in identifying individuals who have learning disabilities. In Britain, 'learning disability' is the term used instead of 'mental retardation'.

IQ level 50–55 to approximately 70	Mild mental retardation
IQ level 35–40 to 50–55	Moderate mental retardation
IQ level 20–25 to 35–40	Severe mental retardation
IQ level < 20 or 25	Profound mental retardation

(DSM-IV: APA, 1994)

Causes of learning disabilities

There are four broad areas in which learning disability can occur.

Chromosomal and genetic abnormalities

Abnormalities may occur at the time of cell division and can include extra chromosomes or translocation of chromosomes. One of the most common of the variable forms is Down's syndrome which has an incidence of 1 in 600–700 live births and may be related to maternal age. Genetic abnormalities can be produced by the presence of abnormal dominant and recessive genes or by the absence of genes responsible for essential enzymes. One such gene deficiency is manifest in cases of phenylketonuria where the enzyme responsible for converting phenylalanine to tyrosine is absent. This results in toxic levels of phenylalanine in the blood, which causes damage to the developing brain.

Infections

The illness may be the result of a primary infection by an organism attacking the brain or central nervous system (CNS), as in the case of encephalitis, or a secondary complication of one of the common childhood illnesses such as measles. Sometimes the contributing factor is the degree of raised temperature that is characteristic of such infections and which can lead to brain damage.

Trauma

Injury to the baby can occur during labour or at the time of birth and is thought to account for 1 per cent of all cases of learning disability. Anoxia may be caused by pinching of the umbilical cord, stopping the blood flow between the placenta and the baby, or mechanical injury from forceps delivery.

Socioeconomic factors

These may include alcohol abuse by the mother. The term 'fetal alcohol syndrome' was coined in America in 1973 to describe a range of specific mental and physical abnormalities observed in babies born to alcoholic mothers that were particularly related to deficiencies in performance and growth such as microcephaly (Fraser et al., 1995; Shanley and Starrs, 1995; Gates, 1997).

In practice, however, clear-cut diagnoses of causes such as these account for less than a quarter of those with learning disability. Most of those who have severe or moderately severe learning disability are, however, affected by chromosomal abnormalities or severe and rare genetic conditions, or clinically manifest brain damage. They often show evidence of physical signs of CNS disorder, biochemical abnormalities or sensory impairment. However, this group has a prevalence of only about 3 or 4 per 1000 of the population (Sims and Owens, 1993).

There is a prevalence of mental health difficulties among those with learning disabilities: dementia (3%), schizophrenia (3%), affective disorders (10–15%), obsessive–compulsive disorder (4%) and personality/behavioural disorder (25–30%) (Bloye and Davies, 1999). The Mental Health Foundation (1993) said that it is well recognised that individuals with learning disability are vulnerable to mental health difficulties, but the majority do not come to the attention of the health professions.

Learning disability is generally considered a lifelong condition but the course and prognosis will vary depending on the cause(s) of the disability. The complexity of needs presented by individuals with profound multiple learning disabilities means that it is inevitable that several agencies will be involved throughout their lives (Lacey, 1998).

Most cases of learning disabilities are non-progressive, although early identification and intervention are essential to increase the child's ability to grow and develop to his or her maximal capacity (Gordon et al., 1996). Identification of a chromosomal or genetic disorder may help to explain or predict various impairments. Conversely, knowing that a child has a specific condition poses two dangers: not all available information about such disorders is accurate; and, if the child is deemed to have limitations, there is a risk that correspondingly low expectations may lead to functioning below full potential (Sims and Owens, 1993). Clancy and Clark (1990) suggest that the general objective is to provide management that will enhance the child's acquisition of skill in: caring for him- or herself, engaging in appropriate social behaviour and interpersonal relationships, and participating in activities that are valued by the community.

Impact of the condition on the child

Most aspects of the child's activities are affected by learning disability. The impact of the condition on the child's occupation will depend on factors such as the presence of additional medical diagnoses and the severity of the disability. Children who have, for example, physical disability in addition to learning disability will have some difficulties in their sensory integration, neuromuscular and motor skills (Hansen and Atchison, 2000). Other individuals with learning disabilities will have reduced ability to understand new information, learn new skills or cope independently (Department of Health, 1995).

Occupational therapists who work with children with learning disabilities will be influenced not only by the philosophy of the profession but also by social role valorisation. Wolfsenberger (1983) believed that individuals with a learning disability should be given the same basic human rights as others in the community based on a shared humanity. Central to his thinking was the concept of integration. All people should relate to one another as equals and have mutual respect.

O'Brien's (1987) five accomplishments help to extend further the concept of integration. He suggests:

- ensuring that individuals with a learning disability are present in ordinary places
- supporting them to make informed decisions
- developing skills to increase their independence
- giving them respect
- enabling them to establish relationships with their family and the community.

Dolan (1995) said that activities or goals selected should reflect normal learning and, wherever possible, activities should take place in ordinary, accessible, community facilities where the individuals can be given the necessary support to achieve access.

Assessments

Our assessments are concerned with occupations: self-maintenance or self-care, productivity or work activities, and leisure or play activities; occupational performance skills consisting of sensorimotor, cognitive and psychosocial skills; and the impact of the environment on the child's occupation (Reed and Sanderson, 1992).

Briefly, our aims have been outlined in Chapter 1. First, we carry out an initial assessment which usually consists of interviews with the child and the parents about their concerns and observations of the child's performance in carrying out occupations and occupational performance skills as illustrated in Table 9.1.

We may, however, use the Canadian Occupational Performance Measure instead (Law et al., 1994), which is an individualised measure in the form of a semi-structured interview designed to measure a child's self-perception of occupational performance.

Table 9.1: Initial assessment interview

Environment
Who is the main carer for the child?
What support does the family get?
How does the family support each other?
Is the child's environment conducive for his/her development?

Occupational performance skills
Sensory motor skills
Can the child see? Does he/she look at and follow an object?
Can he hear? Does he listen?
Does he respond to smell, taste and touch?
Can he reach for, grasp and release objects?

Cognitive skills
Can he concentrate on an activity long enough to achieve a goal?
Does the child cooperate in activities?

Psychosocial skills
Does the child initiate social interaction and communication?
How does the child express his feelings?

Occupations
Self-care occupations
Can the child change from one position to another? Is his movement well-controlled?
How much can the child do in basic self care activities?

Work occupations
What does he do during the day?

Leisure occupations
What does the child like to do?

Having ascertained the overall needs of the child and his family, we may then use some of the specific assessments listed below:

- AAMR Adaptive Behaviour Scales (Nihira et al., 1993)
- Behaviour Assessment Battery (Kiernan and Jones, 1982)
- Guide to Early Movement Skills (GEMS) (White et al., 1994)
- The Caring Person's Guide to Handling the Severely Multiply Handicapped (Golding and Goldsmith, 1986)
- The Next Step on the Ladder Developmental Assessment Scale (Simon, 1981)
- Sensorimotor Integration Inventory (Reisman and Hanschu, 1992)
- Vineland Adaptive Behaviour Scales (Sparrow et al., 1984).

Finally, we find it necessary to analyse the skills needed to perform occupations that the child has difficulties with, e.g. eating.

There are a number of considerations that need to be taken into account: some children with profound multiple learning disabilities have difficulties with attention. Kiernan and Jones (1982) suggest that we select objects that are of interest to the child. For some children, their physical disabilities obscure their underlying cognitive abilities. Appropriate positioning and seating are therefore important for children who rely on these to achieve manipulative skills. In other children, the child's physical difficulties will impede his or her speed of response. Some consideration should be given when using and interpreting the use of timed assessments in children who have a physical disability (Cogher et al., 1992). Micro-technology enables maximum use to be made of minimum responses. Any voluntary movement that the child can produce can be used to access a touch screen or to operate a mechanism by means of simple switches or joysticks. Useful clinical tools include videotaping functional tasks such as seating and fine motor activities. This technique provides qualitative evidence of change when numerical scores do not reflect change or progress (Cogher et al., 1992).

Application models

We use the following application models:

- Behaviour modification
- The Bobath concept
- Sensory integration.
  Other 'application models' include the following.

Creative approaches

The aims of creative activities are to help children to enrich their experience, develop their creative potentials, and experience new feelings and dimensions, e.g. in the early stage of art activities, it is likely to be about giving the child the experience of handling materials and, at a later stage, of making marks. As progress is made, there are opportunities to enable art to relate to something outside that immediate experience, e.g. the child can be encouraged to make pictures about things that he or she has seen and found of interest. Creative activities such as art, drama, music, movement and play are also useful tools in the development of relationships (Peck and Hong, 1994).

Perceptual motor function

This is defined as perceiving information and responding with a judgement, followed by a coordinated motor response. Cratty (Goldstein, 1978) suggested that there was an interrelationship between judgement and motor expression, and that both are related to the intellectual growth of the child and have a positive effect on intellectual development. Price (1978) pointed out that there is a great emphasis on sensory input to enhance the function of the neural systems concerned with perception. Intervention consists of gross motor activities, including structured games, balancing activities and motor planning, and components of academic work.

Sensory motor stimulation

According to Seifert (1973), the body is the instrument for the child's kinaesthetic–tactile impression, e.g. finger feeding gives the infant the sensation of texture and shapes. This provides the opportunity to establish inner language and the beginning of body image which forms the basis of spatial concepts such as distinguishing left from right. As meaning is given to sensation, this becomes perception. Chu (1990) suggests sensory stimulation as techniques to help the child become aware of his or her basis senses and body.

In practice, most occupational therapists use a combination of application models (Table 9.2). This is supported in the literature. Norton (1979) reported a 9-month study of three children who have profound multiple learning disabilities aged under 5 years who were treated by neurodevelopmental and sensory integration approaches. The children showed improvements in their postural, emotional, perceptual and cognitive development. Edwards and Yuen (1990) examined a twin with Down's syndrome incorporating neurodevelopmental therapy (NDT) techniques and vestibular and tactile stimulation. The team created an intervention programme with home-based treatment. This study suggested that the proposed intervention programme decreased the rate of decline in development for a child with Down's syndrome.

Practice settings

Most occupational therapists who work with children with learning disabilities work in the child's home, child development units, community teams for individuals with learning disabilities and special schools (Chia, 1987, 1997a, 1997b).

Table 9.2: Strengths, needs and plan checklist

After the assessments, consider strengths, needs and plan checklist:

Strengths	Needs	Plan
What are his strengths?	What are his needs?	What should he be doing to enhance his overall developmental needs? Plan a general programme of activities What should he be doing to enhance his specific needs? Plan a specific (individual or group) activity programme Which application models should be used to enhance his development?

Pre-school

Occupational therapists usually work with pre-school children and their parents at home because this enables assessment and therapy to take place in a realistic environment. Melton (1998) considered that individual or group work sessions based on small activities, facilitated by an occupational therapist and focused around individual needs, can also assist the therapist to gain a thorough understanding of an individual's motivations and skills. This knowledge will help the occupational therapist to advise on adaptations to the individual's environment and enrich teaching sessions with the individual's carers. The College of Occupational Therapists Research and Development Group (1998) point out that individuals with learning disabilities need support and rehabilitation to enable them to integrate into the community, and their carers should be provided with advice and support.

School

Therapeutic work may be divided into two categories: direct and consultative therapy. In the former, each child is seen for intensive therapy on a regular basis either individually or in a small group. In the latter, the children are taught by teachers who use activity programmes devised by the occupational therapist. This enables the occupational therapist to disseminate the skills among a larger group of children than would have been possible using a face-to-face approach.

A literature review before the study undertaken by Thress-Suchy et al. (1999) found the following: Giangreco et al. (1997) explored the attitudes of parents and found that most parents preferred direct occupational therapy services and agreed with the statement 'direct individual provision of related services is the most appropriate way of providing related service support for students with deaf–blindness and other severe disabilities'. When examining teachers' perceptions of occupational therapy services, Cole et al. (1989) found that teachers felt that occupational therapy services provided directly by the occupational therapist in the classroom were the most beneficial to their students. Dunn (1990) compared direct and consultative occupational therapy services in the school setting. She found that the percentage of goals achieved throughout the year were similar for both groups of children. However, in this study, teachers felt that consultative occupational therapy services were more effective.

As a result of these differences, Thress-Suchy et al. (1999) undertook a study to assess the perceptions of mothers, fathers and teachers about the effectiveness of direct and consultative occupational therapy services in meeting children's needs in a pre-school setting. Mothers, fathers and teachers perceived occupational therapy services to be somewhat effective. In addition, there was no major difference among mothers, fathers and teachers about their perceptions of direct versus consultative occupational therapy. Although the order of priority was different, mothers, fathers and teachers all indicated activities of daily living and fine motor skills as areas where occupational therapy is effective. Teachers also identified provision of help in the classroom, incorporation of sensory integration in the classroom and sharing of information as ways in which occupational therapy was effective in meeting the needs of their students. All of these areas of occupational therapy practice may assist teachers in managing the classroom and engaging each student to his or her potential in all classroom activities, even when the occupational therapist cannot be in the classroom. The primary reason for occupational therapy being perceived as ineffective was 'not enough therapy'. Mothers and fathers felt that occupational therapists need to provide more recommendations for the home. In a recent study, McCall and Schneck (2000) found that parents reported that they were generally satisfied with their child's occupational therapy services. However, they also requested improved communication between therapists and parents and between occupational therapists and other professionals. By enhancing better communication and parental involvement, occupational therapists can begin developing positive parent–therapist relationships that can enhance optimal therapy for the child.

Case study

Charlie is a 4-year-old boy. He lives in a well-furnished two-bedroom bungalow with his parents in an inner city. His dad is a greengrocer. His mother is a full-time housewife who is also the main carer for Charlie. Both his parents appear to be supportive of each other and are extremely interested in providing stimulation for their child at home. He has been diagnosed as having profound multiple learning disabilities (severe learning disabilities and cerebral palsy). He attends a special school 5 days a week. Charlie and his parents receive intervention and support from the multidisciplinary team.

We interviewed Charlie's parents and used the following assessments:

- Next Step on the Ladder
- Behaviour Assessment Battery
- Qualitative assessment based on the Bobath concept
- Reed and Sanderson's work (1992) formed the structure of the assessment process.

The assessments were completed over four 1-hour sessions.

Occupational performance areas

Sensory skills

When Charlie was comfortably seated, the assessment process began. Charlie turned his head and eyes and looked towards the torch light when it was presented about 6 inches (15 cm) in front of his face at eye level and gradually moved out to a distance of about 2 feet (60 cm). He also watched and followed toys shaken in front of him. Charlie blinked and turned his head when an object was brought towards his eyes. When a small bright rattle was placed on the table, Charlie was able to fixate it for up to 3 seconds. When presented with two objects successively, Charlie alternated his glance between the two objects. He did not inspect the occupational therapist's face. He did not watch when the occupational therapist drew and scribbled on a piece of paper. Charlie followed a moving object when presented vertically and horizontally. He was not able to follow a moving object through the major part of its irregular path. Charlie looked at a person when an individual moved across his visual fields. Charlie was able to follow an object moving rapidly in a horizontal or vertical plane, and relocate it when it was dropped in full view on to a soft pad. He was unable to do it when the object was moved in a series of curves and angular movements. He did not adjust his position in such a way that he was able to relocate an object that was slowly passed from sight behind a screen.

Charlie showed a startle response when a drum was banged out of sight at a distance of 6 feet (1.8 m). He appeared to still at familiar sound, e.g. saying hello. He did not turn in the direction of a sound or appear to appreciate differences in tone of voice. He did not show much response to smell, taste and touch.

General programme of activities (Chia, 1996a)

- Fill your child's day – find lots of things for your child to: look at, e.g. mobiles, listen to, e.g. clock ticking, feel, e.g. furry mat, smell, e.g. fruit, think about and do, e.g. playing with electronic toys.
- Talk about everything you do.
- Find ways of enjoying each other's company.
- Reduce the help you give as and when appropriate.
- Make time for rest.

Motor

While lying on his back, Charlie attempted to move his limbs. He was not able to bring his hands from side to side and keep his head in the centre. When pulled up to sitting, he made an effort to lift his head.

When placed on his tummy, Charlie turned his head to one side. He was not able to lift his head up even for a moment or two. When held in a sitting position, Charlie was able to hold his head erect and steady and turn his head to either side. Charlie was able to roll back from lying on either side. He was not able to roll from back to stomach and vice versa. Charlie was able to take up a sitting position when supported by an adult. A qualitative assessment of movement based on the Bobath concept was carried out.

Charlie showed undue resistance to any change of posture and delayed adjustment if he made any at all. Charlie resisted when his arms were elevated, abducted horizontally and arms moved to the sides of his body. When pulled to long sitting with abducted legs, there was resistance to abduction and extension of his legs. There was resistance to abduction and outward rotation of legs and extension of knees. Briefly, Charlie's basic postural tone was hypertonic and the influence of the extensor tone was strongest when he lay on his back and stood with a support. His movement was influenced by a number of reflexes, in particular asymmetrical tonic neck reflex.

Charlie opened and closed his fists when the backs and palms of his hands were touched. He was able to hold two objects, one in each hand.

He was not able to reach for toys or release objects. He had a grasp reflex.

Charlie played with his fingers and appeared to be interested by his hand movements. When a cube was placed in each of Charlie's hands, he grasped them reflexively. He could not release them. When an object was presented close to Charlie's hands and in the same visual field as the hand, Charlie would move his hand and tried to grasp the object.

General programme of activities

Supine

Externally rotate the legs and flex Charlie's knees, bringing one foot up to touch the opposite side hand. Encourage Charlie to take off socks and shoes while in this position.

Use a floor wedge so that Charlie is in a better position for observing his surroundings. Provide toys such as mobiles.

Side-lying

Continue the above activity in supine position, flexing and crossing one hip and knee well over the other side, and prompting Charlie to roll on to his side.

Use a side-lying board to help him maintain his position.

Prone

Place Charlie over a wedge. Make sure that his forearms are abducted from the body, with the elbows at right angles if possible. The shoulders and arms should be externally rather than internally rotated, the head and trunk aligned, legs apart and externally rotated at the hips. Introduce visual and auditory toys to encourage Charlie to raise his head and to look at and follow the toys and/or sounds.

Sitting

Sit Charlie on the floor or on your knee with your hand supporting him behind the shoulders. Move Charlie from side to side as well as forwards and backwards.

Encourage Charlie to sit in the special chair. Provide a range of toys.

Standing

Kneel down, sitting on heels and sit Charlie on your knee. Place your hands on Charlie's knees and, as you rise to an upright kneeling position, press downwards and outwards, bringing him to a standing position.

When standing, make sure that Charlie's feet are flat on the floor and his weight is equally distributed. His legs should be slightly flexed at the hips and knees, apart and a little out-turned; the trunk should be upright.

Use the prone board to assist his standing. Provide some toys to look at and touch.

Handling techniques

Roll Charlie on to his side and 'curl' him up until his knees nearly touch his chest. Keeping his head well forward, lift Charlie in this position, supporting him under this thighs and across the back. Keep the knees and hips flexed as Charlie is carried or, if the legs abduct together, carry Charlie with his legs astride.

Kneel on the floor and lift Charlie into a sitting position by supporting his shoulders and keeping his legs around one of your knees. Turn Charlie to either the right or left, supporting him under his thighs and across the back, keeping his knees and hips flexed at all times. Make sure that his head is kept free.

Before getting Charlie to play, use a facilitation technique for his hands. Get an extension of the spine with abduction, outward rotation of the arm, together with extension of the elbow, supination of the forearm and extension of the wrist with abduction of the thumb.

Cognitive skills

Charlie showed general awareness of and interest in his surroundings. Charlie was able to look at and follow a moving object, but was unable to locate it when it was slowly passed from sight behind a screen. He watched adult actions. His attention span was short and he needed prompting to complete an activity, e.g. knocking down a tower of bricks.

Specific (individual) activity programme

Name of child:	Charlie
Activity:	finding objects
Long-term aim:	Charlie will develop object permanence
Current aim:	Charlie will find half-hidden objects
Related aims:	develop attention
	increase tactile awareness
	develop interaction
	enhance the feeling of achievement
Equipment:	you will require the beanie bear and a towel and a side-lying board

Activity (Table 9.3)

If appropriate, use the facilitation technique. Encourage Charlie to lie on the side-lying board. Partly cover the bear with a towel so that its feet, head and ears remain visible. Encourage Charlie to pull the towel. If he does, praise him and mark a tick on the chart. If he doesn't, help Charlie to pull the towel away. Praise him and mark a tick with a circle on the chart. Do it five times per session.

Table 9.3: Result of activity

5	✓	✓	✓	✓	✓
4	✓	✓⃝	✓	✓	✓
3	✓⃝	✓	✓	✓	✓
2	✓⃝	✓	✓	✓	✓
1	✓⃝	✓⃝	✓⃝	✓	✓
	Mon	Tues	Wed	Thurs	Fri

Comments

Charlie's parents are encouraged to play activities such as peek-a-boo and hide and seek.

Psychosocial skills

Charlie responds with pleasure to friendly handling and cuddling, and recognised familiar people and demonstrated affection towards them. He loved adult attention. He made several different non-specific sounds. Charlie cried when he was unhappy or wanted attention. Charlie's parents reported that their son was a cooperative boy. They attend a local support group.

Self-maintenance occupations

Charlie was dependent on his self-care activities. He showed awareness of routine activities and appeared to anticipate sequences.

Charlie had difficulties in taking food from a spoon because his lips did not close around the spoon properly. His tongue was small and did not move much, although at times it was curled and pushed up against the roof of the mouth. He took food, particularly liquids, in a sucking pattern. He had bite reflexes. He was spoon fed with a small plastic spoon.

Charlie drank but sometimes failed to keep the fluid in his mouth because his lips did not close for swallowing. He used a doidy cup. Charlie was doubly incontinent. He cooperated passively while being washed and groomed, dressed and undressed.

General programme of activities

Talk with him about the nature of the activity. Encourage Charlie to be involved in the activity as much as he is physically able. Read general hints listed earlier.

For toileting, Charlie needs to be placed on the special toilet seat at regular times.

Specific (individual) activity programme

Eating

Sit Charlie on a chair with a table. Encourage Charlie to place his forearms on the table.

When spoon feeding Charlie, the handle of the spoon should be kept horizontal and not raised to scrape the food off the spoon against his teeth nor should food be dropped into the mouth from the spoon. The aim is to encourage the upper lip to move down and remove the food from the bowl of the spoon, and neither of the procedures described earlier helps in the development of this skill. Positioning small amounts of food on alternate sides of the spoon will also encourage tongue mobility and chewing.

Encourage Charlie to finger feed small portions of food and later to bite portions of food from a bigger piece, e.g. eating an apple or a piece of toast.

Drinking

Prompt Charlie to sit at a table with his elbows securely resting on the table in front of him and using a two-handled cup, then move his head slightly forward to meet the cup. If more help is needed, stand to one side or behind Charlie, cupping his jaw firmly in one hand, while supporting the cup in the other.

Productivity occupation

Charlie attends a special school 5 days a week. The school maintains an extensive curriculum and organises weekly creative arts activities with the local junior schools.

Specific (group) activity programme

Name of children: Charlie and friends
Activity: growing tomatoes
Long-term aim: Charlie is given opportunities to participate in groups
Current aim: Charlie will increase his tactile awareness
Related aims: develop attention
     develop interaction
     enhance the feeling of achievement
Equipment: you need:
     pots filled with seed compost
     seed tray
     tomato seeds
     water drainage tray

Activity

In the series of sessions, Charlie and his peer groups are encouraged to:

- arrange the pots in the seed tray
- put one or two seeds in the centre of each pot
- push a little of the compost over the seed
- water gently
- place on the drainage tray in a warm place, covering with plastic
- when the seedlings grow, remove the plastic and place the tray on a sunny windowsill; water when necessary
- transplant into big pots preferably 12 cm filled with potting compost in June
- grow in a sunny spot.
  A summary of the children's performance is presented in Table 9.4.

Table 9.4: Results of children's overall performance during session

Results of children's overall performance during session
Each child's overall performance is rated as indicated in the key below: see Appendix I

Name	II	IG	A	P	C	Comments
Ali	3	3	3	3	4	Enjoyed putting the compost over the seed
Charlie	2	2	2	1	2	Enjoyed watering and the feel of water
Lizzy	2	2	2	1	2	Enjoyed watering
Mary	2	1	2	1	2	Enjoyed putting the compost over the seed
Tony	1	1	1	1	2	Showed a little awareness of the session

Comments:
Most of the children appeared to enjoy the tactile nature of the group work. The children do need time to see the end-products.

Leisure occupations

Charlie shows interest in his surroundings by looking and listening. He likes messy play, playing with beanie babies and robots, and experiencing the multisensory room.

Specific (individual) activity programme

Name: Charlie
Activity: playing with electronic toys
Long-term aim: Charlie will be able to operate electronic toys
                             for play, school work and leisure
Current aim: Charlie has to roll as he places his hand on the
                             pressure switch of the robot toy
Related aims: Develop attention
                             increase tactile awareness
                             develop interaction
                             enhance the feeling of achievement
Equipment: You need the robot
Activity: If appropriate, use the facilitation technique.

Place Charlie on a mat on the floor. Place the switch at shoulder height to the side of him at his right, so it will move in his field of vision. Hold his right leg straight with light pressure on the knee using your left hand, with your right hand bend his left knee and bring it over his right leg so starting the rolling movement. Hold it there when his knee touches the floor. Then hold your left hand near the switch and say 'Charlie, give me your hand'. If he brings his hand over and places it on the switch, say 'Good boy' and let him watch the robot. If Charlie does not bring his hand over, return him to supine and begin the movement again. Again, holding your left hand near the switch, say 'Charlie, give me your hand'. Then with your left hand bring his right hand over and help him press the switch. Say 'Good boy' and let him watch the robot. Repeat it five times per session.

Result

Charlie is normally able to place his hand on the pressure switch of the robot toy after the third trial. The facilitation technique appears to help his movement.

Comments

Charlie and his parents are encouraged to borrow electronic toys from the local toy library.

Conclusion

Charlie continues to make progress in his overall development. All his needs are monitored and reviewed on a regular basis.

Appendix I

Key to groupwork plan/record sheet (Chia, 1995)

II = interaction with individuals
IG = interaction with group
A = attention
P = participation
C = cooperation

Interaction

Interaction with individuals

1. Resists contact with other students, e.g. when approached, moves away

to

4. Establishes and maintains contact/relationships with students

Interaction with group

1. Resists joining in with group

to

4. Joins group without prompting and plays an active part

Attention

1. Attends for less than a quarter of the time

to

4. Attends for more than three-quarters of the time

Participation

Participates mainly with:

1. Physical prompt

to

4. No prompt

Cooperation

1. Is actively uncooperative – resists help in tasks or refuses to cooperate

to

4. Is actively cooperative, e.g. follows simple instructions when asked, or initiates own activities and needs little guidance as to what is the appropriate action in most circumstances.

Conclusion

The process of occupational therapy with children who have learning disabilities has been outlined. Occupational therapists have an important role to play in the assessment and implementation of individually designed programmes in order to help each child to develop to his or her maximum potential.

Chapter 10
Children with autism/Asperger's syndrome

Joan O'Rafferty

> ... the same principle applies to autistic children – work with them instead of against them. Discover their hidden talents and develop them.
>
> Grandin (1986, p. 142)

Autism and Asperger's syndrome are developmental conditions that pervade every aspect of a child's life and for which there are no known cures.

This chapter intends to inform the reader about autism and Asperger's syndrome. Each condition is described separately initially; then the term 'autism' is used throughout for ease of reading, except where there is a difference between the conditions that needs highlighting.

Presentation

Autism and Asperger's syndrome are grouped together as part of the pervasive developmental disorders, which also include Rett's syndrome, childhood disintegrative disorder and pervasive developmental disorder not otherwise specified (*Diagnostic and Statistical Manual of Mental Disorders*, 4th edition – DSM-IV; APA, 1994). The most commonly used criteria are the DSM-IV and ICD-10 (*International Classification of Diseases and Related Health Problems*; World Health Organization, 1992). Readers are referred to these manuals for a differential diagnosis of other conditions.

Autism

The core features originally noted by Kanner (1943) continue to guide diagnosticians in their recognition of the disorder.

Impaired or abnormal social interaction/behaviour

This is manifested in an inability to form and maintain peer relationships which can range from a lack of empathy to using other people in a mechanistic fashion. Non-verbal skills, including eye contact, gaze, facial expression and awareness of the space of others, are often lacking or impaired. The desire or need to seek out others to share experiences is often absent.

Impaired or abnormal social communication

This can range from no speech to echolalic or stilted speech. There may be the presence of idiosyncratic speech. An ability to use gesture to compensate for lack of spoken language or to accompany language is often lacking. More subtle but none the less socially isolating difficulties are seen in higher functioning autistic people, such as an inability to take turns in conversation.

Restricted repetitive and stereotyped behaviour which interferes with day-to-day/normal functioning

This can include a fixed and in-depth fascination for an area of interest. Stereotyped motor behaviours such as hand flapping, jumping, flicking fingers or total body postures may be present. Often there is a need to carry out rituals or routines which have no apparent significance. Any imaginative play is often stilted and tends to have been learned rather than being a spontaneous expression of the person's ideas. A fascination for parts of an object rather than appreciating the whole is often noted.

For a diagnosis of autism to be made, the child must have significant impairment in each of these three areas, with a greater impairment in the social interaction category. The impairments should be inconsistent with the child's developmental level. Onset of the condition must be evident before the age of 3 years in at least one of the major areas.

Other impairments that have been noted but are not included in the core features are cognitive inflexibility, poor motor planning, poor sensory processing and perceptual difficulties (Chu, 1997). There may also be unusual responses to sensory stimuli, e.g. apparent deafness to most sounds, over-reaction to noise and light, and abnormalities in sleeping and eating, and the presence of behavioural difficulties including self-injurious behaviours, hyperactivity, impulsivity and short attention span (DSM-IV; APA, 1994).

Asperger's syndrome

The presentation of Asperger's syndrome has much in common with autism; however, diagnosis centres on two core features only:

1. Impaired or abnormal social interaction/behaviour
2. Restricted repetitive and stereotyped behaviour which interferes with day-to-day/normal functioning.

The distinguishing feature for differentiating Asperger's syndrome from other pervasive developmental disorders is the lack of clinically significant delay in language or cognitive development. ICD-10 (WHO, 1992) also notes that these children often display evidence of clumsiness and a delay in achieving motor milestones, although these are not diagnostic features.

Autism versus Asperger's syndrome

There is ongoing debate about whether there are two separate conditions or whether they should be viewed within a spectrum of disorders that have impaired social interaction as its core deficit. Some studies indicate that there is a difference between high functioning autism and Asperger's syndrome (Manjiviona and Prior, 1995), whereas others have found this not to be the case (Szatmani et al., 1989). Both DSM-IV (APA, 1994) and ICD-10 (WHO, 1992) classify them as separate disorders, although there is much overlap. A summary of the similarities and differences detailed by Howlin (1998) is presented below.

Similarities

- Abnormal communication skills
- Abnormal social skills
- Desire for sameness
- Repetitive and stereotyped behaviour
- Poor imaginative play
- Mainly seen in male population
- Hypersensitive to noise and sensory stimuli
- Incoordination.

Differences

The differences are shown in Table 10.1.

One of the difficulties in understanding both conditions is the small but significant differences between the two major diagnostic criteria, i.e. DSM-IV (APA, 1994) and ICD-10 (WHO, 1992). Children diagnosed using DSM-IV are excluded from a diagnosis of Asperger's syndrome if they meet criteria for autism; this is not the case with ICD-10, which gives more attention to clumsiness – not specifically mentioned in DSM-IV.

Table 10.1: Diferences between autism and Asperger's syndrome

Autism	Asperger's syndrome
Strong link with low IQ	Generally normal or high IQ
No speech often or, if present, is very limited	Verbal although difficulties with abstract concepts
Avoidance of social contact	Disinhibited in social situations
Poor outcome re independence and social functioning	Better outcome for some individuals who can use special interests in work situation
Prevalence 5 per 10 000	Prevalence 30 per 10 000
Sex is 4 : 1 male : female	Sex is 10 : 1 male : female
Onset often noted in first year but definitely before 30 months	Often noted later in life as problems only apparent then

The use of the terms 'autism' and 'Asperger's syndrome' continues to be debated. Asperger's syndrome appears to be used increasingly with children who have mild or no cognitive impairment. Asperger's syndrome has only recently been brought into the limelight with the rediscovery of Asperger's writings (Wing, 1981). It may be an easier term to accept because it does not carry the history of psychogenic theories on cause that were linked with autism (see Causes below).

Prevalence

The prevalence of autism varies depending on how wide the disorder is taken to be and whether it includes those diagnosed with Asperger's syndrome. There was some concern that the condition was increasing; however, it is now felt that changes in the diagnostic criteria in DSM-III-R (APA, 1987) included too wide a spectrum which gave a false impression of a sudden increase. DSM-IV (APA, 1994) and ICD-10 (WHO, 1992) are now more closely aligned to the initial criteria set out by Kanner and the subsequent prevalence has fallen to the levels existing in 1987. The current estimates for the UK are 4.5 per 10 000 and a sex ratio of 4 male : 1 female (Trevarthen et al., 1996).

Causes

Autism is defined as neurodevelopmental disorder (Trevarthen et al., 1996). Much research into autism has been carried out in recent years and there are many theories about the cause(s). At present, there is no single theory that has gained general acceptance.

There is strong evidence from twin studies to suggest that autism has a genetic component (Folstein and Rutter, 1977; Le Couteur et al., 1996). Other studies have shown that siblings have an increased risk of communication disorders of a pragmatic nature (Bolton et al., 1994).

Autism has strong links with organic factors, most notably epilepsy which tends to occur in the early teens (Bailey et al., 1996). Autism is strongly associated with a low IQ, with up to 70% of autistic children having a dual diagnosis of autism and a learning disability (Piven and Folstein, 1997). The level of cognitive ability in a child has a major impact on the presentation of autism. Although there are strong links between autism and low IQ, it is not yet clear from the research whether the link is causal or associative.

Current theories on cause suggest structural changes (anatomical), chemical changes (neurochemistry) and/or changes in the processes/functions of the brain (neurophysiology/neuropsychology).

Anatomical

Bauman (1991) found fewer Purkinje cells in the cerebellum; however, this may have been as a result of an associated condition of epilepsy. Priven et al. (1996) noted that autistic patients had a larger brain.

Neurochemistry

Involvement of neuropeptides and monoamines in autism has been observed by Anderson (1997); both influence the limbic system functions. Elevated rates of serotonin have been found in autistic people (Bailey et al., 1996).

Neurophysiology

From his studies on vestibular dysfunction, Ornitz (1985) hypothesised that autism resulted from disordered sensorimotor integration, which stemmed from brain-stem dysfunction. Others suggest that the disorder is seated within the core of the brain, with responsibility for focusing attention and learning (Trevarthen and Aitken, 1994). Involvement of the limbic system receives much comment because the areas with which it deals, e.g. arousal, emotion and sensory thresholds, are affected in autism (Bauman and Kemper, 1997).

Neuropsychology

Studies indicate deficits in executive functions which appear to occur mainly within the frontal lobe (Prior and Hoffman, 1990; Hughes and

Russell, 1993). Others point to an inability to establish a theory of mind (Baron-Cohen, 1989). Dawson et al. (1998) discussed impairments of attention which are apparent in autism, especially shifting attention for social stimuli and sharing attention with others.

Most of the research has limitations which prevent any firm conclusions being drawn from it. Most of the studies are small. They are looking from one perspective, i.e. the neuropsychologists are examining only the neuropsychology. There is a limited use of control subjects. As a result it is difficult to combine many of the studies to form a meaningful understanding of autism. It may well be that some of the research is looking at the symptoms of autism and helping in the understanding of the processes that occur, rather than leading to a discovery of the cause(s). Some theories may indicate specific treatments to follow; however, caution needs to be exercised because no one theory has yet been proved conclusively.

It is worth mentioning the earlier psychogenic theories on autism which have now been found to be untrue. In the 1950s and 1960s, it was suggested that parents who were aloof and uncommunicative were responsible for the presentation of autism (Trevarthen et al., 1996); these theories were being explored in a climate of psychotherapy. Although it is easy to point out the errors of previous researchers, it is important to see how they were trying to make sense of what they saw in the context of current ideas. It may well be the case that the aloofness they saw in the parents was a symptom of a communicative disorder, as has been indicated in recent genetic studies by Bolton et al. (1994).

Referral to occupational therapy

Increasing numbers of autistic children are now referred to child development centres (CDCs), whereas in the past they would most probably have come through Child and Adolescent Mental Health Services (CAMHS) and/or learning disabilities teams. The change in referrals has occurred as a result of increased understanding of the condition (which is now viewed as a neurodevelopmental one) and a broadening of the criteria to include children with minimal or no cognitive impairment. The occupational therapist may, however, come into contact with autistic children in any of the above venues, depending on his or her specialism. In some settings, the CAMHS and CDCs work jointly to assess and treat autistic children, and some areas provide a specialist assessment team which may include occupational therapists. A referral to occupational therapy may come from a number of sources depending on the referral procedures and policies that exist.

Impact of condition upon child's occupation

The impact of autism on a child's life can be devastating because it pervades all aspects of a child's life. It affects one of the core features of humans – namely, the desire to communicate with others for the inherent pleasure that it brings rather than purely as a means to an end. For autistic people the desire and need to communicate are impaired even in the most able.

The autistic child needs to be viewed in the context of his or her family because the condition also has an immense impact on other family members. The overall impact of autism on a child's life and on his or her family will also vary, depending on the presence of other conditions, e.g. low IQ, epilepsy.

In seeking to break down or separate different elements of the child's life, there is a risk of losing sight of the whole child and the overall dysfunction that permeates into every social contact. However, such an exercise is necessary to obtain a real impression of the difficulties that the child faces and to establish appropriate intervention (Kramer and Hinojosa, 1993).

Impaired or abnormal social interaction/behaviour

By nature, humans seek out and interact with other humans even from birth. An autistic child does not have the social skills that are used continuously when engaging in conversation, e.g. raising the eyebrows to accentuate meaning or indicate irony. These often subtle skills, when lacking, result in an oddity of behaviour that is not always easy to define. As a result, even if the child seeks out to engage in social contact, others may turn away or avoid his efforts.

Impaired or abnormal social communication

Although an inability to speak is a significant impairment, it need not be a handicap with the invention of alternative forms of communication. Unfortunately for the autistic person, the same problems will affect communication whatever media are used.

Restricted repetitive and stereotyped behaviour which interferes with day-to-day functioning

The presence of ritualistic behaviours, whether simple or complex in nature, takes up time that might otherwise be spent engaging in purposeful activities. Autistic children lack variety of play, as well as having limited social and imaginative play. As play is the fundamental way in which a child explores, makes sense of and learns about his or her environment, any condition that adversely affects play will have a major impact on the child's learning abilities.

A further breakdown of the child's function into its major components indicates the effect autism has on all areas.

Motor

- Poor motor planning
- Poor coordination
- A lack of desire to explore his surroundings.

Sensory

- Poor sensory registration, modulation and discrimination
- Poor attention to sensory cues
- Difficulties with perception of all sensory pathways (vestibular, proprioceptive, tactile, auditory and visual)
- Presence of tactile defensive behaviours.

Cognitive

- Difficulties with executive functions
- Carries out ritualistic behaviours which prevent or impair opportunities for other learning
- Increased risk of associated learning difficulties.

Interpersonal

- Lack of spontaneity
- Lack of reciprocation
- Lack of empathy, inability to see situation from other's perspective
- Lack of cooperation in many situations
- May be easily led astray by others
- Poor non-verbal skills
- May have limited or no speech
- Often isolated
- Lack of social understanding to 'fit in to society'; therefore, may not wash appropriately, understand social rules at mealtimes
- Difficulties working with others
- Obsession with limited interests which may be foisted on to others.

Intrapersonal

- Often presence of obsessions

- High levels of anxiety and fear, especially around changes in environment and routines
- Poor motivation to carry out activities of self-care
- Faddy eater, often restricted food intake which can affect health
- Difficulties coping with change
- May work best in structured work situations
- Inability to occupy self because carrying out ritualistic behaviours.

Assessment

Occupational therapists assess autistic children for a variety of reasons: as part of the diagnostic procedure, to obtain a baseline from which any intervention can be measured, to identify deficits that require occupational therapy input, and to evaluate progress or the lack of progress.

The model or frame of reference used will inevitably guide the choice of assessments, but whatever approach is followed the following areas benefit from inclusion:

- Motor skills:
  - muscle tone
  - gross motor
  - fine motor
  - postural control
  - balance
  - motor planning/praxis
- Sensory skills:
  - sensory processing
  - registration
  - modulation
  - discrimination
- Social skills:
  - interaction
  - communication-verbal/non-verbal
  - emotional organisation
- Occupational skills:
  - activities of daily living
  - basic play and learning
  - types of play, e.g. social, parallel
  - activity levels
  - stereotyped behaviours which interfere with function
- Cognitive skills:
  - perception
  - problem-solving

- ability to see the whole (gestalt)/reasoning
- attention/concentration
- academic skills.

Types of assessments

There are a number of checklists and questionnaires that enable practitioners to make a diagnosis of autism (Trevarthen et al., 1996). Most of these come from the USA; however, CHAT (Checklist for Autism in Toddlers – Baron-Cohen et al., 1992, 1996) is a British one. The occupational therapist may use such material, usually with other team members to aid in diagnosis, and may extract useful observations that will guide her or his input.

To date, there are no standardised occupational therapy assessments for autistic children that are geared to the particular problems that they encounter or the ways in which they may best respond to assessment procedures. Therefore, occupational therapists use a variety of assessments depending on the initial presentation/information about the child and their previous experience about which tests might be suitable. Occupational therapists who have focused on the motor planning difficulties and the stereotyped behaviours have used tests such as the Movement ABC (Henderson and Sugden, 1992), Bruininks–Oseretsky Test of Motor Proficiency (Bruininks, 1978) and Sensory Integration and Praxis Test (Ayres, 1989). However, many of these tests are not generally useful as a result of the high degree of cooperation required, and the level of cognitive ability needed to understand and follow test instructions.

Ermer and Dunn (1998) and Kientz and Dunn (1997) have used a sensory profile to determine differences between autistic children and other non-disabled/disabled children, which may be useful to highlight areas needing input.

Often the occupational therapist relies on non-standardised methods to build up a profile of the autistic child and determine the areas of difficulty where she or he can intervene. Such methods can be valid as long as they are carried out in a rigorous fashion. One such method is the use of parental interviews and questionnaires which are invaluable with autistic children because their performance is often adversely affected by unfamiliar surroundings.

Before an assessment, the occupational therapist needs to have knowledge about normal and autistic development and occupational therapy theory. This is required in order to analyse the autistic behaviours that are interfering with occupational performance and thereby formulate appropriate input.

Some practical guidelines that may aid in the assessment process are:

- Assessment may need to take place over more than one session, particularly if the environment is new to the child because change or novelty often produces extreme anxiety in the autistic person.
- Assessment in the home environment may be more desirable, although care needs to be taken that the observed performance of the child is not just learned patterns of behaviour, which work well at home, but are not transferred to other situations.
- Within the assessment, the therapist may need to use verbal commands accompanied by physical gesture. Often such clients need to be physically guided through the movement before it can be reproduced.
- Some children may need a longer time to respond to a command because there appears to be a delay in processing the information; a lack of allowance may result in an incorrect assessment.
- Isolated areas of ability are often seen, e.g. the child may have excellent manipulative skills in putting together a complex jigsaw puzzle, but be unable to point to items within the picture or use the manipulative skills in other situations, e.g. to put a lid on a bottle.

Therapeutic approaches

As a result of the nature of autism, the condition will present in each person differently, so an individual approach to intervention is required. Intervention may be provided to modify the symptoms of a condition or to tackle the underlying processes. In the case of autism, occupational therapists do not claim to cure the condition but aim to improve the child's functional abilities. As a result the occupational therapist aims to lessen the impact of the core features on the child's ability to function in everyday situations. Small changes are important (Cammisa and Hobbs, 1993) and can make a big difference to the child and family on a daily basis, thereby improving the quality of life. Some approaches have focused on changing the underlying processes, namely the use of sensory integration to deal with the sensory modulation difficulties experienced by many autistic children (Ottenbacher, 1982b; King, 1992; Chu, 1997).

The choice of approach used by the occupational therapist is often as a result of a number of factors. These usually include the therapist's training and experience, the philosophy and milieu of the working environment, and the presenting features of the child. Care needs to be taken when adopting an approach to ensure that current research continues to espouse such an approach or, at least, has not indicated that such an approach is no longer valid.

A number of approaches for use with autistic children have been cited in the literature. Within the USA, the occupational therapist's role is viewed either as a specialist as in sensory integration therapy or in a broader role of development of occupational performance (Stancliff, 1996).

The most commonly used approaches are presented here with a brief explanation of the reasoning behind their choice.

Approaches used

Sensory integration

Most of the occupational therapy literature for autistic children discusses a sensory integrative approach (Ayres, 1980; Ayres and Mailloux, 1983; Larrington, 1987; Sanders, 1993; Stancliff, 1996; Gorman, 1997). But how effective is a sensory approach and on what premise is it used?

Individual case studies have yielded some good results: a decrease in self-stimulation (Ayres and Mailloux, 1983), increase in activities of daily living, improved interaction (Sanders, 1993) and a calmer state (Ayres and Mailloux, 1983; Larrington, 1987). The main premise for the use of sensory integration is a belief that the autistic child has a problem in modulating sensory input; therefore autistic children may over- or under-respond to sensory input. It is hypothesised that the presence of stereotyped behaviours is the child's way of attempting to regulate or make sense of sensory information (Baranek et al., 1997).

Unfortunately, because many autistic children have learning difficulties associated with frank brain damage, the use of sensory integration with autistic children is at odds with the theory lying behind sensory integration. In addition, current literature on the efficacy of sensory integration for the group for which it was originally intended suggests that any intervention is as effective as sensory integration (Vargas and Camilli, 1999), so it may not be the actual intervention that is working. A sensory integrative approach, however, provides the occupational therapist with a framework from which to give meaning to some of the behaviours seen, such as stereotyped behaviours; thus, it may provide some explanation about the processes that occur in autistic children.

Sensory stimulation

A number of articles in the occupational therapy literature indicate the use of sensory stimulation for autistic children. The major difference between sensory stimulation and sensory integration is how it is provided to the child: sensory stimulation is applied passively, whereas the child directs his or herself in a sensory integration session. Different types of sensory stimulation have been used: the use of splints to reduce self-stimulation and stereotyped behaviours (McClure and Holtz-Yotz, 1991; Zisserman, 1992) vestibular stimulation (Slavik et al., 1984) and deep pressure (Edelson, 1998). Results indicated decreases in self-stimulation (Zisserman, 1992), increase in overall function (McClure and Holtz-Yotz, 1991), increased eye contact (Slavik et al., 1984), and a calmer state and decrease in anxiety (Edelson, 1998). Again, in common with the use of sensory integration, the premise appears to be one of assisting the child to modulate sensory input by providing specific types of sensations.

Behavioural approach

A behavioural approach has been used, often in combination with other approaches, to obtain a baseline of the child's behaviours and as a way of establishing clear goals. Intervention has targeted inappropriate behaviours and promoted desired behaviours through positive reinforcement. Occupational therapists tend not to use a purely behavioural approach but a cognitive-based one (Hagedorn, 1992).

Other approaches

Other approaches cited by occupational therapists in the literature are: play therapy (O'Rafferty, 1998), developmental therapy (Bloomer and Rose, 1989), occupational role (Stancliff, 1996) and psychoanalytical therapy (Bloomer and Rose, 1989a, b).

Combination of approaches

A combination of approaches has often been recommended for autistic children in order to deal with the complexity of difficulties that they face (Stancliff, 1996; Bloomer and Rose, 1989). Frequently, sensory integrative techniques are combined with a behavioural approach (Fisher et al., 1991; Sanders, 1993). In these case studies, the behavioural approach was used to get a baseline of the behaviours and to reinforce specific desired behaviours, e.g. tolerating a greater variety of food. The sensory integrative techniques were aimed at enabling the child to modulate sensory input as described above.

When a combination of approaches is used it should be ensured that they are compatible. Some combinations recommended in the literature, such as sensory stimulation and sensory integration (Gorman, 1997), are contentious because they require a different locus of control, i.e. sensory integration is child led whereas sensory stimulation is adult directed.

When a combination is under consideration, the occupational therapist needs to be aware of possible conflicts and be able to justify and explain her or his reasons in using them together. The therapist should also be conscious that confusion can arise when two approaches explain the symptoms in different ways, e.g. stereotyped behaviours are viewed as inappropriate and need to be reduced from a behavioural view whereas a sensory integrative approach would see them as a necessary function of the child's attempt to deal with the sensory input in his or her environment.

Specific areas of intervention

Another way of approaching intervention with autistic children is to examine the performance areas that indicate dysfunction. These can then be dealt with through a variety of approaches, e.g. the occupational therapist may use a problem-solving approach to deal with a number of difficulties that interfere with functional abilities; the approach may not be directly linked to any of the above approaches, but it may use elements of some. The solutions to many problems are often found through a process of collaboration and problem-solving with the child, his family and other agencies.

The following areas give some indication of the kinds of interventions that an occupational therapist may use; these are examples and are not exhaustive.

Social skills

Intervention can range from developing turn-taking in simple games (e.g. rolling ball to each other, passing toys down a tube to each other) to running social skills groups for more able children. Social skills for older children may use role-playing to portray situations, although caution is required to retain a connection with real life because there can be more difficulties dealing with such abstract concepts and generalising practice to real life.

Communication

Although this area is the remit of the speech and language therapist, occupational therapists are often involved in assessing for alternative forms of communication, such as the use of symbols or pictures. Signing can be used but its success is often limited because people tend to use it to have needs met rather than for sharing information. One of the difficulties with communication is seeking out ways to encourage the autistic person to communicate in a spontaneous situation or to share a thought rather than as a means to an end. Occupational therapists are often involved in finding motivators for communication.

Functional independence

This area is vast and covers a host of skills necessary for everyday life. The areas chosen will depend on each child's specific needs, his cognitive abilities and the environment in which he lives.

One of the difficulties for autistic people is dealing and coping with unexpected changes to the routine. The occupational therapist needs to allow for variability when teaching a skill and incorporate coping strategies to deal with change where possible. It is, however, beyond the scope of an occupational therapist to deal with every contingency.

Rigid behaviours and habits can interfere with many everyday tasks and make the performance of daily tasks a struggle for the child and his family. Often a behavioural approach is recommended, e.g. to increase the child's repertoire of food.

Play

Play is fundamental to a child yet it is severely restricted even in the most able autistic youngsters. As a medium, play is used by paediatric occupational therapists to achieve specific goals. However, in autistic children, the concept of play itself needs addressing. Bundy (1993) noted that occupational therapists do not generally assess play and are lacking in thorough assessments that define play. Restall and Magill-Evans (1994) suggest that play can be used both to determine 'developmental delay or deviancy' and as a 'therapeutic medium'. They cited the main areas of play that require intervention as social, imaginative and encouragement of a variety of play. These children are often lacking in the intrinsic value of playing for play's sake, except when engaging in more repetitive behaviours that do not allow the opportunity for development. The encouragement of spontaneous play is therefore required. It is postulated that promotion of play in the autistic child may facilitate increased interactions with peers (Restall and Magill-Evans, 1994). Play and its role in learning for autistic children are a subject that has not yet been thoroughly explored by occupational therapists; it would benefit from further study to assess the effect that limited and stereotyped play has on the overall functioning of the autistic child.

The family

The autistic child needs to be viewed in the context of his or her family who are usually severely affected by the impact of the condition on a daily basis. The occupational therapist needs to be aware of the stage that the family are at in terms of their understanding of and coming to terms with the condition. The values and beliefs of the family will dictate the kinds of therapy to which they are receptive. Often, as autism is such an enigmatic disorder, families are searching for a cure and may seek out a number of therapies. The occupational therapist needs to respect the family's actions, while not compromising her or his profession.

The occupational therapist may also work with the family, teaching them how to play with their autistic child. Often the usual patterns of play have disappeared because the family has not received any feedback from the child. The occupational therapist can assist in developing new forms of play in which family expectations are more in keeping with the child's level of development, and show them alternative responses to look out for which indicate that the child is enjoying the experience.

The occupational therapist may provide the explanations for the child's behaviour, e.g. stereotyped behaviours, and assist the family in developing strategies to deal with such behaviours.

Conclusion

Children with autism are complex in their presentation and their response to interventions; the occupational therapist needs to be flexible to respond to the different needs of each child. Experience of even a small number of children will provide the occupational therapist with a wealth of strategies that she or he can use with other autistic children. Whatever approach is used, the occupational therapist will benefit from spending some time getting to know the child before engaging in treatment; this is required if there is any hope of achieving a positive outcome.

As the efficacy of many interventions has not been proved, it is important that occupational therapists keep accurate records of interventions applied and any changes (positive or negative) that have occurred. She needs to keep up to date with the literature on autism and ongoing research which will guide her interventions on the use of current best practice.

Case study

Luke was a two-and-a-half-year-old boy who attended the Child Development Centre. There had been ongoing concerns about his development since his screening at 18 months, when it was noted that he showed no response to speech. He was sent for a hearing test but this was clear. Luke had been late to reach his milestones, walking at 18 months and, at the time of referral, he had no speech.

His parents had been concerned for some time that he did not play with his siblings or other children. He did not relate to adults either, although he used them in a mechanistic way to have his needs met, e.g. he would take them by the hand to the fridge when he wanted a drink. They were confused about his hearing because he did not respond to his name, yet he would scream when the Hoover was turned on or at planes flying overhead. They were having difficulty going out with Luke because he showed no awareness of danger and would run straight out on to the road; he also climbed everything, including the shelves in supermarkets. Another problem with shopping was the way people starred at Luke when he ran on his tiptoes down the aisles flapping his hands.

Assessment

The occupational therapy assessment took place at home and at the centre over four sessions. The assessment consisted of:

- A parental questionnaire.
- A developmental checklist to determine current level of fine and gross motor skills.
- A combination of structured and unstructured play opportunities were provided to build up a profile of Luke's level of play.

Findings

Motor

Luke displayed almost age-appropriate skills in gross motor activities and was adept at climbing and getting into small restricted places. However, he lacked the safety awareness to go alongside such skills and was therefore a danger to himself while performing such activities. His stumbling over toys and equipment was also a result of his poor attention. Luke was delayed in fine motor skills; manipulation lacked precision and Luke tended to grasp objects with his whole hand. He rarely held on to objects for more than a few seconds, except toys to which he was particularly attached.

Sensory

Luke appeared to be very unresponsive to sounds, especially speech. He displayed a mixed picture during the assessment where some noises caused him discomfort (Hoover, planes) whereas he sought out others (play phone).

Luke did not like being touched and found being dressed/undressed and bathtimes particularly disturbing. He had a preference for holding/touching solid objects and avoided soft materials such as sand, play doh, soft toys. He spent much time walking around the room touching the furniture and hard surfaces. His sensory behaviour indicated that Luke had severe tactile problems and difficulty modulating sensory input.

Social skills

Luke tended to use adults as tools, e.g. he would take an adult's hand and place it on to a toy when he needed help to turn it on. He showed no interest in other children and did not appear to notice them, although occasionally it was noted that he seemed to watch others playing out of the corner of his eye.

He would quickly move away if an adult approached him, although as the assessment progressed he tolerated some parallel play alongside a familiar adult. Even though he did not show any social attachment towards people, he was attached to a toy train which he took everywhere with him.

He did not use eye contact as a means of communication.

Occupational/play skills

Luke demonstrated little use of objects. His play was primarily at the pre-relational stage where he explored objects in a number of limited ways, i.e. mouthing, turning objects, occasional banging. He had difficulty coping with any intervention in his play, so joint attention towards a toy and turn-taking were difficult.

All self-care skills were performed by parents which was quite a struggle because Luke usually reacted adversely at most dressing and bathtimes. They were having difficulties at mealtimes because Luke would not hold any utensils and tolerated only a limited variety of foods.

His parents were particularly concerned about Luke's safety: he showed no awareness of danger. Although he had not been walking long, he had mastered climbing and could scale the wall in the back garden.

Cognitive skills

It was difficult to get a true impression of Luke's functioning in this area because he did not attempt any of the cognitive tasks in standardised tests. Within the assessment, he demonstrated some problem-solving skills to have his needs met, e.g. moving a chair to the cupboard so he could get himself a drink. Assessments from other professionals were suggestive of moderate learning difficulties.

Diagnosis

The occupational therapist was part of an interdisciplinary team which provided a complete assessment of Luke and diagnosed him as being autistic. He was also diagnosed as having moderate learning difficulties. At 30 months Luke was functioning between 9 to 12 months for most areas; his speech was more delayed and was not following a normal progression. Although his gross motor skills were in line with his chronological age, he did not have the safety and social awareness to be independent in this area. Luke was enrolled in a special school for autistic children from the age of 3.

Intervention

Luke required a structured environment where he could feel safe and secure as a starting point. Occupational therapy input was used to address the specific issues set out below. A consistent approach by all people working with Luke was important to make his environment as secure and predictable as possible. Once this was achieved, Luke was able to channel his energies into more productive learning. Occupational therapy input was initially in Luke's home centring around mealtimes and in joint sessions with the speech and language therapist at the CDC, where Luke had begun to attend some nursery sessions to prepare him for school.

- Advice on early turn-taking activities to build up opportunities for meaningful communication.
- Motivators to assist in establishing the need for communication were sought: Luke particularly liked bubbles and bouncing on a large therapy ball. These activities were used initially to encourage Luke to look at the therapist in order for activity to be repeated, and later to make a sound before activity commenced.
- Safety issues at home were addressed; Luke's bedroom window was replaced with shatterproof glass and window locks put on. Access to the garden required supervision.
- Activities to reduce Luke's tactile defensiveness were incorporated into Luke's day. Tactile activities were provided at Luke's developmental level.
- The benefits of providing some deep pressure to calm Luke before self-care tasks was instigated by his parents. Initially they concentrated on mealtimes and also worked on providing tactile input with a hand-over-hand approach to hold and manipulate feeding utensils.

Conclusion

By the time Luke had a place at school he had shown some positive changes in his behaviour. He was using increased eye contact when he wanted his favourite activities repeated and had said 'again' on a few occasions when playing on the therapy ball.

He tolerated turn-taking activities with a familiar adult, although he did not initiate them and had not generalised this concept to everyday situations.

He was more able to tolerate being handled while engaged in self-care activities. His parents had introduced a therapy ball and trampoline at home which he had access to after dressing and bathtimes; this resulted in these activities taking less time. Luke was also actively seeking out rough-and-tumble play from his dad; during these times he was heard to utter some new words which was a great boost for his parents.

Luke's play skills were slowly progressing; during structured play under adult guidance, Luke was able to complete form boards and shape sorters, and was beginning to point to favourite television characters in books/comics. His own play continued to be at an early relational stage. Structured activities were interspersed with time to run in the garden because Luke needed to release the pressures he experienced from more formal activities. The parents had put prickly bushes near the wall as a deterrent for Luke which had worked well.

Another change that had occurred as a result of intervention was the way the parents were now dealing with Luke both at home and outside. They felt they now had the language to explain why Luke behaved in the way he did. In fact they became involved in promoting a better understanding of the condition in their locality.

When Luke started school, the occupational therapist shared her findings with the staff and provided some possible explanations for Luke's tactile and auditory dysfunction. She provided literature to back up these explanations and a programme to assist Luke in being able to function in a more productive manner. Luke's needs are reviewed on a regular basis.

Chapter 11
Children with fragile X syndrome

DIDO GREEN

Fragile X syndrome (FXS) is the most common cause of inherited learning disability (intellectual impairment) and the second most common cause after Down's syndrome. FXS affects between 1 in 4000 and 1 in 6000 births compared with Down's syndrome which affects 1 in 800 (Jacobs et al., 1993; Turner et al., 1996a, b). Despite enormous variability in expression, FXS creates a distinct pattern of physical, cognitive and behavioural features.

Original descriptions of an X-linked chromosomal learning disorder were presented by Martin and Bell in 1943. In 1991 the fragile-X mental retardation gene (*FMR-1*) was identified and sequenced as a fragile site on Xq27.3 (Hagerman, 1996). Genetic mutation/variance in FXS affects a polymorphic triplet region of nucleic acids (cytosine, guanine, guanine or CGG) of the gene. This triple repeat occurs within the general population at levels between 5 and 50 repeats. The syndrome is identified through chromosomal (cytogenetic analysis) or molecular testing, showing this CGG region to be expanded to between 200 and 2000 triple repeats. This is associated with methylation of the gene and subsequent failure of the FMR-1 protein to be transcribed, resulting in loss of gene function. The full mutation (expansion of the CGG region beyond 200 repeats and methylation) is associated with clinical manifestation of the syndrome (Hagerman and Cronister, 1996). Individuals who possess a moderate increase in repeats (between 50 and 200 repeats) – an intermediate stage between the normal and fully mutated gene (the 'pre-mutation') – account for the 'carrier' status (Cornish, 1996).

The X-linked inheritance of FXS in families is atypical, i.e. different from that anticipated between carrier mothers and unaffected fathers.

The typical mendelian mode of sex-linked inheritance of genetic mutations among offspring results in a 50 per cent chance of transmitting

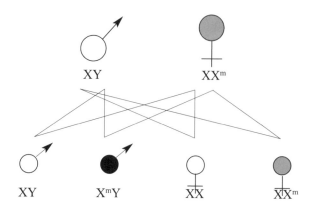

Key: X = female sex chromosome
Y = male sex chromosome
X^m = X chromosome carrying mutation
◯ = carrier
● = affected

= male

= female

Figure 11.1: Mendelian mode of X-linked inheritance.

the anomaly, with equal risk of its presence to a male or female offspring. However, in FXS the actual incidence of affected males is slightly less, at approximately 40 per cent (Black, 1992). In addition, up to one-third of carrier females (an unusually high percentage) are affected to some degree with the learning difficulties, behaviour disorders and social–communicative difficulties seen in affected males. The frequency of expression of the fragile site in carrier females may reduce with age which creates further difficulties in identification. In addition, the frequency and severity of FXS increase from generation to generation. However, FXS has been noted infrequently to skip generations when males are 'silent carriers', i.e. they show no clinical evidence of the syndrome. Despite the fathers being cytogenetically negative, all their daughters would be obligate carriers with receipt of an X chromosome from their father, and therefore their offspring may be affected (Black, 1992; Hagerman, 1996). Despite advances in molecular testing providing more detail of repeat numbers and distribution of the mutation through a family (superseding older and less reliable chromosomal analysis), more is still to be learnt about how the gene works and its impact on fetal maturation, development and behaviour.

What is known about the expression of the FXS gene supports a profile of strengths and needs, resulting in distinctive characteristics of language, learning style and behaviour, and significant physical morphology. The most common of these are set out in Table 11.1.

Descriptions of children with FXS (and often the presenting features) frequently include: poor attention and concentration, with or without hyperactivity, impulsivity, social and linguistic difficulties. In addition, difficulties with transitions, poor sleep patterns, hypermobile joints and single palmar creases, idiosyncratic behaviours including gaze aversion, hand-flapping and hand biting, and sensory hyperresponsivities, especially to tactile (touch), auditory (hearing) and visual (sight) stimuli, have also been documented (Hagerman, 1996; Miller et al., 1999). These deficits may compound and contribute to difficulties with learning. A limited number of FXS children present with more autistic features, such as social withdrawal, restricted interests and peculiar obsessions (Hagerman, 1991a; Turk and Philip, 1997). In contrast these children are frequently described as having above-average imitation skills, vocabulary, reading skills and contextual memory (when any attentional requirements are reduced), and they also demonstrate a sense of humour (Schopmeyer and Lowe, 1992; Hagerman, 1991b, 1996).

Sensorimotor profile

Connective tissue dysplasia with hypermobility of joints and hypotonicity can create significant problems for children with FXS and will be discussed in more detail when considering the impact on function of various features. A number of FXS children suffer from anomalies of joint alignment with scoliosis and flat feet (Hagerman and Cronister, 1996). The skin of individuals with FXS is also notable in its softness and smoothness, particularly of the hands (Hagerman and Cronister, 1996). A single palmar crease, either a simian crease or a Sydney line (Simpson et al., 1984, cited in Hagerman, 1996, p. 22), may be present with calluses often occurring as a result of hand biting. Gross and fine motor skills are generally on a par with intellectual level and early gross motor milestones tend to be unremarkable. However, joint laxity and hypotonicity may disproportionately influence postural alignment, postural stability and balance, as well as delaying the use of the hands for precision in grasp and fine motor resistive actions (Anderson, 1992). The acquisition of motor skills may also be

Table 11.1: Common features of fragile X syndrome

Physical/medical	Behavioural
Long face	Reduced attention
Prominent ears	Poor concentration
High-arched palate	Hyperactivity
Connective tissue dysplasia:	Anxiety
Hypermobile finger joints	Mood lability:
Hernia	Aggression
Hypotonicity	Obsessiveness
Flat feet (pes planus)	Sleep disturbances
(joint dislocation/orthopaedic intervention)	Gaze avoidance
Double-jointed thumb	Hand mannerisms
	Hand flapping
Macro-orchidism (large testicles)	Hand biting
	Hand stereotypies
Skin: Single palmar crease	Stereotypies/tics
(simian crease or Sydney line)	Social impairment:
Hand calluses	Approach–withdrawal
Soft and smooth	Shyness
Increased ridge breadth	Psychosis
Sensory hypersensitivities	**Language/communication**
	Immature articulation
Epilepsy	Rapid speech
Heart murmur/apnoea history	Dysrhythmic speech
Otitis media	Perseveration and repetition of
Visual disorders:	parts or whole words
Strabismus (lazy eye)	Word retrieval difficulties
Refractive errors (myopia/hyperopia)	
Amblyopia	
Diagnosis of autism or ADHD	
Unusual growth patterns/failure to thrive in infancy	

Cognitive
Learning disabilities (mental impairment)
Specific learning difficulties
Poor sequencing functions

Strengths	Weaknesses
Single word vocabulary	Symbolic language
Visual matching	Visual motor coordination
Verbal labelling	Arithmetic/digit span
Comprehension	Abstract thinking
Long-term memory(emotionally/	Short-term memory (including
contextually cued)	visual motor and auditory
	processing)
Perceptual closure (gestalt)	Spatial memory

influenced by poor sensory processing functions underpinning the development of body scheme, spatial awareness and motor performance (Stackhouse, 1994).

A variety of sensory processing deficits have been identified in children with FXS (Hickman, 1989; Hagerman, 1991b; Anderson, 1992; Stackhouse, 1994; Miller and McIntosh, 1998; Miller et al., 1999). Miller et al. (1999) have documented the electrodermal responses to sensory stimuli in individuals with FXS, showing increased magnitude of response, more responses per stimulus and poor habituation. Vestibular functions that enable us to perceive, adapt to and tolerate changes in the position of the body in relation to gravity are frequently poor in the child with FXS. A higher incidence of otitis media (middle-ear infection) has been noted; however, it is unclear whether the proximity of structures may have an impact on the development of vestibular functions. Language and cognitive deficits can be worsened as a result of recurrent otitis media (Kelly, 1995; Hagerman, 1996).

Poor somatosensory functions, the perception of tactile (touch) and proprioceptive (body position) information received through the skin, joints, muscles and tendons, are frequently seen in FXS. Individuals with FXS are more likely to have tactile hyperresponsivity (tactile defensiveness) (Lachiewicz et al., 1994; Miller at al., 1999). Although visual disorders (see Table 11.1) are common, it is believed that the features of gaze aversion and impaired eye contact may in part be related to sensory hyperresponsivity (sensory defensiveness). Hypersensitivities in the auditory system have also been documented, which may interfere with learning and behaviour (Hagerman, 1991b; Anderson, 1992; Stackhouse, 1994; Miller et al., 1999).

Cognitive

Neuropsychological testing in individuals with FXS is somewhat complicated by the decline in measured intelligence quotient (IQ) in males around adolescence and the variability in expression of the fragile site in females (Bennetto and Pennington, 1996). Research is somewhat inconclusive regarding syndrome specific features that are independent of general intellectual impairment and/or features of anxiety or autism (Garner et al., 1999). Bennetto and Pennington (1996) have reported more specific difficulties with sequential processing among individuals with FXS. In contrast, strengths with contextual and long-term memory, vocabulary and visual matching can support learning. FXS children have particular difficulty with abstract reasoning and persistence in tasks that are not immediately viewed as meaningful. Therefore these children frequently demonstrate difficulty with number concepts and under-standing arithmetical processes (Gibb, 1996).

There is inconclusive evidence with respect to a relationship between measured cognitive ability and number of CGG repeats (Baumgardner et al., 1995; Bennetto and Pennington, 1996; Cornish, 1996). Mazzocco (1998) found that the perceptual/organisational factor score on IQ testing was a strong predictor of mathematics performance in girls with FXS. The independence of IQ from behaviours characteristic of FXS suggests that the behavioural profile is specific to the syndrome and not a function of cognitive development (Baumgardner et al., 1995; Garner et al., 1999).

Speech and communication

The conversational styles of children with FXS have a somewhat distinct profile when compared to other conditions involving impairments of speech, language and/or communication (Ferrier et al., 1991). Poor articulation of an immature nature, rather than being truly atypical, is common (Schopmeyer and Lowe, 1992). Lack of fluency, notable fast and dysrhythmic speech ('cluttered'), tangential comments and frequent digression in conversation are typical, along with frequent verbal perse-veration and delayed 'echolalia' – repetition of parts of words, whole words and/or phrases (Lachiewicz et al., 1994; Gibb, 1996; Turk and Philip, 1997). Motor planning deficits and poor sequencing functions may impair oral–motor skills and respiratory timing for adequate articu-lation and phonation (Schopmeyer and Lowe, 1992). Hypotonicity will also affect intelligibility and articulation and poor lip closure may contribute to drooling. McClennon (1992) has argued that perseveration may be used as a strategy to buy time when word-finding difficulties and anxiety occur, especially when responding to direct questions. Subsequently, and despite a relatively strong vocabulary, children with FXS have difficulties sustaining a conversation, turn-taking and using non-verbal skills such as body position, eye contact and gesture to support communication.

Oral–motor behaviour of hand-to-mouth actions and mouthing of objects beyond infancy may be evident, especially with decreasing IQ. Noticeable among FXS children are the more sensory-related behaviours that are socially inappropriate and may interfere with communication, such as rubbing of the face with saliva, biting and pressing the mouth or forehead firmly. Hypersensitivity in the oral area, particularly tactile defen-siveness, may exacerbate difficulties during mealtimes with restricted or adverse eating habits being evident.

Behavioural characteristics

Hyperactivity is one of the most noticeable features of childhood (becoming less apparent after puberty). Parent and teacher ratings have also shown a significantly higher incidence of hyperactivity, stereotypical movements and unusual speech in FXS boys (Baumgardner et al., 1995). A higher incidence of attention deficit (hyperactivity) disorder (ADHD) symptoms in FXS boys has been reported (Turk, 1998). Although less frequent in girls, impulsivity and short attention span can be significant factors and coexist with shyness and social withdrawal.

There is some discrepancy in the literature regarding the prevalence of autism and autistic features in FXS. This is complicated by the fact that specific screening for fragile X in populations of children presenting with learning disabilities/difficulties and autistic features has become more commonplace only relatively recently. Adding to this confusion is the variance in criteria for diagnosing autism. Studies using rigorous diagnosis procedures, and that take into account specific cytogenic/molecular testing, suggest a prevalence of the fragile X anomaly in cases of autism at a rate of between 2.5% and 16% which is above general population figures (Gillberg, 1995; Bailey et al., 1996; Hagerman and Cronister, 1996). Autism in females with FXS is uncommon and represents the most severe end of the spectrum of social anxiety and social withdrawal (Hagerman, 1996). Although features of gaze avoidance, stereotypical actions, language deficits and problems with social interaction (particularly peer interaction) and unusual non-verbal communication are common in FXS, a more pervasive lack of related-ness (theory of mind) is rare (Baron-Cohen et al., 1993; Hagerman and Cronister, 1996; Garner et al., 1999). There is some evidence to suggest that FXS speech patterns differ from those of autistic spectrum (AS) disorders with a greater degree of perseveration of words and phrases and less echolalia in children with FXS than in children with AS alone (Sudhalter et al., 1990). Children with FXS also seem to demonstrate more meaningful and functional use of language with a greater degree of emotional perception than children with AS disorders (Turk and Cornish, 1998).

Males with FXS (and females in a more subtle way) do not usually show a disinterest in social interaction but demonstrate social behaviours more suggestive of social anxiety. A distinct pattern of approach and withdrawal is seen through poor greeting skills, inappropriate timing of social initiation and difficulty sustaining interaction. They will be seen to make a social approach, yet they are ineffective in following this through with conventional social behaviour, e.g. in Western societies, after an initial approach they may turn their body and head away and avert gaze in a shy manner. FXS individuals seem to have few skills in identifying and responding to non-verbal cues (McClennon, 1992). Carrier females were found by Sobesky et al. (1995) to have discomfort with interpersonal contact, social oddities and social isolation, with this being more apparent as learning disabilities increase.

The frequent occurrence of psychiatric symptoms, including attention deficits, depression, tics and autistic features, has been identified (Weidmer-Mikhail et al., 1998), although Baumgardner et al. (1995) suggest that these stereotypies may well be environmental and relate somewhat to the imitation capabilities of FXS children, when exposed to other children demonstrating these behaviours. Clinical experience suggests that complex hand stereotypies such as hand flapping or posturing may in part be related to aspects of sensory hypersensitivities and an internal drive to inhibit irritable sensations by seeking out more calming/inhibitory stimuli such as joint compression or deep pressure touch (Reisman and Hanschu, 1992). These behaviours can be exacerbated by anxiety.

Obsessiveness and mood fluctuations are relatively common and may contribute to aggressive outbursts; however, destructiveness and temper tantrums seem to be features associated more with learning disabilities (Turk and Philip, 1997). Aggressiveness in FXS may be a consequence of over-stimulation, which is aggravated by exposure to perceived noxious stimuli, especially tactile ones (Hagerman, 1996). There is excess worrying and anxiety in some carrier mothers of children with FXS (Sobesky et al., 1995). Significantly increased levels of anxiety disorders, bipolar disorders, mood lability and social phobia occurring in carrier women may affect the therapeutic relationship and family–child relationship. Depression may be common; however, distinguishing between this and the depression occurring in parents of children with disabilities is difficult. Wright-Strawderman and Watson (1992) showed that there was an increased prevalence of depressive symptoms in children with specific learning difficulties; therefore this may also be a factor contributing to depression within FXS. Psychoses can occasionally occur and are important to recognise because pharmacological intervention can be helpful (Hagerman and Cronister, 1996). However, there is no evidence that psychosis is more common in individuals with FXS than in non-FXS individuals with similar degrees of learning disability. When present, the psychiatric process will usually involve a deterioration in independence in daily skills functioning requiring regular monitoring of ability.

Various mechanisms have been postulated about the influences of the *FMR-1* gene on function. Summarising the literature presented by Hagerman (1996) suggests that FMR protein (FMRP) expression is involved with modifying synaptic structure in response to environmental stimuli. The FMRP is known to be concentrated in areas of the brain associated with short-term memory and emotion (hippocampus/temporal lobe), learning (cerebral cortex) and inhibition, sequencing and control of movement (cerebellum). These structures are most notably atypical on neuroimaging of individuals with FXS (Peterson, 1995). Lack of cholinergic innervation, particularly in the limbic system, may be contributing to the over-reaction of the sympathetic nervous system to stimuli, leading to anxiety, mood lability and sleep disturbances. Dysregulation of the modulatory mechanisms of sensory processing may further contribute to difficulties coordinating adaptive behaviour in children with FXS.

Impact of fragile X syndrome on children's occupations

The broad spectrum of involvement from fragile X genetic expression and the pervasiveness of functions potentially influenced by the syndrome result in a complex profile of strengths and needs of individuals with FXS despite some overall similarities. Problems processing tactile, vestibular, visual, auditory, olfactory and gustatory stimuli frequently occur in FXS children. In combination with physical characteristics of joint laxity, language difficulties and cognitive limitations, they can have a wide-ranging effect on the occupations of childhood – those of play, child–adult role, school work, and development of independence in activities of daily living. Table 11.2 outlines the impact of some of the features of FXS on play.

The various characteristics of FXS listed in Table 11.2 have a multiplicative effect rather than a purely additive one, whereby each characteristic interacts with and exacerbates the difficulties of other contributory features. Attention deficits reduce orientation to salient cues during play and are exacerbated by poor visual motor and fine motor capabilities to manipulate objects and participate in play. Poor speech and communication coupled with social anxiety add to the difficulties in relating to play partners and achieving success in collaborative ventures.

The physical features most likely to affect function are hypotonia and ligamentous laxity influencing joint stability and proximal control. This can have an effect on the acquisition of motor milestones and more notably on qualitative aspects of movement. The child with reduced strength and control at the shoulders may use distal stabilising postures such as propping on wrists or elbows, with a resultant lack of fluency in arm/wrist movements during manipulative tasks. Poor balance and difficulties in hopping, skipping, jumping and fine motor skills are frequently affected, with many FXS children seemingly presenting as children with

Table 11.2: The impact of characteristic features of FXS on play

Feature	Influence on play behaviour
Attention deficit	Decreased orientation to differences between objects, e.g. bigger/rounder, etc. with failure to succeed in constructional tasks
	Problems focusing on salient information of objects or conversation to maintain focus on play theme
Tactile defensiveness	Heightened distractibility and discomfort during messy play or physical contact games
	Decreased in-hand manipulation of objects as a result of sensitivies of palmar surface for development of fine manipulative skills
Poor visuospatial skills	Difficulty orienting objects and/or self in space for participation in games or social play
	Difficulty recognising changes in facial expression of playmate
Anxiety	Poor ability to adapt to change with increased arousal and distress (tantrums) with change of either environment or topic
	Difficulties adjusting to the dynamic interplay during social exchange and creative play
Hypotonia/hypermobile	Poor stability for developing gross and fine motor skills that support play behaviour
Speech and communication	Difficulties in articulation, word retrieval, interpretation and use of non-verbal social cues reduce understanding, resulting in misunderstandings about topic/activity

developmental coordination disorders (DCD; see DSM-IV – APA, 1994). Thenar and hyperthenar muscles may be poorly developed in influencing fingertip-to-palm action, thumb opposition, grasp and in-hand manipulation. Motor skills and adaptive behaviours are considered to be poor not only because of joint laxity and hypotonicity related to an underlying connective tissue disorder, but also because of poor sensory integrative processing (Anderson, 1992; Stackhouse, 1994).

FXS children seem to have particular difficulties using sensory information to support productive behaviour. The sensory systems support behaviour in two main ways:

1. Discrimination – which supports knowledge about analytical aspects of sensations, e.g. size, shape, texture, colour, depth, and speed and direction of movement, etc.

2. Protection – which acts to prevent harm and maintain homoeostasis and comfort in response to sensory input, whether internally or externally derived.

The ability to discriminate between types and dimensions of sensory input provides valuable information about ourselves and our environment, and works closely with mechanisms that alert us to the possibility of danger in order to assist us in coordinating appropriate responses (Royeen and Lane, 1991; Bear et al., 1996). For example, when walking along an uneven surface with our postural base displaced, the vestibular, proprioceptive and visual systems work together to support spontaneous adjustments for postural realignment. If our postural base is displaced suddenly and our vestibular system alerts us to the impending danger of falling forward, we automatically extend our arms forward in a protective response, at times before we have registered consciously the fact that we are falling.

The ability to orient towards novel stimuli and habituate to non-essential background stimuli allows us to attend to salient information while maintaining an appropriate level of arousal to support necessary actions (Cermak, 1988). If this balance is disturbed, it is difficult to interpret sensory information in a meaningful way. The inverted U curve represents the extent to which an optimal level of arousal is required to achieve a good standard of performance (Figure 11.2).

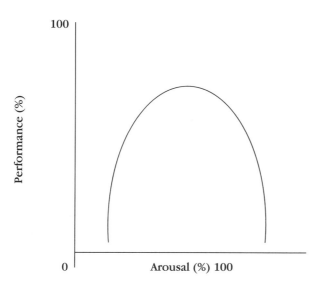

Figure 11.2: Schema of the relationship between arousal and performance.

If an individual is placed in conditions of persistently high levels of stress, arousal levels are too high to sustain performance. The FXS child who consistently perceives non-noxious, common stimuli as threatening will find it difficult to orient towards more relevant stimuli and learn from their response to support success in a task. Heightened responses to stimuli and failure to habituate to repeated non-threatening stimuli can have implications for behavioural arousal and inhibition (McIntosh et al., 1999).

Many FXS children seek out and require additional vestibular input (body movement stimuli) and seem to be perpetually on the move. However, discriminative capabilities that help them distinguish between aspects of movement such as speed and direction may also be reduced, which restricts their opportunities to learn from their experience. Some FXS children seem to experience disproportionate fear to body changes in relation to gravity – gravitational insecurity – thus reducing their desire to participate in movement activities (Hickman, 1989; Stackhouse, 1994).

Children with FXS are frequently seen to have tactile defensiveness, i.e. they show an aversive reaction to tactile stimuli or the perceived threat of tactile stimuli that would normally not be considered noxious or irritable. Ferri et al. (1994) studied the somatosensory-evoked potentials in 10 males with FXS and found sufficient evidence to suggest hyperexcitability in the supplementary motor area (SMA) of the cortex. The SMA is particularly important for integrating sensory and motor information for motor planning and coordination. Miller et al. (1999) report large electrodermal responses with poor habituation after tactile stimulation in children with FXS. There is a risk that children with FXS may have both discriminative and modulatory difficulties in processing tactile stimuli.

Deficits in processing auditory, visual, gustatory (taste) and olfactory (smell) stimuli are also documented among FXS children (Hagerman, 1991b; Anderson, 1992; Miller et al. 1999). Either in isolation or in combination with other sensory processing deficits, skilled, adaptive behaviour can be influenced by hyper-responsiveness to sensory input.

Frustration and repeated failure or discomfort in activities may cause children to run away or avoid circumstances that expose them to failure and/or 'sensory irritants'. On the other hand, children may find strategies to reduce the noxious element such as 'rubbing out light touch'. Williams and Shellenberger (1992) provide extensive examples of how 'normal' individuals undertake actions to modulate the amount of a particular sensory input received, either to 'calm' or 'alert' themselves when required to maintain an optimal level of arousal. These behaviours may range from biting their fingernails or chewing gum, to going for a jog, etc. Children with FXS frequently have difficulties with self-regulation, including disordered sleep cycles, attention deficits, difficulties maintaining appropriate levels of alertness and arousal, and difficulties modulating emotional intent and affect which may relate to global sensory processing problems (Stackhouse, 1994). The child with FXS may not always develop socially acceptable methods of 'calming', e.g. chewing may not be limited to fingernails or the ends of pens and pencils.

The tendency for FXS children to become overwhelmed by increasing amounts or types of stimuli reduces their chances of learning from more subtle sensory experiences. This may be the result of poor discriminative functions as much as it is of inadequate modulatory/protective mechanisms, whereby information about dimensions of sensory stimuli is poorly processed. This lack of knowledge about sensory stimuli can place individuals in a 'heightened' state of alertness. The child may endeavour to seek out additional information to provide a reference for learning and/or to 'control' perceived aversive aspects of stimuli. These children require additional opportunities for practice and experience to develop discriminative functions, yet may simultaneously avoid direct contact with some stimuli as a result of defensive reactions. Figure 11.3 illustrates the interaction between sensory processing and behaviour.

The ability both to discriminate and to modulate sensory input is required to support adaptive behaviour and achievement in complex tasks.

The learning difficulties of the FXS child may have a significant impact on how they acquire knowledge. Deficits with abstract concepts and sequential processing affect the child's ability to learn in environments, with a strong emphasis on symbolic reasoning, calculations and sciences. These children also have difficulty in settings that encourage the child to be autonomous and independent in how they organise themselves within the classroom.

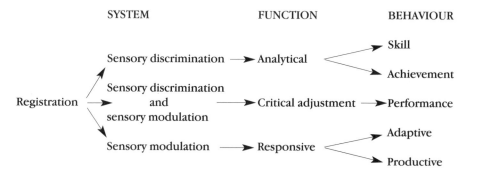

Figure 11.3: Interaction between sensory processing and behaviour.

To date there is no evidence that the sensory deficits of the FXS child dissipate over time. Ligaments are known to stiffen with age and reduce one of the variables contributing to poor performance. Cognitive deficits are purported to increase in FXS males with age, although this may be a testing artefact because 'older age'/adult IQ tests have a greater emphasis on abstract concepts (Bennetto and Pennington, 1996). Intervention can help to modify and change the behavioural responses to sensory stimuli. In-depth assessment is therefore required to identify areas of both strength and weakness for the best understanding of the child's learning style, sensory profile and motor capabilities.

Assessment

Careful analysis of individual needs within the context of their environment is essential when attempting to address the individual concerns of children with FXS and their families. Assessments should provide information on how best to help a child rather than just define the extent of any difficulty. Research scientists may wish to identify precise levels of intellectual, speech and language, sensory, motor and/or functional and educational attainments. However, most occupational therapists will be concerned with promoting independence, quality of life with improved skill level and/or reducing the burden of care on families in which more severe levels of disability occur. The pervasiveness of problems within FXS requires the collaboration of a multidisciplinary team to identify the strengths and weaknesses of FXS children and address their individual medical, learning, speech and language, and functional performance needs. The assessments and approach adopted will be guided by theoretical and clinical reasoning and relate, in particular, to sensory processing, neuromotor development and behavioural learning theories.

The assessment process may involve a number of routes with formal and informal channels all providing useful information. Standardised assessment tools, clinical observations, informal observations, clinical history, questionnaires and checklists will all serve a purpose, as well as providing the opportunity to listen to the concerns and comments of the child and his or her family and teachers. First and foremost is the consideration of the effects of novelty and anxiety when a child with FXS is confronted with unfamiliar adults, different environments or changes to routines. It is important to schedule more than one visit and across venues, both clinical and functional, to identify areas of strengths and weakness and the impact of these on functional skills. Although the presenting problem may be specific to one environment, e.g. toileting at school, it will be important to identify when and how the child is able to achieve particular skills and the compensatory strategies that he or she may employ. Observations during 'prime time' – the optimum period during the day when the child is able to perform at his or her best – are equally important as 'fragile' times – periods during which the impact of deficits is likely to be most pronounced.

Length of session, venue, participants and time of day are all important and should be documented, with antecedents and consequences also noted. When formal assessments are undertaken, it may be necessary to incorporate 'calming' techniques and/or include familiar materials or equipment such as a 'bean bag chair' to reduce anxiety. Careful liaison with family/carers before meeting the child can help to identify activities/objects that provide motivation for the child and may encourage the child during the session, particularly by providing contextual cueing where appropriate. During any observation (formal or informal), identifying the exact nature of a response can be helpful in guiding intervention, e.g. when pouring milk from a carton to a glass, is the child able to ensure that there is no spillage during pouring, but unable simultaneously to monitor the height of the mounting liquid in the glass, which subsequently overflows? Formal testing may require some adaptation to discriminate between the ability to perform that test versus the underlying construct (Stackhouse, 1994), e.g. when testing visual–perceptual functions, avoid tests that have tabulated responses, select those that have responses presented in a straight line and preferably those that only have one picture per page (McClennon, 1992, cited in Schopmeye and Lowe, 1992). The Test of Visual Motor Skills may be preferable to the Developmental Test of Visual Motor Integration (VMI), in view of the fact that there is only one stimulus and response required per page with the former. If using the VMI, or similar tests with more than one picture per page, it may be necessary to prepare a template to cover extraneous stimuli to help the child focus his or her attention. It may then be helpful to undertake a similar test to compare the child's response with and without the adaptation. Using the previous pouring task as an example, it may be useful to have a clear glass with a coloured line demarcating the maximum level versus a non-transparent glass.

Table 11.3 sets out some examples of observations and instruments for gaining information regarding functional skills and underlying components. It outlines aspects of assessment and tools that may assist analysis of performance and behaviour. If available it is helpful to have knowledge of cognitive capabilities, particularly as poor motor coordination is associated with learning disabilities (Sugden and Wann, 1987). It is important to bear in mind that characteristic behaviours of hyperactivity and poor attention, impulsivity and anxiety, combined with the need for meaningful

Table 11.3: Assessment of the child with fragile X syndrome

Domain	Observation	Measurement/Tool*
Play	Ability to occupy self Playfulness Participation with others Manipulation of materials Enjoyment/Humour Creativity/Imagination Purpose/Construction	Knox Preschool Play Scale (Knox, 1997) Test of Playfulness (Bundy, 1997) Autistic Diagnostic (Lord et al., 2000) Observation Schedule Narratives (Bryze, 1997) (Burke and Schaaf, 1997)
ADL	Dressing Toileting Bathing Feeding Community independence	PEDI (Haley et al., 1992) Wee Fim (UDS, 1991) AMPS (Fisher, 1995)
Social	Physicality Social reciprocity Conversation/Communication Timing skills Life role development	SBS (Green, 1997) CCC (Bishop, 1998)
Functional	Task attainment Tool usage Pre-vocational/leisure activities	ETCH (Amundson, 1995) Peabody (Folio and Fewell, 1984) AMPS (Fisher, 1995) Vineland Adaptive Behaviour Scales (Sparrow et al., 1984)
Sensory integrative	Aversion or extreme sensitivity to touch, sound, movement or visual stimulation Toe walking Low muscle tone	Sensory Profile (Dunn, 1999) Sensory Inventory for Individuals with Developmental Delay (Reisman and Hanschu, 1992) TIE (Royeen, 1991)
	Delays in gross/fine motor skills Poor balance Discriminative ability/matching Poor motor planning skills Discriminative ability/matching Resistance to change/transitions	DeGangi Berk Test of SI (Berk and DeGangi, 1983) SIPT (Ayres, 1989) Kinesthetic Sensitivity Test (Laslow and Bairstow, 1985)
Motor	Balance Postural alignment Joint range/stability	Movement ABC (Henderson and Sugden, 1992) Bruininks–Oseretsky (Bruininks, 1978)

Table 11.3: (contd)

Domain	Observation	Measurement/Tool
	Grasp and prehension	MAP (Miller, 1988)
	Palmar creases	Peabody (Folio and Fewell, 1984)
		Erhardt (1982)
		Bayley (1991)
		COMPS (Wilson et al., 1994)
		HELP (Parks, 1994)
Perceptual	Visuospatial	VMI (Beery, 1989)/TVMS (Gardner,
	Figure–ground	1986)
	Visual closure vs gestalt	DVPT (Hammill et al., 1993)
		MFVPT (Colarusso and Hammill,
	Visual memory	1995a)/TVPS (Gardner, 1982)
	Body awareness	WRAML (Adams and Sheslow, 1990)
	Sensory–perceptual functions	Draw-a-Man (Goodenough and
		Harris, 1963)
		SIPT (Ayres, 1989)
Learning	Consultation with psychologist	WRAML (Adams and Sheslow, 1990)
	Memory	VMI (Beery, 1989)/TVMS (Gardner,
	Sequencing functions	1986)
		MFVPT (Colarusso and Hammill,
		1995a)/TVPS (Gardner, 1982)
	Visuospatial skills	DVPT (Hammill et al., 1993)
Attention	Distractibility/Fidgeting	Sensory Profile (Dunn, 1999)
Self-regulatory	Arousal/Calming	Brazelton (Brazelton and Nugent,
	Orientation to novel vs	1995)
	irrelevant stimuli	Sensory Inventory (Reisman and
		Hanschu, 1992)
		Sensory Profile (Dunn, 1999)

*Assessment instruments are listed in Appendix: PEDI, Paediatric Evaluation of Disability Inventory; Wee FIM, Wee Functional Independence Measure; AMPS, Assessment of Motor and Process Skills (personal activities of life measures in preparation); SBS, Social Behaviour Scale; CCC, Childhood Communication Checklist; ETCH, Evaluation Tool of Children's Handwriting; TIE, Tactile Inventory for Elementary Children; SIPT, Sensory Integration and Praxis Tests; COMPS, Clinical Observations of Motor and Postural Skills; HELP, Hawaii Early Learning Profile; MAP, Miller Assessment for Preschoolers; VMI, Developmental Test of Visual Motor Impairment; TVMS, Test of Visual Motor Skills; DVPT, Developmental Test of Visual Perception; MFVPT, Motor-free Visual Perception Test; TVPS, Test of Visual Perceptual Skills; WRAML, Wide Range Assessment of Memory and Learning.

contexts, can confound results of any standardised or formal testing. Parents and teachers commonly report a higher level of skill attainment at home or school than is demonstrated clinically. Tests or situations that allow for some flexibility of administration and offer practice trials providing familiarity with the materials are to be preferred. Many of the sensory and motor tests currently available use materials that children do not necessarily play with regularly, e.g. nuts and bolts, pegs and pegboards, balance beams, etc., and the novelty of these assessments may increase anxiety and affect performance.

Establishing the child's perception of his or her abilities and identifying skill areas is critical when working with children with FXS, to support meaningful contexts for intervention. The Canadian Occupational Performance Model and the Canadian Occupational Performance Measure ([COPM] Law et al., 1994) attempts to ascertain clients' perceptions and satisfaction with performance in activities that they deem important to them. The COPM may be a useful adjunct to assessment but requires some adaptation for children with FXS, in view of its use of numerical (abstract) coding to represent the level of importance of a task and feelings of competence and skill. Experience indicates that the occupational therapist's role when assessing a child with FXS is to ascertain the impact of deficient skills on adaptive behaviour, particularly the relationship between discriminatory and modulatory (protective) sensory functions, motor planning, learning style and self-regulatory 'calming' abilities.

Intervention

An integrated approach is imperative if the complex needs of the FXS child are to be adequately addressed. Environments and approaches for both assessment and intervention need to offer some flexibility to cater for this diversity and help reduce anxiety. Highly motivating materials are required to help a child focus attention and concentration and develop maximum capabilities. Treatment approaches which may be adopted in occupational therapy for children with FXS include neurodevelopmental, sensory integration, neuropsychological and behavioural with environmental adaptations following on from these. Discussing any of these independently is rather artificial as each of these must be integrated to address the complexity of deficits. For academic purposes a summary of the main approaches and examples of implementation will be given.

Neurodevelopmental approach

A neurodevelopmental therapy (NDT) perspective considers the central mechanisms for control of posture and movement and analysis of patterns of movement. Joint laxity and hypotonicity are important features that limit functional attainments of the FXS child. It may be relevant to focus on establishing central stability, to enable greater dexterity in distal/fine manipulative actions. Working against gravity will not only enhance proprioceptive feedback, but will develop strength in sustaining muscle contractions against a constant force.

Figure 11.4 illustrates a treatment for postural stability while using picture reinforcers. When recommending any activity with a motor emphasis, it will be important to consider the sensory components of the task, especially if undertaken in a public facility such as swimming baths in which the novelty of the environment and echoing, slippery, wet rooms may overwhelm the child with FXS.

Sensory integration

Sensory integrative therapy helps the FXS child to process sensory information more effectively, to elicit an appropriate adaptive (motor, speech or behavioural) response as opposed to becoming confused, frustrated, overwhelmed or defensive. Treatment should also help the FXS individual acquire self-regulatory mechanisms to maintain an equilibrium between protective and discriminative functions in order to support an adequate level of arousal for learning and success.

The ability to discriminate between qualitative dimensions of sensory stimuli and to modulate sensory input allows individuals to plan and coordinate their responses. Sensory integrative therapy can help the FXS child

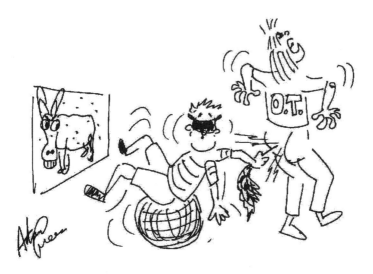

Figure 11.4: Illustration of intervention for postural stability.

process and analyse sensory information more effectively in order to be less sensitive to noises, sights, physical contact and movement in the environment (Hickman, 1989). The techniques of sensory integration that promote the organisation of sensory stimuli for use can be helpful, in particular the calming/inhibitory techniques for when the child is over-aroused or distressed (Hickman, 1989; Hagerman, 1991b, 1996).

The Alert Program for Self-Regulation of Williams and Shellenberger (1992) helps children recognise and expand the number of appropriate self-regulation strategies in a variety of tasks and settings, based on the principles of occupational therapy and sensory integration. Wilbarger and Wilbarger (1991) have defined a specific intervention programme for addressing sensory defensiveness. Oetter et al. (1985) have designed the MORE programme to improve the sensory integrative and sensory motor problems associated with oral–motor, respiratory and postural skills (MORE = motor components, oral organisation, respiratory demand and eye contact). Auditory integration training, a specific auditory sensory intervention rather than a sensory integrative approach (Brown, 1999), may be helpful in desensitising the child's response to auditory stimuli in order to modify behavioural responses.

Incorporating a sensory integrative approach when working alongside speech and language therapists and psychologists will enhance overall intervention to promote speech and language development, play and learning. The 'calming' techniques, such as deep pressure, protective spaces, rhythmic activities and slow linear vestibular stimulation, can be implemented in the home and educational settings to facilitate learning. Merrill (1990) has compiled a useful reference for examining the environment from an occupational therapy perspective, which incorporates sensory integration theory. Environmental strategies may be included that support orientation and re-focusing on salient information, such as the use of visual and auditory contextual cueing. Scharfenaker et al. (1996) have demonstrated the feasibility of implementing a sensory integrative approach for FXS children when working together with educationalists and speech and language therapists in an educational setting. Liaising with psychologists and parents/carers will also be helpful in providing advice on sexual education and moving towards adult life. Consideration of the sensory nature of activities and environments, including the intensity, frequency, duration and relative contrast between sensory modalities as well as within a specific sensory domain, may help the FXS child develop more organised interactions with their physical and social environments. Recruiting a sensory integrative approach within an overall treatment programme may contribute towards life role development as a family member, friend, student or worker (Stackhouse, 1994).

Neuropsychological

The FXS child's strengths in vocabulary, 'gestalt' learning and contextual understanding should be taken into consideration when compiling a programme to support learning. FXS children benefit from structured activities which are clearly demarcated to focus attention and placed within a meaningful context. Verbal rehearsal, the process of telling oneself what to do, can use a child's strengths in verbal memory, particularly contextual, to assist the child in following instructions. Visual memory strengths will support the use of pictures representing completed tasks ('gestalt'), with number-coded instructions of individual stages of the activity provided. The child can be encouraged to tick off each step when completed, developing autonomy for moving on to the next sequence. It may be necessary to place one step per page, providing arrows or colour coding, e.g. green to start, red to finish, to encourage the child to turn each page on completion. McClennon (1991) has provided some useful tips for teaching time management with picture schedules, and recommends incorporating real objects within educational settings to provide relevance for referencing the relationship of objects to each other. The PACE-Math programme developed by Grumblatt and McClennon (McClennon, 1991) focuses on problem-solving real objects rather than non-contextual learning. These strategies can be particularly helpful for developing money management and community skills.

The use of computers will be dependent in part on whether the child finds a computer a motivating and meaningful object. The visual presentation of microtechnology may build on the strong visual skills of children with FXS (Scharfenaker et al., 1996). Many children with poor attention find the computer useful in focusing their visual and listening skills. Observing how the child responds to visual changes and types of auditory feedback will be an important consideration in the choice and use of software. Lane and Ziviani (1999) have provided a detailed analysis of the visual–motor demands of software designed for children. They suggest that the use of computers would be a useful adjunct for teaching and leisure time for children, in view of the reduced motor demands when using a mouse for access to compensate for poor coordination. Software programmes that use visual presentation may support the sequencing elements of tasks.

Behavioural approach

Strengths in imitation support the use of modelling to demonstrate an action or skill. This process builds on the FXS child's ability to use visual (contextual) cues and on the children's positive interest in others (Schopmeyer and Lowe, 1992). Equally important to remember, however, is the effect of 'role models' (peer environment), as noted by the increase in swearing or coprolalia when the child with FXS is placed in environments in which use of swear words is more frequent (Baumgardner et al., 1995). Motivators and conditional learning, i.e. the positive reinforcement of desired behaviours and actions, will support any intervention approach. For more able children, using star charts and accumulative positive reinforcers, including attempts to respond appropriately, may be helpful. The number of attempted responses before the receipt of a reinforcer will depend on the child's tolerance of delayed gratification, a particular problem for children with ADHD, and one that may need to be considered in programmes for FXS children (Sonuga-Barke, 1994; McClennon, 1992). Various programmes such as the TEACCH (Schopler et al., 1984) and Lovaas (1977) have been developed from behavioural theories to structure reinforcers within teaching models and on a 24-hour schedule. However, it remains unclear whether these intensive programmes are required in their entirety or whether certain specific components are sufficient.

Specific skills teaching may be appropriate; however, consideration must be taken of the reasons why skill is poor, e.g. with poor memory for data that are not immediately apparent, the over-rehearsal of a skill using positive reinforcers may be required. Also, it may be necessary to reinforce various aspects of tasks such as lacing shoelaces or learning to buy extras of frequently used items before you run out, and then reducing or delaying rewards as the child acquires successive skills (McClennon, 1992). Using strategies such as picture-cued books to deal with events/things that go wrong may also be helpful.

Goal attainment scaling (Young et al., 1995) has been shown to be successful as a method of identifying and measuring the outcomes of occupational therapy with individuals with learning disabilities. The ability to evaluate individual increments that use a variety of approaches will be essential when working with the FXS child. Goal attainment scaling offers a client-centred approach to evaluation and can incorporate a photo survey to obtain the child's view of therapy. This method of monitoring intervention may also prove helpful as a means of promoting multiprofessional teamworking and integrated goals.

Table 11.4 details the approaches implemented in Figure 11.5. This illustrates an integrated intervention approach, which combines neurodevelopmental, sensory integrative, behavioural and neuropsychological theories in supporting communication for a child with FXS. Table 11.4 details the approaches implemented in Figure 11.5.

Table 11.4: Example of an integrated treatment for a child with fragile X syndrome

Approach	Target behaviour	Intervention
Neurodevelopmental	Fine motor pinch grip (thenar/hyperthenar strength)	Pinching clothes pegs
	Shoulder stability	Working against gravity by placing picture line above shoulder height
Sensory integration	Sensory defensiveness	Use proprioception/heavy work, e.g. pinching pegs, holding basket
	Reducing inadvertent stimuli	Wearing tighter fitting clothes
	Integrating vestibular, tactile and proprioceptive stimuli	Multiple sensory demands of task
Neuropsychological	Visual memory	Use of pictures for communication
	Sequencing	Development of left–right sequence placement in picture
	Communication	Use of PECS
Behavioural	Positive reinforcement	Reinforcing successful attempts to place picture

PECS, Picture Exchange Communication System.

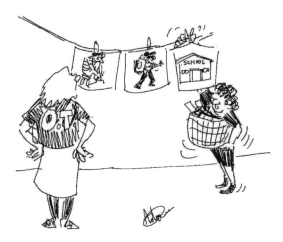

Figure 11.5: Illustration of integrated treatment approach.

Implementing treatment – a case study

Background information

Thomas was aged 2 years and 10 months when he was referred to the consultant paediatrician by his GP as a result of concerns about what appeared to be some regression of skills over the preceding 6 months. Thomas was the first child of unrelated parents born after a reasonable pregnancy, labour and delivery. His medical history was insignificant, although he had had a number of intercurrent infections. There were no concerns about early development until the age of about 27 months. Thomas's mother felt that he had been using phrases since 2 years old, but these had become more stereotyped in fashion. Behaviour was generally withdrawn with irritability and infantile behaviours (e.g. tantrums, smearing of food, pica) evident. When friends visited, Thomas preferred to be on his own. Once placed in a play group Thomas began to develop some skills in response to routines and cues, such as placing his coat on a hook with his picture above it. However, he tended to get very agitated by the other children and would frequently need to be withdrawn from the main group.

Neurological examination at age 3 found Thomas to have no dysmorphic features and normal palmar creases. There was no strabismus and other CNS examination was insignificant, although muscle tone was mildly hypotonic and his gait was slightly immature. His play was generally unproductive and, when being examined, he tended to scream relentlessly when approached. It was felt at this point that, although Thomas showed features of autism, this diagnosis would not be appropriate. Despite a short attention span and immature play skills (over-focusing on the physical attributes of objects), Thomas was able to sustain good eye-to-eye contact with his parents and assist with dressing.

Play and adaptive behaviour continued to be significant problems for Thomas and he was referred to occupational therapy, speech and language therapy and a developmental paediatrician for further opinion. By this time Thomas had developed a more extensive vocabulary, but would generally communicate his needs by retrieving related objects or undertaking actions such as taking his mother to the door when he wanted to go out. Speech and language assessment conferred with developmental assessment and it was concluded that Thomas had general learning difficulties with an autistic pattern of development, which was nevertheless somewhat atypical of autism. It was felt that Thomas would benefit from special education with a structured, picture-based, learning environment. Occupational therapy input at this stage addressed the difficulties Thomas was experiencing in daily tasks, particularly feeding and toileting. A skills training programme was implemented with behavioural reinforcers to develop toileting and self-help skills.

Following this, results of chromosomal analysis became available which showed that Thomas had a full expansion mutation, which was fully methylated consistent with fragile X syndrome. His mother was found to be a premutation carrier. A Statement of Thomas's Special Educational Needs detailed his deficits in communication skills, both expressive and receptive, poor social interaction, poor play skills, decreased attention, difficulties with transitions and adult-led activities, problems with symbolic reasoning (pre-literacy and pre-numeracy) and delays in independence in activities of daily living. In consultation with the local educational department, a special school for children with moderate learning disabilities was chosen by Thomas's parents to address Thomas's need for structure and motivational incentives, in order to meet his educational objectives. A behavioural system was in place within the school following the TEACCH approach and incorporating picture-based learning. Thomas's statement also stipulated, as part of non-educational provision, that continued assessment and monitoring by the consultant paediatrician, occupational therapy services and clinical psychology were required. This was put into place when Thomas was 5 years old.

Progress had been slow and further occupational therapy advice was sought when Thomas was 6 years old about tactile stimuli and how to tackle inappropriate responses to tactile stimuli. Staff changes in the occupational therapy department in the interim had resulted in a therapist being available who had been trained in the use of sensory integrative therapy. In view of the current parental concerns discussed at length over the telephone, it was felt that a detailed sensory history was required and the Sensory Profile (Dunn, 1999) was completed by Thomas's parents. On receipt of this questionnaire, a home and school visit was undertaken and Thomas attended an informal clinical setting, which provided the opportunity to see him interact with various sensory-based activities.

The Sensory Profile (Dunn, 1999) was designed specifically to measure six sensory domains of function with two additional behavioural sections: (1) auditory; (2) visual; (3) taste/smell; (4) body position/proprioception; (5) movement; and (6) touch as well as (a) activity level and (b) emotional–social skills. The checklist was designed to highlight clusters of reactions to types of sensory input across environments, which may be indicative of regulatory disorders and/or discriminative difficulties contributing to learning and sensory processing disorders. It is not a specific indicator of a child's developmental functioning; however, it can be used in conjunction with other developmental tests to support decisions about a child's developmental status.

Thomas's sensory behaviour, as indicated by the checklist and clinical observations, reflected the significant difficulties he had in organising and processing information from the different sensory channels in order to emit an adaptive motor response. Thomas was found to have both tactile defensiveness (intolerance to touch or the fear of contact) and poor tactile discrimination. He noticeably withdrew from tactile input imposed by others/materials as if they were an aversive stimulus. In what appeared to be an attempt to 'dampen down' the effects of persistent tactile irritants (e.g. sleeve edges, collars, textures, etc.), which constantly influenced his underlying level of arousal, Thomas seemed to have adopted several strategies. Self-mediated deep tactile pressure (e.g. pressing hands together, firmly stroking objects, etc.) and 'heavy work' pressure to joints and muscles (e.g. maintaining finger joints rigidly in hyperextension, squeezing objects such as a ball and pressing objects firmly to mouth and forehead) appeared to be used in an attempt to override irritable tactile input. In addition, Thomas had difficulty discriminating different aspects of tactile input, such as the differences between buttons and coins in his pocket or different textures when pulling up his underpants and trousers. He could also be seen actively to seek out additional input either in an attempt to control his tactile environment (tactile input we give ourselves is more comforting than that received inadvertently and randomly from the environment) or to gain more information about objects and materials. The conflict between these two aspects of tactile processing resulted in a greater degree of behavioural disorganisation. Of note during observations of Thomas's play were the difficulties he had resolving his need to control his tactile world without becoming over-stimulated and confused by the variety of touch sensations experienced. The stereotypical posturing and hand mannerisms further interfered with his ability to engage in more productive play and learning activities. However, when proprioception was included within a game, such as when playing with a vibrating cushion, improved spontaneous turn-taking, joint gaze and social interaction were noted.

Thomas was also seen to be mildly hypotonic, with difficulties grading the force and direction of movement. Although the parents had no concerns about acquisition of motor milestones, Thomas was seen to seek out an excessive amount of movement stimuli and yet to have delayed responses in adjusting to changes imposed by the environment, e.g. when transferring from a stable to an unstable surface. The increased activity and movement sought by Thomas would generally heighten his arousal level, with resultant difficulties discriminating more subtle cues for organising adaptive (appropriate) responses.

As a consequence of the initial assessment, a sensory diet was adopted, as recommended by Wilbarger and Wilbarger (1991), in combination with neurodevelopmental strategies to support postural and fine motor skills. Figure 11.5 illustrates how these approaches were combined and incorporated within Thomas's educational and communication programme. *The Alert Program for Self-Regulation* by Williams and Shellenberger (1992) has also been implemented to help Thomas develop greater autonomy in self-regulation. Initial environmental adaptations were undertaken to reduce exposure to perceived 'irritating' stimuli, with a gradual reintroduction of these during activities that were calming. For example, when slow, rhythmic vestibular input was provided via a rocking chair, the textures of supportive cushions were changed to increase variety and experience of tactile stimuli and postural challenges while in a supportive and calming activity. The introduction of new tasks, which had previously been avoided as a result of tantrums, was then possible, using either a bean bag or rocking chair for comfort. Sensory 'time-out' periods have been built into Thomas's schedule to allow him periods free from having to analyse excessive sensations. A small quiet space within a tent with dense foam cushions and squeezy 'stress' balls was set up within Thomas's home and classroom and every 2 hours he was able to retreat into this 'womb' environment to reduce sensory overload. Thomas learnt that this was the place for him to retreat to for brief periods when agitated and distressed. He was subsequently able to attend for increasing times to instructional lessons and is now able to copy letters, sequence size and shape, categorise objects and assist with stacking groceries, sorting laundry and playing a greater variety of games. In addition, he is able to enjoy time with his family in activities such as cycling and shopping, watching TV sitting next to others and participating in mealtimes without getting distressed.

Today, Thomas's programme continues to change and be modified as his skills develop and task demands are altered to optimise his physical, behavioural, communication and learning abilities. His school has more recently incorporated the Picture Exchange Communication System, which has been modified for Thomas to include a greater proprioceptive component to the reward system. An integrated treatment approach that addressed Thomas's needs across a variety of perspectives has proved beneficial in supporting calm and organised behaviour at home and in the community.

Chapter 12
Children with Duchenne muscular dystrophy

PHILIPPA HARPIN, TERRY ROBINSON AND JENNY TUCKETT

The muscular dystrophies are a group of inherited diseases in which various genes controlling muscle function are defective. In certain types of muscular dystrophy, the basic defect is already known. There are over 60 different neuromuscular conditions, varying widely in terms of severity, age of onset, type of muscle affected, pattern of genetic inheritance and their effect on life expectancy (Carter and Dearman, 1995). The common features of the conditions are that they are:

- progressive
- muscle wasting
- disabling.

At the time of writing there is no known cure or treatment, although significant advances in medical research are being made.

Muscular dystrophy affects 20 000 people in the UK, both adults and children. The most common and usually most severe form of muscular dystrophy is Duchenne muscular dystrophy.

What is Duchenne muscular dystrophy?

Duchenne muscular dystrophy (DMD) is caused by a mutation on the X chromosome and is inherited as an X-linked recessive condition (Gardner-Medwin, 1999) (Figure 12.1). The gene defect causes a deficiency in the protein dystrophin. Usually, only boys are affected; there is an incidence of 1 in 3500 live male births. In approximately two-thirds of all cases, the mother carries the defective gene, but she is not usually affected by it herself; such women are carriers. Genetic counselling is important in helping family members to understand the implications of X-linked inheritance and to consider the options available.

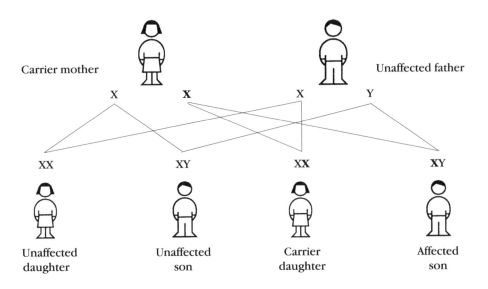

X normal gene on X chromosome   **X** abnormal gene on X chromosome

With each pregnancy, this couple has a 25% chance of having an unaffected daughter, a 25% chance of having a carrier daughter, a 25% chance of having an affected son, and a 25% chance of having an unaffected son.

Figure 12.1: X-linked inheritance.

Most affected boys show the first signs of mobility problems between the ages of 1 and 3 years. The symptoms may vary and include delayed walking, abnormal waddling gait, frequent falls, difficulty with stairs or running, reluctance to walk, toe walking, an inability to hop, skip or jump, cramp in the legs (usually calves) and difficulty getting up from the floor, which is achieved using Gower's manoeuvre: the boy turns on to all fours, and rises by pressing on his thighs and 'walking' his hands up his legs until he is able to extend his hips and back. There is often pseudo-hypertrophy of the calf muscles and a waddling gait with a lordotic posture, which becomes more obvious as the disease progresses. Some boys may present with speech and language difficulties or global development delay. There may be a varying degree of intellectual impairment, which may be reflected in poor reading ability, comprehension and memory skills.

Weakness of the arms is a later symptom, but may be found on clinical examination at an earlier date. The distribution of muscle weakness in both upper and lower limbs is initially mainly proximal and symmetrical; as the disease progresses distal weakness develops.

Inability to walk, in most affected boys, occurs between 8 and 12 years. Loss of ambulation is complicated by the development of joint contractures at the hip, knee and ankle, and spinal deformities; in addition, the elbow and wrist may be affected by contractures.

The prognosis is universally poor and, although a few boys survive into their late 20s, the average age of death is about 19 years. The cause of death is usually respiratory failure, often following a chest infection, although about 10 per cent die suddenly and unexpectedly of cardiac failure.

Occupational therapy input

Occupational therapists have a very important role in the management of boys with DMD and, because the deterioration is stereotyped, it can be divided into three predictable stages. However, as the rate of deterioration is variable, it cannot be linked to age; the stages are, therefore, discussed in relation to the level of disability, as follows:

Early stage: diagnosis → to difficulty in climbing stairs.
Middle stage: difficulty in walking → to use of powered wheelchair out of doors.
Late stage: use of indoor/outdoor powered wheelchair → to terminal stage.

At each stage, the help needed can be divided into:

* mobility
* school
* home, including emotional support and (in the later stages) medical/care support.

Leisure is equally important and discussion of the appropriate activities for all the stages is included as a separate section later in this chapter.

Early stage: diagnosis → to difficulty in climbing stairs

Mobility

The most effective way of delaying deterioration in muscle strength is active exercise, although care must be taken to ensure that the child is not over-fatigued. He should be encouraged to walk for as long as possible to maintain muscle tone; however, his walking may be laboured. As mobility decreases, it is important that a low-fat diet is encouraged to prevent excess weight gain, which would increase the management difficulties.

Provision of bike/buggy/transit and/or lightweight self-propelled wheel-chair

A low-geared tricycle may be useful as an interim mobility aid, provided that the child is not too large and still has trunk support. However, some children never achieve the ability to ride a tricycle. A powered tricycle, used under supervision, may be helpful for enjoyment and to provide both active and passive exercise. In this respect, it may be particularly satisfactory used in the school playground as an alternative to unsuitable PE activities.

In view of the early mobility problems, a boy with DMD may use a baby buggy for much longer than his unaffected peers. However, the appropriately timed supply of a properly assessed, lightweight, active-user manual wheelchair, from the local statutory wheelchair service, is a more suitable option. In addition, there will be the psychological advantage of independence, better support and positioning, and the opportunity of playing safely while actively exercising his arms (Harpin, 1999).

Passive exercises and night splints

From the time of diagnosis, passive stretching exercises are taught by the physiotherapist to minimise the development of contractures in upper and lower limbs, which can cause functional problems. At every stage, liaison with the physiotherapist is very important, particularly as the physical management will influence the provision of equipment. The wearing of night splints or ankle–foot orthoses in conjunction with passive stretching is the most effective way of reducing the development of contractures (Hyde, 1993). It is essential that the night splints fit properly, and are comfortable and lightweight. Early introduction is likely to result in greater compliance.

School

Statement of special educational need.

'Up to a third of boys with Duchenne Muscular Dystrophy have some degree of intellectual impairment . . . this intellectual impairment is not related to muscle weakness and is not progressive' (Emery, 1994). Some affected boys may show challenging behaviour. All affected boys have progressive muscle weakness, causing increasing functional and mobility problems.

In view of these difficulties, it is important that the procedure for providing a Statement of Special Educational Need is in place, preferably before the boy starts school, so that the appropriate level of support is available.

The practical issues to consider are access to buildings, in order for the child to partake in the curriculum and extracurricular activities, in addition to the provision of a classroom learning support assistant and specialised equipment. The child should receive physiotherapy treatment at school, monitored by a physiotherapist. Suitable transport in which the child can travel to and from school in his wheelchair will be necessary.

Other issues to consider are the child's and his parents' concerns and wishes, liaison with the school staff and other professionals, acknowledgement of changing needs, focus on achievement and disability awareness. These issues will inevitably result in discussion in relation to mainstream versus special education.

Planning and provision of adaptations

If at all possible, the child should remain with his peer group so that he has their support during the transition from walking to wheelchair use (Turner et al., 1996b). Since the implementation of the 1981 Education Act and the most recent 1993 Education Act, this will often mean planning within the context of the child's local mainstream school.

Angled writing surface and suitable pens and pencils

The proximal weakness of the shoulder girdle and the deterioration of posture both affect handwriting, leading to fatigue and reduced control. Consideration should be given to spreading throughout the day those activities that require manipulation and handwriting skills, to minimise fatigue (Charlton and Kavanagh, 1994).

There is evidence to suggest that use of a sloping desktop can improve posture for writing in the general primary school population (Charlton and Kavanagh, 1994). Children with DMD are at risk of developing asymmetries and spinal deformity; therefore, introduction of an angled writing surface can help to promote good posture for writing at an early stage. A sloping desktop can also assist in overcoming the early effects of shoulder girdle weakness, because it raises the working surface slightly and assists in giving proximal stability.

Consideration should be given to the provision of either a fatter pen or pencil, or a grip to enable the child to hold and control it more easily.

Seating

Suitable seating should be provided in school from an early stage. The school chair should be supportive and fully adjustable, providing adequate back, arm and foot support. When sitting, it is important that the ankle is kept at a right angle to prevent plantar foot deformities; where necessary, this can be achieved by introducing a simple wooden block. In the context of writing, attention to seating is important on the basis that, if the pelvis, lower limbs and trunk are not supported, upper limb function will be compromised. In addition, there is the previously mentioned risk of developing asymmetry and spinal deformities; although good seating will never prevent these problems, the age of their onset and their severity can be influenced.

Introduction of keyboard skills

Difficulties with handwriting arise when deterioration in proximal stability at the shoulder girdle begins to influence motor control, affecting the quality and legibility of written work. Proximal muscle weakness in the upper limb may also lead to fatigue where sustained handwriting is required. Specific learning difficulties can sometimes be an additional factor.

The occupational therapy treatment plan should include preparation of the child and his family for decrease in motor ability and provision of a means of recording on paper that requires a minimum of motor effort, before that provision becomes essential. It is advisable to learn keyboard skills while handwriting is still a useful skill (Penso, 1990). Ideally, introduction to keyboard skills should be initiated as part of the child's individual education plan, with liaison between teaching staff and the occupational therapist. There is an ever-increasing selection of computer software available, ranging from keyboard familiarisation games to touch-typing programmes, which allow the child to progress at his/her own pace. Children generally find this style of learning more acceptable and enjoyable than formal typing tuition. It can easily be accommodated in most schools and carry-over into the home is often possible.

Provision of IT support

Initially at primary level, and later at middle school level, additional use of the existing classroom/school computers may meet the child's needs. However, the work surface must be at a suitable height, and the keyboard must be positioned to allow the child to stabilise his forearms on the work surface, or his ability to function will be severely compromised. This cannot always be readily achieved, because school computers are frequently positioned on standard computer trolleys, which are often not adjustable in height and do not allow for wheelchair access. Where environmental factors, such as physical location or class size, preclude use of the existing school computers, or where the degree of need or volume of work dictates, provision of a personal alternative to handwriting should be considered: ideally, this should be a laptop, which has the convenience of being easy to move between classrooms.

Each local education authority (LEA) will have its own procedure for undertaking assessment. Independent assessment at a specialist centre may be recommended if one exists locally. A multi-agency assessment is advisable, with advice from the occupational therapist on the child's physical and (possibly) perceptual needs, advice from the school's special educational needs co-ordinator on the child's educational requirements and subsequent recommendations from an IT specialist with regard to the most appropriate hardware and software to meet these needs. The LEA should then consider provision of the equipment.

If an application is made to the Joseph Patrick Memorial Trust (JPMT), which is the grant-funding arm of the Muscular Dystrophy Campaign, complementary equipment can be supplied for home use. JPMT supply some funding, and then refer the application to the Aidis Trust, who subsequently consider provision of the equipment.

In the early stages, difficulties within the school environment usually present as:

- unsteady gait
- frequent falls and problems in rising from the floor
- tiredness on moving from one part of the school to another (e.g. classroom to school canteen)
- problems in rising from the toilet
- inability to carry a lunch tray
- difficulty in dressing/undressing including, at a later stage, dealing with orthoses such as calipers and spinal jackets
- difficulty in participating in PE activities.

Initially these difficulties may be overcome in the following ways:

- providing a classroom learning support assistant to help with mobility and personal care (e.g. when using the toilet or at lunch times)
- where possible planning the school timetable to limit the need to move between rooms, and avoiding rooms approached by steps or stairs
- providing handrails adjacent to the toilet, or the use of a toilet that has already been adapted for disabled people
- allowing extra time to move between rooms, thus enabling the child to leave before his peers, in order to avoid busy corridors and the risk of being knocked off balance
- adapting the child's role in PE activities so that he does not feel excluded (e.g. using him as a scorekeeper or referee).

Home

Emotional support

The stress caused by the diagnosis of DMD and the subsequent progression of the condition can cause widespread problems in the family. There may be feelings of guilt, particularly in the mother if she is a carrier. The initial shock of the diagnosis may be followed by feelings of anger, anxiety and depression.

Parents may attempt to compensate the child for their feelings, by over-protection and indulgence; consequently, the child may be restricted in his emotional development and become timid and hesitant. In some children this over-protection only adds to the frustrations caused by the physical disabilities and their behaviour may become aggressive or unco-operative. The parents should be encouraged to express their problems openly and discuss their feelings. Contact with other families may be helpful to some parents and referral to a counsellor may be appropriate at this stage. In addition, the Muscular Dystrophy Campaign employs family care officers to provide support, and to refer children and their families to other appropriate professionals and sources of help. Contact can be made through the Muscular Dystrophy Campaign office in London. Paediatric occupational therapists must be aware of the importance of developing their own counselling skills and, where possible, in arranging to attend an accredited course.

Benefits advice

The Disability Living Allowance is divided into two components – the care component and the mobility component. The care component may be awarded at low, middle or high rate, depending on the amount of help needed; the mobility component may be awarded at low or high rate, depending on the level of mobility. Eligibility is based on the child having more difficulty and needing more assistance than an unaffected child of the same age. Parents may apply for the care component as soon as the diagnosis is confirmed. The child must be 3 years old to be eligible for the mobility component.

Planning and provision of major adaptations

Adaptations should be planned sufficiently early for the facilities to be available by the time that the child cannot climb the stairs. Usually, this will mean that a referral should be made to the Social Services Department when he is 6 years old. It is not too pessimistic to anticipate that the whole process will take an average of 2 years. The aim should be to plan for the long term, and to have the adaptations ready by the time that they are needed. However, if there is a delay, it may be helpful to provide the following three items in the interim period:

1. Additional banister rail: the child will find it easier to lean on a rail with downward pressure than to reach up, and the optimum height should be determined for each individual child. He will climb and descend with one foot at a time, placing both feet on each tread; without an additional banister, when he goes down the stairs he will lean on the wall for support.
2. Bath aid: getting in and out of the bath independently will become impossible without help and, if he is heavy to lift (particularly out of the bath), a means of getting him up from the bottom of the bath will be a great help. There is an extensive choice of elevating bath seats, but it is usually adequate to use the model that the Social Services Department holds in stock.
3. Toilet rail: this should be horizontally and vertically adjustable, so that the rail can be positioned as close as the child needs it and at the optimum height. However, the rail is unlikely to be needed in the long term and eventually will restrict circulation space around the toilet.

Middle stage: difficulty in walking → to use of powered wheelchair out of doors

Mobility

Physiotherapy

There should be an emphasis on the need for ongoing stretches to both upper and lower limbs. If a growth spurt occurs, there should be a regular review of splints.

Ischial-bearing calipers

At the stage where the child is finding it difficult to walk, walking and standing may be prolonged for periods of up to 2 years or more, by the use of ischial-bearing calipers, which stabilise the lower limb. This can delay the development of contractures and scoliosis, maintain independence and be of psychological benefit. In addition, assisted transfers between a chair and toilet or bed are easier if the knee joint is stable. However, the use of calipers will increase the risk of falling, particularly in the school environment, and supervision will be essential. Alternatives, such as dynamic elastic bracing, may be considered. Sometimes a small surgical procedure is required to release the Achilles' tendon (heelcord) before rehabilitation in a knee–ankle–foot orthosis (KAFO).

Standing frame

The use of a standing frame should be introduced before a child is no longer able to walk, and is an integral part of the management of DMD. It is important that the frame promotes symmetry and, as several different types of standing frames are available, advice should be sought from a physiotherapist experienced in the treatment of children with neuromuscular conditions. Provision of an adjustable table for use with the standing frame is recommended.

Means of getting the child into a standing frame

Children are encouraged to use their standing frames at home. To avoid the need to lift the frame from the floor manually, consideration should be given to the provision of an electric standing frame or a powered tilt table. The latter option has implications for adaptations: there must be sufficient space in the child's bedroom to use the ceiling hoist to lift him on to the tilt table, and also a suitable place for storage when not in use.

Powered indoor/outdoor wheelchair with postural support/pressure relief

At this stage the child should be referred to the appropriate wheelchair service for the assessment of an indoor/outdoor powered wheelchair for independent mobility. This chair will be needed in addition to his manual chair, because it is likely that he will be finding it difficult to propel himself very far indoors, and virtually impossible to do so when outdoors. In addition, a seating assessment should be carried out and an appropriate seating system (which includes a seat and backrest) provided, so that a good postural position can be achieved while ensuring comfort and maintaining function.

Transport

It will become increasingly difficult to lift the child into and out of the car, or for him to travel in comfort. Many families will consider the need for a wheelchair-accessible vehicle in which the child can travel in his wheelchair; the headroom available, particularly when entering the van, will be crucial. A wheelchair ramp or a tail lift will be required, together with a safety harness and suitable floor-fixing clamps for the chair. A headrest on the wheelchair is essential to prevent a whiplash injury in the event of an accident.

If the child is receiving the high rate of the mobility component of the Disability Living Allowance, this may be used towards the provision of a vehicle through the Motability Scheme. Help may also be available, from Motability's Equipment Fund, to adapt the vehicle.

School

Adaptations

In some situations it will be necessary for adaptations to be carried out in a primary and/or secondary school when the parents have chosen to retain their child within mainstream education. The nature and course of the condition make forward planning and preparation for wheelchair use around the school essential (Turner et al., 1996b). Planning takes time, and the cost may have to be built into the budgets. It is important that the school environment is made suitable before the child becomes dependent on a wheelchair for mobility.

Planning for major adaptations to a school should take a collaborative approach. The ideal solution is to set up a planning team consisting of the young person, his parents, school staff, special needs coordinator/adviser, representation from the Education Department (preferably from the Buildings Department), the school medical officer, a moving and handling assessor and the occupational therapist. The role of the occupational therapist will be to advise on facilities required by the wheelchair user and on the adaptation of the environment to accommodate a wheelchair (Hyde, 1993). Consideration may need to be given to the following.

Wheelchair access

Ideally, wheelchair access should be provided to all areas of the school. This may involve provision of ramps, levelling of floors, widening of doorways and a lift. For a child to attend the local school, families often accept limited routes of access and a restricted curriculum, but this is not recommended. Semi-permanent ramps can sometimes solve the problems posed by single steps into school buildings or classrooms.

Lift or stair climber

Provision of a ramp, short-rise lift or through-floor lift are the optimum solutions to overcome the physical barrier of steps or a flight of stairs. In schools where one lift will allow access to otherwise inaccessible areas, it will be the most appropriate choice. However, in some cases this is not practical, either because the layout of the building is not suitable or because more than one lift is needed, making the cost prohibitive (Harpin, 1997). A stair-climbing wheelchair may be an alternative.

Any stair-climbing chair can present a potential hazard; the features and safety of the individual products must, therefore, be assessed carefully by potential users, their families and professional advisers.

Most stair climbers operate slowly and are not suitable for use in an emergency. Where lifts or stair climbers are in use, provision of suitable evacuation equipment should be considered and an emergency evacuation procedure must be put in place.

A secure area will also need to be provided for charging and storage of stair-climbing equipment.

Disabled-toilet facility

Long-term provision for a child with DMD will need to incorporate sufficient space for the following:

- the child's wheelchair and a carer
- a mobile or overhead tracking hoist
- a changing plinth/table (for adjusting clothing)
- wall-mounted/drop-down rail adjacent to toilet
- a height-adjustable washbasin with lever taps.

Many existing disabled-toilet facilities in schools are designed for independent wheelchair users and do not take into account the additional requirements of a child with DMD. As a result, many boys have a tendency to restrict their fluid intake, which may eventually lead to medical problems including dehydration. If a school purports to have a disabled toilet, it will be necessary to check that this will meet the child's needs. Ideally, facilities should be planned for multi-use to cater for any level of disability, by using a wall rail that allows the fittings to be moved laterally and with height adjustment (Harpin, 2000).

Hoist

A mobile hoist should be considered if the child needs to transfer to and from his wheelchair in more than one area of the school. Where space is restricted and/or transfers are confined to a specific area of the school, an overhead-tracking hoist may be a better option. Models that can be user operated by a hand-held remote control allow the child to maintain some independence in the transfer.

A sling that, if necessary, includes head support will be needed. A secure area must be provided for charging and/or storage of the hoist.

Height-adjustable table/table raisers

In the primary school, where lessons tend to be confined to one classroom, a height-adjustable table will be an advantage. It allows wheelchair access, provides arm support at the correct height, and also can enable the child to use a standing frame while accessing curriculum activities.

In a secondary school, where the curriculum may be spread throughout a number of classrooms, use of the child's wheelchair tray or less-expensive table raisers (which can be applied to existing classroom tables) is recommended to provide a working surface of appropriate height. As muscle weakness progresses to the trunk and pectoral girdle, table height will become increasingly important in assisting functional activities.

Home

Adaptations

Major adaptations should be carried out at this stage. The priority is to assess the needs and to establish eligibility for a Disabled Facilities Grant (DFG) or Home Improvement Grant. It is important that therapists are aware of the sources of funding and are able to support the family through the adaptation process, which can be very traumatic.

Wheelchair access

A non-slip ramp with a safety flange will be needed for the wheelchair and a gradient of 1:15 will be suitable for the powered model. Doors will need to be widened to provide a clear opening of 900 mm, although it may be satisfactory for existing external doors to be narrower if the approach is in a direct line without the necessity to turn the wheelchair. When boys get older, they need wheelchairs that have sophisticated features – including reclining backrests, elevating legrests, and tilt-in space seat and backrests – and these chairs are usually large; it is, therefore, important to plan for a 1700mm turning circle in order to provide adequate space (Harpin, 2000).

Ground-floor bedroom/bathroom extension or through-floor lift

There are many factors to be considered and these are discussed in the 'Lift vs extension' chapter of the *Muscular Dystrophy Adaptations Manual* (Harpin, 2000). Essentially, the decision will depend on the size of the existing house and its facilities. The issues to be considered can be identified by clarifying the priorities: these are for the child to have an en-suite bedroom and bathroom, use of a ground-floor toilet, an easily accessible room on the ground floor in which he can use his computer and entertain his friends, in addition to adequate space within the house for the circulation of his wheelchair. If the existing house is sufficiently spacious for the floor area taken up by the lift not to be missed, and if the priorities discussed above are either available or can be provided with additional building work, then a lift may be the best option. The reality is that not many houses are able to accommodate these facilities, but they will be available with the building of a ground-floor extension, with the added advantage of increasing the space within the house. The only disadvantages of an extension are (1) that it may take up space in the garden that the family would prefer not to lose, (2) if the child needs help in the night his parents will have to go downstairs and (3) he will not have access to the rooms upstairs. However, many families have found an extension to be a very successful solution and the only possible drawback is that, if he is timid, he might feel isolated when he is alone downstairs at night.

Hoisting (bedroom/bathroom)

A hoist will be needed to lift the child in and out of bed and to transfer him from one wheelchair to another and, if necessary, to a bath chair on a chassis or to a shower/toilet chair. Unless the hoist is needed in other rooms in the house, a ceiling hoist is likely to be more satisfactory than a mobile hoist, because it does not require space in which to be manoeuvred, is easier for the carer to use and places less strain on the back. If a shower toilet (previously known as a combined WC/bidet) is needed, it is more satisfactory for the child to sit directly on the seat and the tracking for the hoist should, therefore, extend into the bathroom. In these circumstances, the track should be supplied with a ceiling turntable to allow the bathroom fittings to be placed in the optimum position and the hoist used for both the shower toilet and the specialist bath. The track should pass from front to back over the centre of the seat to allow the child's position to be adjusted.

Level-access shower or bath

A level-access shower is unlikely to be the optimum solution for anyone with muscular dystrophy who cannot shower independently, because it is difficult for a carer to remain dry when helping, and the use of a shower screen makes it impossible to get down to wash the child's feet. In addition, a shower does not allow the child to soak in the water and relax his muscles. However, it is important that the child and his family consider both options and the factors to be considered are discussed in the chapter 'Bath vs shower' in Harpin (2000).

For a bath to be satisfactory for a child with DMD, there must be a method of support. Specialist baths are available with an electrically-operated integral seat that allows the child to recline with good head and body support and with supportive chair arms in front and to the side. In addition, the base of the bath is contoured to provide support behind the knees; this will be important in the later stages, if he has knee contractures. The bath must have either an integral shower or a wall-mounted shower for hair washing or for a quick shower over the bath in the summer. The boys love the spa facility; if the DFG, Home Improvement Grant or charitable funds can cover the cost, this should be included in the bath specification when it is ordered.

Height-adjustable washbasin

To maximise good hand function it is important for a child to be able to get right under the basin until his chest is up against the front edge. To make this possible (because he cannot bend down to lift up the footrests on his wheelchair), the basin must measure 600 mm front to back. The child needs the basin low enough to be able to get his hands into the water and high enough to be able to rinse out his mouth when cleaning his teeth, without leaning forwards, which would make it difficult for him to get back into his wheelchair. This can be achieved only with a basin that is height adjustable, and for independence this must be controlled electrically; this also enables the basin to be used as a mobile arm support to bring the child's arms up to the level of his face for cleaning his teeth, washing his face, etc. As a result of his difficulty in reaching, the basin should be supplied with remote-control electronic taps operated by a touch-sensitive switch, and automatic control of the strip light over the mirror.

Shower toilet

This combined toilet and wash/dry bidet will be necessary when the child can no longer clean himself and he wants privacy and independence. There is the option of plinths to raise the pan, but these are not usually necessary, because a standard height will enable him to get his feet squarely on the floor to help to stabilise himself. Shaped supportive toilet seats that will help with balancing are available and the operating switch must be touch sensitive.

For a shower toilet to be effective, the user must sit directly on the seat; if a chair is superimposed, the washing and drying action will be less effective. It is important, therefore, that the unit should be used with a ceiling hoist in conjunction with a special frame to provide the support needed. As previously mentioned, the hoist should pass over the pan from front to back to allow the child's sitting position to be altered as his body shape changes, to ensure maximum washing and drying efficiency.

Height-adjustable work surfaces

A wheelchair-accessible work surface should be installed in the bedroom. If this work surface is L-shaped, it allows the child to sit close into the right angle and support his forearms on the two adjacent surfaces; this will be particularly important when he is using his computer keyboard. The height adjustment will ensure that the optimum height can be achieved, irrespective of the height of the wheelchair seat and armrests.

It will be essential for a 'standing' surface 600 mm or 800 mm wide to be included, to allow the child access to purposeful activities while he is using a standing frame.

Electric light switches and sockets

The height and position of light switches is crucial to enable them to be reached by a boy with DMD. The *Muscular Dystrophy Adaptations Manual* (Harpin, 2000) includes a wide range of information relating to all the issues around adaptations; the information officers should be contacted for details.

Referral for environmental control

The purpose of an environmental control for a child with DMD is to ensure that he maintains maximum independence. The equipment allows him to unlock the front or back door, switch on lights and use the telephone, and it also provides an intercom within the house and to the front and/or back door.

Criteria for supply from the NHS depend on the local arrangements; a designated medical consultant assesses the need. Occupational therapists should make a referral when a child is no longer able to carry out these functions and when it is felt that he needs the independence and will be sufficiently motivated to use the control.

Intercom

During the years before a child with DMD will qualify for an environmental control, it will be necessary for his parents to buy an intercom to be plugged into 13-amp sockets between his bedroom and their bedroom and the sitting room. This will be particularly essential if he needs to call for help during the night.

Electrically-operated bed

An electric bed will be needed when a child cannot sit up in bed or when he finds it difficult to get out of bed (Harpin, 2000). The elevating backrest will raise him into an upright sitting position; if the bed is height adjustable, this will help him to stand up from the edge of the mattress. This height adjustment will be invaluable also for the carers, so that each one can work at the optimum back height when dressing him in bed and working at the bedside. Beds should be supplied through the health authority (to fulfil a nursing need) or, on occasions, by Social Services (to increase independence). Specific models are recommended for boys with DMD to provide the optimum head and leg action on the bed, and reference should be made to the information provided by the Muscular Dystrophy Campaign (Harpin, 2000).

Replacement mattress or mattress overlay

Many boys who are unable to turn over or move in bed need frequent attention in the night. The number of times that a parent or carer is disturbed can be influenced by the surface on which the boy is sleeping and by his level of comfort. There is a wide range of alternative mattress overlays or replacement mattresses, ranging from a simple foam or polyester low-pressure mattress overlay to sophisticated alternating air-pressure mattresses. A survey to find out whether any particular type is universally successful has been carried out in Newcastle upon Tyne and the results will be available from the Muscular Dystrophy Campaign.

Supportive easychair

Some children like a change from sitting in their wheelchair at home, but ordinary furniture is usually unsuitable because it does not provide adequate trunk support. The provision of a wheeled, adjustable and supportive easychair in which a variety of positions can be achieved is recommended; for independent use, this should be controlled electrically.

Provision of small aids

As upper limb strength and hand function begin to deteriorate, provision of a few basic small aids to daily living can assist the child to participate in practical subjects at school and may be useful at home also. These may include:

- non-slip mats
- bean-bag tray (the advantage is that it enables him to work on his lap without the need to raise his arms and the beans allow the surface to be tilted to the most convenient angle)
- spike boards/buttering boards (for food preparation)
- easy-grip peeler

- large-handled and lightweight cutlery
- L-shaped knives
- spring-assisted or easy-grip scissors.

Emotional support

Continuing emotional support for the boy and his family is important as the condition progresses. Consideration should be given to facilitating supportive counselling for the child and his family.

Late stage: use of indoor/outdoor powered wheel-chair → to terminal stage

Mobility

Physical management

Physiotherapy treatment, including stretches to the upper and lower limbs, continues to be important and good liaison between therapists is invaluable to a family. From time to time the issues relating to splinting of the arm to prevent ulnar deviation and wrist flexion contractures may be discussed; although, currently, this practice is not generally used because of the lack of compliance, it may be appropriate in some cases.

Spinal surgery

A scoliosis often develops in boys who have DMD, soon after they become unable to walk. Eventually, this results in pelvic obliquity and deformity of the chest, which will restrict the capacity of the lungs. It is important to keep the child walking for as long as possible, and then to consider a spinal support or spinal surgery. The issues to be considered in spinal surgery are as follows (Muscular Dystrophy Campaign, 1994):

- When is the correct time?
- What does the operation entail?
- What are the risks?
- What may be the results?
- What are the disadvantages?
- Who makes the decision?

Before surgery, it is important for the occupational therapist working in either the specialist neuromuscular clinic or the orthopaedic clinic to liaise with the community occupational therapist to ensure that the necessary equipment is in place. If equipment has been provided at the appropriate stages, this should not present a problem; this underlines the need to plan ahead and thereby to avoid a crisis after surgery, which may culminate in a delay in discharge from hospital.

Spinal surgery results in a number of issues that affect the boy's function; therefore, without suitable equipment, some independence can be lost. The relevant issues are as follows:

- As a result of the fixation and rigidity of the spine the boy can no longer compensate for his shoulder weakness by flexing his spine and bringing his head down (e.g. for eating); there therefore appears to be a reduction in upper limb function.
- The length of the spine is increased and the boy sits more upright in his wheelchair, making height-adjustable equipment vital.
- Although the initial loss of head control is usually regained within a few weeks, there may be persistent difficulties with head control if the boy is tipped away from a vertical position (e.g. in a hoist) – hence, the need for head support in a sling.
- The inability to flex forwards and 'dip' his head when entering a wheelchair-accessible van will result in the need for greater headroom, in the height both of the door and of the roof of the van. As a van may be bought several years before spinal surgery is carried out, this need must be anticipated in advance.

The following equipment is needed:

- a hoist with a sling which provides a stiffened back support and head support
- an electric bed
- support on the toilet
- a wheelchair (which may need modifying to provide armrests of the correct height) and a head support
- a height-adjustable table or work surface that can be adjusted to provide wheelchair accessibility, irrespective of the height of the armrests
- a height-adjustable washbasin.

Mobile arm support

In addition, increasing upper limb weakness can cause difficulties with feeding. Manual dexterity frequently remains good in many children until a fairly late stage. The provision of a mobile arm support to counteract the force of gravity can be useful in ensuring maximum independent upper limb activity for as long as possible.

The current development of a powered mobile arm support, which is attached to the wheelchair and powered by a separate battery, is an exciting concept and should enable even very severely disabled children to feed themselves.

Reclining backrest/comfort in wheelchair

Despite the provision of a good postural position in the wheelchair achieved by a suitable seating system, backache and pain associated with increasing deformity make it essential to be able to alter the pressure on the body.

At this stage of the condition, the following wheelchair features are necessary:

- a reclining backrest
- a seat and backrest that tilt back from the horizontal
- legrests that can be raised and lowered independently of each other.

All these functions should be controlled electrically, to allow the young man complete independence to move within his chair (Harpin, 1999b). At present, the supply of sophisticated wheelchairs is limited through the statutory wheelchair service; fortunately, however, there are charities that will help with the funding of mobility equipment.

School

At this stage the factors to be considered should be divided into those relevant before or after the child reaches the age of 16 years (pre- or post-16).

Pre-16

Technical support

Consideration must be given to the support required for all the technology subjects, including food technology, science, metal/woodwork and IT.

Examinations

The necessity for extra time and/or a scribe or a separate room to use voice-activated software must be assessed.

Post-16

The opportunities can be categorised as follows:

- educational
- employment
- occupational.

Educational

Opportunities at 16+ will depend on the young man's academic ability, his level of functional ability, and his interests and skills. Options for consideration at the transition stage may include:

- 6th form at special school
- 6th form college
- further-education college
- vocational college
- residential college
- home-based opportunities
- university and a place on a degree course.

The use of ' high-tech' computer equipment, including voice-activated software and on-screen keyboards, will enable young men to compete on equal terms with their peer group. As previously, before external examinations, it will be necessary for the teachers or lecturers to assess the need for extra time or the use of a scribe.

Careful assessment of all the care needs is important at this stage to ensure an adequate level. Most young men will need 24-hour support if they are residential at college or university, or if they leave home to live independently; furthermore, such support is increasingly necessary for boys who choose to remain living with their parents, to relieve the latter of the caring role.

Employment

The young person should be referred to the disability employment adviser of the Employment Service for advice about the range of schemes available to assist (even severely) disabled individuals into employment or training.

Occupational

Occupational activities should be considered for boys who do not wish to remain at school beyond the age of 16 or to progress to further education at the age of 18. Options include the following:

- home-based activities
- day centre
- leisure activities, either at home or away from home
- contact with disabled and able-bodied peer groups.

Home

Medical support

Medical support may be necessary for the relief of respiratory distress, with nocturnal ventilation, bowel and bladder care, the relief of pain, and discussion about emergency resuscitation. At this stage it may be necessary to refer to a dietitian for appropriate advice to improve nutrition, and food supplements may be recommended. Nasogastric feeding and gastrostomies are used in some centres.

Emotional/care support

In addition to further emotional support, increased care support (day and night), may be needed. The specialist mattress or mattress topper should be reassessed to increase comfort, to eliminate any pressure problems, and to try to reduce the number of times that the young man needs to be turned in the night.

Continuing respite care is important for the young person and his family. It may be necessary to offer pre-bereavement support to the family and an opportunity for the boy to talk about his death, if he wishes. This is a very difficult time for the whole family.

Environmental controls

Referral for this equipment should be considered if it was not included when the home adaptations were carried out.

Automatic door opener

It is essential that boys are supplied with indoor/outdoor wheelchairs to provide independence, and it is equally important that they can get into and out of the house without having to ask someone to open the door. When the adaptations are carried out there is usually a lack of funding, and the recommendation would be to install the electrical socket for the unit to be supplied at a later date. This can be funded privately, or an application for an additional grant can be made.

Leisure activities

Impact of DMD on social and leisure activities

Care must be taken to ensure that students in mainstream schools do not become socially isolated from their unaffected peer group, because it may be harder to maintain interaction with their peers than in a school for physically handicapped pupils.

Therapists should encourage parents to see the direct benefits of leisure activities – and not only as secondary needs to education and physical treatment. The pursuit of hobbies and interests will give the child or teenager pleasure and enjoyment, and may help overcome feelings of apathy and depression. The child should be encouraged to develop new skills while at the same time being realistic about present and future functional abilities.

Children should be discouraged from taking part in any repetitive muscle-building type of exercise that is likely to damage muscle tissue further.

Playground activities for young children

Affected children should be encouraged to take part in the everyday activities of childhood, within the limit of their functional ability. In the early stages, lower limb muscle weakness makes such children unable to hop, jump, skip, run or walk distances, as their unaffected peers can do. The child with DMD may have problems in riding a tricycle or playing on apparatus such as slides or swings. These difficulties can limit social interaction with the peer group, both in and out of school, and the level of fatigue can lead to social isolation.

Swimming

Swimming is an excellent all-round activity, providing exercise and fun. It is important that a child with DMD should learn to swim on his back, because a suitable float can support the back of his head when he can no longer lift it. Other possible activities include: riding, fishing, pets, breeding small animals, model making, painting/drawing, music making, joining uniformed organisations, outings and bowling.

Computers

Computers and computer games have enhanced the leisure activities of many disabled children. The use of the Internet will increase the information available to users and offers social interaction with others sharing the same interests. In the late stage, severe upper limb weakness may cause problems with the use of a conventional mouse/keyboard, and voice-activated software or finger pad control of an on-screen keyboard may be appropriate solutions.

Conclusion

Working with boys with DMD and their families is very rewarding for an occupational therapist, whose skills and expertise will be invaluable in increasing the boy's independence, thus making life easier for his parents and carers, and (even more important) ensuring that the quality of life enjoyed by other children is shared by boys who are affected by this very disabling condition. The Muscular Dystrophy Campaign offers a wide range of literature and employs information officers, family care officers and a national occupational therapy advisor, all of whom can be contacted if any advice is needed.

Duchenne muscular dystrophy: a case history

Peter has Duchenne muscular dystrophy which was diagnosed when he was 4 years old, after a history of problems with his mobility. Although his mother is a carrier of the defective gene, his younger brother is not affected.

Peter's parents were told that he would be dependent on a powered wheelchair by between the ages of 8 and 12 years; life expectancy, on average, was between 14 and 24 years and there was no cure or treatment available. They were devastated at this news and his mother felt very guilty that she had passed on the faulty gene to her son.

As soon as the diagnosis was confirmed, Peter was referred to a physiotherapist who taught his parents the importance of regular, active exercise for him (such as swimming) and simple techniques of passive stretching to help prevent joint contractures.

He was due to start at the local infant school in a few months' time, and his parents were very keen that he should go to mainstream school with his peer group. A referral was made to the paediatric occupational therapist, to assess his needs in school at this stage, to liaise with the head teacher, and to make appropriate recommendations regarding any structural alterations required at the school (such as ramps or handrails).

Once Peter had started at school, the occupational therapist was able to advise staff, working with him, on ways of overcoming any difficulties that were presented within the school environment, and to assess his needs regarding suitable seating, writing surfaces, pens and pencils, and computer equipment. The occupational therapist was also involved in the process of providing a Statement of Special Educational Need.

By this time, Peter was having difficulty in walking for distances of more than a few hundred yards and he was provided with a lightweight, manual wheelchair for outings, after assessment by a therapist at the wheelchair clinic.

The family lived in a private, three-bedroomed house with no downstairs toilet. However, there was a large garden and room for a ground-floor bedroom/bathroom extension. Peter was already having difficulty in climbing stairs, especially when he was tired, and it was becoming obvious that he needed suitable facilities as soon as possible. The community occupational therapist was involved in assessing the long-term housing and equipment needs, in conjunction with the specialist recommendations by the national occupational therapy advisor for the Muscular Dystrophy Campaign, and in assisting the family with their application for a Disabled Facilities Grant. Although the adaptation procedure was ongoing, the occupational therapist provided equipment to help with stairs, the toilet and bathing, in the interim period. The whole process took 18 months. However, planning for the future helped the family to be more positive and to come to terms with their son's condition – and Peter was delighted with his increased independence.

Peter's mobility continued to deteriorate and he was reassessed at the wheelchair clinic for his first powered wheelchair with suitable seating, for use at school and outdoors.

The paediatric occupational therapist regularly assessed his changing needs in school, attended annual statement reviews, and was part of the planning team set up to advise on the adaptations required at the secondary school to which Peter would be going in 2 years' time.

Eventually, Peter lost the ability to walk and was re-mobilised in ischial-bearing calipers. The community occupational therapist advised on issues relating to moving and handling at home, and referred him to the health authority for the provision of an electric bed with suitable mattress, to reduce the amount of help he required at night.

Peter was now totally wheelchair dependent. He developed a spinal scoliosis and was due to have spinal surgery. The community occupational therapist was able to liaise with the occupational therapist working in the orthopaedic clinic, before surgery, to confirm that all necessary equipment was in place.

As Peter grew weaker, his functional abilities deteriorated and the level of help he needed increased. To improve his independence, the occupational therapist referred him for the provision of an environmental control system.

Peter achieved well at school, despite his increasing disability. He decided to go on to university, where he would require 24-hour care support. The occupational therapist was involved in assessing his care needs and liaising with appropriate agencies to ensure that care was available and equipment in place.

Peter spent 2 years at university. He made many friends and enjoyed an excellent social life, as well as working very hard at his studies. At the beginning of his final year he became ill with a series of chest infections. He died at the age of 20, before completing his degree.

Acknowledgement

This chapter is produced with the permission of the Muscular Dystrophy Campaign (2000), for which two of the authors work.

Useful addresses

AbilityNet (Computability Centre and the Foundation for Communication for the Disabled)
PO Box 94, Warwick CV34 5WS
Tel: 01926 312 847; fax: 01926 407 425

Dogs for the Disabled
The Frances Hay Centre, Blacklocks Hill, Banbury, Oxfordshire OX17 2BS
Tel: 01295 252 600; fax: 01295 252 668

Disabled Living Centres Council (DLCC)
Redbank House, 4 St Chad's St., Manchester M8 8QA
Tel: 0161 834 1044; fax: 0161 835 3591

Muscular Dystrophy Campaign
7–11 Prescott Place, London SW4 6BS
Tel: 020 7720 8055; fax: 020 7498 0670

RADAR
12 City Forum, 250 City Road, London EC1V 8AF
Tel: 020 7250 3222; fax: 020 7250 0212

Variety Club of Great Britain
93 Bayham Street, London NW1 0AG
Tel: 020 7428 8100; fax: 020 7428 8111

Whizz-Kidz
1 Warwick Row, London SW1E 5ER
Tel: 020 7233 6600; fax: 020 7233 6611

Chapter 13
Children with limb deficiency

Fiona Carnegie

Limb deficiency in children is mostly the result of congenital defects of unknown or genetic origins, but children sometimes have amputations as a result of trauma, malignancy or infections, e.g. meningococcal septicaemia. Both situations are devastating for the families but the response of the children will be different in the two groups. In both groups the personalities of the child and of the parents are of great significance, and must be considered at all times.

The support that the family receive in the early days and weeks will affect their response to the child. The same applies in the way that the need for an amputation is discussed, focusing on the positive aspects while acknowledging the feelings of the parents and child. All the children have the possibility of achieving long-term independence if they and their parents are given the encouragement and advice that they require from an early stage. Some children will use a prosthesis for cosmesis or function; all benefit from contact with a therapist at various points.

Congenital

The reasons for most congenital limb deficiencies remain unknown. Apart from the thalidomide tragedy in the early 1960s the number of children born each year in the UK with limb deficiency remains relatively constant at 1 : 4000 live births. About 30 children are born each year with one limb affected, usually the upper limb. Approximately four children are born each year in the UK with more than one limb affected. These families need support and advice in the early years to understand what the future holds for their child.

There are two main types of congenital limb deficiency: transverse and longitudinal, as defined by International Standard ISO 8548-1.

Transverse

The limb develops normally to a point when the growth is arrested; this occurs mostly in the upper limb.

Transverse arrest at metacarpophalangeal joint

The child will be born without the fingers and thumb but still have a functioning wrist and useful palm. These children may use a cosmetic prosthesis in later life, although this will restrict their function. Some find that a wrist strap or special devices enable them to carry out specific activities, e.g. holding cutlery or riding a bicycle. Many manage very well with no special equipment. These children may benefit from surgery, e.g. a toe-to-hand transplantation. Careful assessment by the surgeon and therapist is essential because the tendons that activate the toe must be functioning well if the toe is to become a useful finger. If the child has no fingers on the hand, it is necessary to consider transplanting two toes. Parents require support in the decision-making process.

Transverse arrest at wrist level

These children are born without their whole hand, but may have some small finger buds and may have movement at the end of the limb as a result of the presence of some of the carpal bones. Initially these children will find a prosthesis unsatisfactory, cosmetically and functionally, because it will have to be longer than their remaining arm. As these children grow, the length discrepancy between the limb-deficient side and the other side usually increases, so it is possible to consider fitting a prosthesis. Some children choose to use no prosthesis; they may find a leather wrist strap or other devices helpful.

Transverse arrest at mid-forearm level

This is the most common level of limb deficiency seen in prosthetic centres because the children often benefit from a functional and/or cosmetic prosthesis (Figure 13.1). There is a clear prosthetic programme for these children: a cosmetic prosthesis fitted when the child is sitting securely (4–6 months), progressing to a functional prosthesis, fitted when the child is walking safely. The child will be seen at the centre at 3-monthly intervals to check the fit of the prosthesis and to help them learn to use it effectively.

Transverse arrest at elbow level, mid-humeral level and shoulder level

Congenital limb deficiencies at these levels are rare. The prostheses require an elbow joint and straps for suspension. They are bulkier and

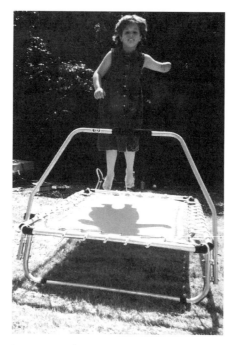

Figure 13.1: Child with congenital terminal transverse arrest at mid-forearm level.

heavier than those for the mid-forearm levels. The prosthetic programme will start later and be less clearly defined. Children with the arrest at mid-humeral level may have problems with bony overgrowth, because the main humeral growth plate is at the epiphysis at the head of humerus. Surgery to trim the humerus may be required during their growing period.

Lower limb congenital transverse deficiencies

Such deficiencies of the lower limb are rare. The primary need is for mobility and a prosthetic replacement will be prescribed as necessary, starting when the child is pulling him- or herself up to standing. Children with a partial foot arrest may require a silicone foot replacement, and they may have leg-length discrepancies as they grow older. Children with an arrest at the mid-tibial level will have problems of bony overgrowth as previously mentioned; as the tibial growth plate is at the knee joint, surgery may be required. Children with an arrest at the knee joint and higher will require a prosthetic knee joint. As with the higher levels of upper limb deficiency, the timing of changing the types of prostheses will vary with each individual child.

Longitudinal

The limb does not develop normally, with the long bones and the distal parts being affected. In describing longitudinal deficiency the absent parts are named. A radial club hand (a radially displaced four-fingered hand, thumb absent) will be described as a 'longitudinal arrest, radius partial, carpels partial, ray 1 total'; the little and ring fingers will be the most functional of the hand (Figure 13.2). This is the most common type of longitudinal deficiency in the upper limb. An ulnar club hand is one where the ulna is partially absent; often the radius is fused to the humerus and there are two fingers and a thumb intact. A central ray defect is where the thumb and little finger are present, but one or more of the central digits are absent; this may affect all four limbs. Children with longitudinal deficiencies may benefit from surgery, e.g. centralising the radial club hand, orthoses to maintain the hand in a functional position, or from special equipment.

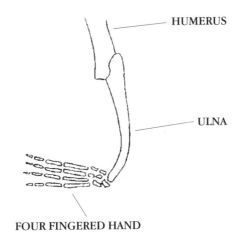

Figure 13.2 Radial club hand.

Some children are born with longitudinal deficiencies of the lower limb, resulting in leg-length discrepancies requiring correction to enable the child to walk, e.g. proximal focal femoral deficiency (PFFD) where the hip may be hypoplastic, the femur shortened, the fibula absent, the foot equinus and the lateral rays absent (Torode and Gillespie, 1991). This requires an extension prosthesis to correct the length difference, which is not satisfactory cosmetically. There are two alternatives: a Symes' amputation and leg-lengthening procedure of the femur, or a knee disarticulation. Both these interventions result in the child being fitted with a more cosmetically acceptable prosthesis.

In some longitudinal deficiencies, the knee joint is unstable and an amputation is essential to enable the child to continue walking.

It is the children with the longitudinal deficiency who are most likely to have genetic reasons for the limb deficiency. These families may benefit from genetic counselling at this stage, and their children will require advice before starting families themselves.

Impact of hearing the news

Parents occasionally know from the antenatal scan that their child will have a limb deficiency. This enables them to gather information and meet relevant people, if they wish, before the birth. It also enables them to separate the giving of the 'good' news (i.e. the birth) and the 'bad' news (i.e. the limb deficiency) to relatives and friends. More frequently, however, the knowledge comes at the time of the birth, with parents and medical personnel feeling equally shocked. The way in which this situation is handled is critical in the weeks and months that follow. There is an important difference between 'you have a beautiful baby boy' as he is handed to the mother, 'but he only has one hand', and the baby is taken immediately away from the mother and a doctor returns alone 'I am sorry your baby is missing his hand'. The first focuses on the positive, giving the information and the baby at the same time, the second on the negative, giving the information in isolation.

Postnatally, the most important professional support will be from the health visitor and the child's GP. The child should be referred to a regional limb deficiency clinic as soon as possible, so the family can gather information about the child's deficiency and the present and future prosthetic and surgical options. It is also necessary for them to gain an understanding of the child's development so that they have realistic expectations of the child at any particular point, and can encourage the child to reach his or her full potential. This information can be gathered from a centre where children with limb deficiencies are regularly seen and from membership of the appropriate self-help groups. Children born with a limb deficiency initially have no concept of being different; later, however, they pick up cues from their parents and other significant adults and their peers.

Questions parents ask

Why did it happen?

The cause of the more common transverse limb deficiency is unknown at present. It is thought that it may be related to an interruption in the blood supply to the limb bud in the first few weeks of pregnancy. In rare cases amniotic bands constrict the limb and lead to an amputation *in utero*. In such cases there are no finger buds and often there are constrictions on other parts of the child's body. Occasionally, there is a genetic cause, which is most likely to be the case in the longitudinal type of deficiency. This includes conditions such as: Holt Oram syndrome which is caused by a recessive gene resulting in bilateral longitudinal upper limb deficiencies of varying severity together with cardiac abnormalities; TAR syndrome (thrombocytopenia and absent radius) is caused by a recessive gene resulting in a blood clotting disorder and radial deficiency that affects the limbs to a greater or lesser extent, with the presence of the thumbs in all cases. There are many other syndromes affecting the limbs and other parts of the body, some also affecting intellectual ability (Evans et al., 1991).

What did I do/not do?

Following the thalidomide tragedy of the early 1960s, it became evident that medication and other factors during pregnancy can be detrimental. Some parents are concerned about medication that they have taken, environments in which they have worked or accidents that they have had in the early stages of pregnancy. There is no evidence that any of these situations have caused the limb deficiency.

What else might be wrong?

In most of the transverse cases there is no reason to expect there to be anything else wrong. However, when the limb deficiency is longitudinal, there may be other factors involved. It is often helpful to the parents if the child is fully assessed by a paediatrician to alleviate any fears that they may have. If the deficiency is genetic the parents may benefit from genetic counselling.

What about the future?

Most children will manage very well in mainstream school, although a few of the children with multiple limb deficiency may attend special schools for some or all of their education. Children with congenital limb deficiency learn to do most tasks with their remaining limbs. Employment prospects will vary; they will be unable to join the Armed Forces or the emergency services. Children with lower limb deficiency have minimal other restrictions, whereas those with upper limb deficiencies will have difficulty where dexterity is of importance, e.g. being a hairdresser. The increase in information technology is of great benefit, enabling jobs to be done that previously were not possible. Many sports and hobbies can be enjoyed and it is important that the child is encouraged to participate in the life of the family fully. University, marriage, driving, child-bearing and caring are as possible for the person with a limb deficiency as for those without.

Amputation

Amputations in childhood are rare, most of them involving the loss of one limb. It is essential that the need for the amputation is presented in a positive way, acknowledging the feelings of the parents and the child.

Causes of amputation

- Malignancy: high levels of amputation, following a period of great anxiety, and possibly difficult treatments which may be ongoing, and uncertainty about prognosis.
- Infection: may result in multiple amputations, again following period of great anxiety and difficult treatments.
- Trauma: probably sudden, no time for preparation, possibly other injuries, skin grafting to residual limb, guilt and blame add to an already difficult situation.
- Deformity: sometimes a congenital deficiency is such that it is considered better to have an amputation, usually of the lower limb.
- Vascular: massive haemangiomas and abnormalities of the lymphatic system can result in the need for amputation; this is very rare.

Levels of amputation

The description of the level of amputation is by naming the severed long bone, e.g. transradial, transfemoral, or the joint, e.g. hip disarticulation. When a child has an amputation, it is advantageous to retain the growth plate if possible. The main femur growth plate is at the knee, so if it is necessary to do a transfemoral amputation the remaining femur will grow minimally and the child will have a short residual limb in adult life. If a knee disarticulation is performed, the femur will grow but slower than the sound limb as a result of less use. When fully grown, the child will have a good length of residual limb for prosthetic fitting (Figure 13.3).

Some children require very high levels of amputation, usually as a result of malignancy. A forequarter amputation means the removal of the clavicle, scapula and whole arm, leaving the chest wall. These children require replacement to the body shape to enable clothing to sit naturally. Initially this will be in the form of a shoulder cap, possibly progressing to a full prosthesis later. A child with a hindquarter amputation loses part of

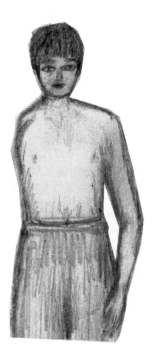

Figure 13.3: Forequarter amputation

the pelvis and the whole leg. They have difficulty sitting, having lost their ischium, and may require special seating for comfort or to prevent scoliosis.

Emotional needs of children and their families

When a child requires an amputation, the child, and the family, need help adjusting to the situation. In the case of amputation after trauma there will possibly be the feelings of blame, directed at family members, medical personnel or other people, or guilt directed at themselves. When the amputation results from a medical problem, malignancy or infection, there may be feelings of anger towards the medical profession and/or anxiety about the prognosis. For children who have the amputation to improve deformity, there is an element of choice and many families prefer to wait until the child is old enough to be actively involved in the decision. Parents of children with amputations are likely to need counselling and may benefit from family therapy.

The age at which the surgery is required is significant in both the emotional response and their future function. A child who has an amputation before the age of 2 years will be emotionally and functionally very similar to a child with a congenital limb deficiency because they have minimal memories of the limb and the surgery. Most of their learning experiences will be as an amputee.

Young children who have amputations will be aware of loss, but may not have the language to express their feelings, which they will need to explore through play. Ideally these children should be involved in discussions related to the surgery in an age-appropriate way. They are often very capable of dealing with such situations.

Adolescents may have considerable difficulty adjusting to an amputation, especially if they are having problems making the transition to adulthood. These children are likely to require counselling.

A child who has an amputation may have phantom sensation after the surgery. This should be discussed openly. For some this sensation may be painful, and medication and other treatment modalities may be required, e.g. TENS (transcutaneous electrical nerve stimulation). Often when the child returns to a more normal lifestyle after surgery, the pain subsides; for some, however, it remains a problem and some children may require active pain management.

Occupational therapy

The occupational therapist may become involved with the child and family at any point, to assess for special equipment, to encourage the child in the use of a prosthesis, to help them in nursery or school, or to teach methods of personal and domestic independence. In the initial assessment, it is essential to assess the child's present function and answer practical questions of how the child will achieve different tasks. It is beneficial to introduce the family to other families and to self-help groups such as: Reach (Association For Children With Hand or Arm Deficiency) and STEPS (Association for Children with Lower Limb Abnormalities); children with multiple limb deficiencies may be able to join the Thalidomide Society. These associations have newsletters, local groups, annual conferences and information databases.

Prostheses

A leg is primarily for mobility; an arm is present to position the hand so that the hand can fulfil a particular task, manipulate an object, express a feeling or explore the environment. A prosthesis is used to replace the body part that is absent. It is relatively easy to replace the function of the leg, but the prosthesis must be weight bearing, so the socket design is critical. No prosthesis can replace all functions of the hand satisfactorily; an upper limb prosthesis may be cosmetic, functional or attempt to be a combination of both. In the case of the lower limb, a prosthesis is essential to enable walking, but an upper limb prosthesis is not essential for functional independence.

For the upper limb there are three main types of prostheses.

Cosmetic

This is the simplest and lightest type available. It consists of a foam-filled glove either fitted directly to the socket or, for children with no elbow, attached to an endoskeletal system with prosthetic elbow joint and socket. Socket suspension for those with an elbow joint is over the condyles and olecranon; babies may require a small cuff over the elbow; those without their elbow joint require a strap around their other arm for suspension.

Body powered

Body movement is harnessed to control the terminal device and/or the elbow. This prosthesis is the most functional. A set of straps harnesses the body movement: biscapular protraction, shoulder flexion and, if present, elbow extension combine to operate the terminal device. The terminal device for a small child is usually a split hook, which has one static and one moving jaw. The grip force is determined by the number of elastic bands that keep the two jaws together. It is possible to remove the split hook and replace it with a cosmetic or mechanical hand or, when the child is big enough, a range of different tools. This prosthesis is a functional tool rather than attempting to be cosmetic.

Electric power

A battery-operated motor moves the hand, wrist or elbow by using switch or myoelectric controls. Rechargeable batteries are supplied, with a remote battery cable and pouch when the child is small and mounted within the prosthesis when the child is older. If a switch control is used the hand is activated by a harness requiring minimal movement. This system may be used by a child aged 2 years old with a transverse deficiency. Touch pads may be used by a child with a longitudinal deficiency using one or two fingers at shoulder level. A myoelectric prosthesis is activated by contraction of the muscles in the residual limb. The micro-volts of electricity are picked up and amplified by the electrodes positioned in the socket. In the simpler single-site system, the child contracts the muscles and the hand opens; they relax and the hand automatically closes. In a more advanced system there are two electrodes, and the child contracts one muscle to open and the other to close the hand.

There are fewer prescription options for <u>lower limb</u> prostheses because the requirement is for mobility and stability. The weight-bearing areas must be considered. The prosthesis for a child with a transtibial amputation or the transverse arrest at mid-lower leg involves weight bearing on the patellar tendon bar; this is called a patellar tendon-bearing (PTB) prosthesis. A child with a knee disarticulation will carry some weight on the end of the residual limb, whereas higher levels will weight bear on the ischium. Children with a longitudinal limb deficiency will weight bear on their foot or knee; the prosthesis is often bulky and uncosmetic.

Children 0–2 years

Babies learn through discovering their environment, and children with limb deficiencies need to be given every opportunity to do the same. Parents benefit from meeting other families with babies and older children similarly affected. Children with one limb affected will reach developmental milestones within normal time scales.

In this early stage of the baby's life the significant people outside the family will be the GP and the health visitor. Their roles depend very much on the early relationship built up with the family. Many of these children should be referred to a regional prosthetic centre at an early age. The rehabilitation consultant should assess with the therapist and prosthetist and refer on, if appropriate, to a surgeon.

Children with a <u>single upper limb</u> deficiency will need toys positioned where they can reach them, e.g. on an activity gym the toys may need to be hung lower on the limb-deficient side. Rattles can be fitted over the residual limb, drawing the baby's attention to this side of their body. Their clothing should, when possible, be pulled up on the deficient side so the baby can use their sense of touch. The baby will be fitted with a cosmetic prosthesis at 4–6 months (Figure 13.4). Babies adapt very easily at an early age. Early fitting enables them to establish a pattern of limb wearing, develops their 'hand'/eye coordination, and helps meet the family's need

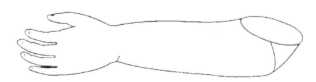

Figure 13.4: Drawing of cosmetic hand for baby with mid-forearm terminal transverse arrest.

for cosmetic replacement. Some babies find the prosthesis helpful for crawling, although others find it gets in the way. The use of the prosthesis can be encouraged by attaching rattles to the hand, giving the child large, light toys to hold with two hands and encouraging them to reach the activity gym with the prosthesis.

Children with a single lower limb deficiency will have minimal functional loss until they try to move about. Most will manage to crawl, those with a knee joint having no difficulty, those without may commando crawl or bottom shuffle. These children will be fitted with the simplest available prosthesis when they are beginning to pull themselves up to standing.

Children with more than one limb affected will be slower to achieve the early developmental skills. This is not a sign of developmental delay, but a result of the difficulties of balance, mobility and dexterity. They require as much experience of their body in space as is possible. They must use everything remaining to them. A child born without arms should wear socks as little as possible so that they can explore the environment with their feet. They may require help gaining sitting balance, in the form of cushions or a corner seat. A child born without legs may need support for sitting in the early stages. A child with all four limbs absent will need a sitting socket and must be encouraged to use their chin, mouth and any other body part to experience their environment. These children benefit from referral to physiotherapy to achieve their greatest physical potential.

Children without one or more limbs have less body surface area than a normal child from which to sweat. They do not feel the cold, so require less clothing. This is helpful for the child, enabling greater freedom of movement. These children are unlikely to be fitted with prostheses at this stage, but each child and family must be assessed individually.

Children in this age group who become amputees will have very few memories of their limb or the surgery, and are unlikely to suffer long-term problems. They are fitted with prostheses once the residual limb is well healed and their development is at an appropriate stage. The parents, grandparents and siblings all require considerable support at the time of surgery and the fitting of the prostheses. They may benefit from counselling to help them adjust.

Children 2–4 years

This is the age when children venture out into society, into play groups and nursery school. Limb-deficient children are proving themselves to be as good and bad as any other child of this age! They are learning and growing very fast and trying to impose their will on the world. It may be during this period that they become aware of being different. This requires careful handling. Children and parents often benefit from meeting others like themselves. The therapist will work together with the parents, play group and nursery staff to enable the child to develop as holistically as possible.

Children with a <u>single upper limb</u> deficiency will be achieving the same skills as their peers; they will be able to undress and may put on some easier clothes. Some may become frustrated with the cosmetic prosthesis because of its limited functional use. The child will progress to a functional prosthesis, when he or she is walking securely, has enough length discrepancy between the residual limb and the sound limb, and is interested in hand function. The first functional limb for a child with a mid-forearm arrest is operated by body movements – extension of the elbow and protraction of the shoulder girdle. It may be a split hook or similar device attached to the socket; the strap to harness the body movement goes around the child's other shoulder (Figure 13.5). Body-powered prostheses are robust and can withstand most toddler's demands. They are very good tools, but cosmetically unacceptable to many parents. An alternative is a small electric hand, operated initially by the same body movement described, and later by myoelectric control (Brenner, 1992).

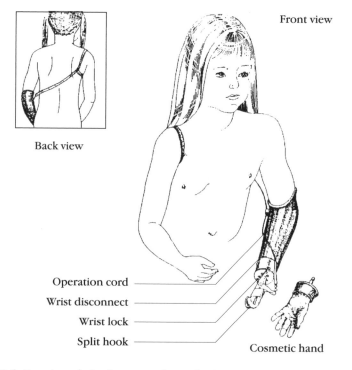

Back view

Front view

Operation cord

Wrist disconnect

Wrist lock

Split hook

Cosmetic hand

Figure 13.5: Drawing of a body-powered prosthesis.

Children with higher levels of limb deficiency will have more complex provision but require similar therapy intervention.

The child and parent require training in the use of the prosthesis to enable its full potential to be realised. This takes the form of half-an-hour to 1-hour sessions of play, initially learning the release method, playing dropping games, e.g. dropping plastic animals into a bowl of water (in the case of the electric hand being careful that it does not get wet), then building the concept of holding, e.g. pushing a doll's buggy (Curran and Hambrey, 1991; Meredith et al., 1993).

It is important that the prosthesis does not become a 'battle ground'. If the child does not want to wear it, and does not respond to gentle but firm persuasion, the prosthesis should be kept in an accessible place, e.g. in the play box at home, brought regularly to the child's attention and the child should attend regular therapy sessions.

As the child gets older the prosthesis becomes more useful. It is the non-dominant assister to the sound hand, e.g. holding paper while cutting out using scissors in the sound hand, holding a bead to thread, card to sew (Figure 13.6).

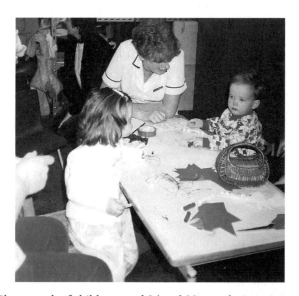

Figure 13.6: Photograph of children aged 24 and 30 months in training session.

A child with a limb deficiency at the wrist or with missing fingers may benefit from a simple leather strap to help with feeding.

The child with a <u>lower limb deficiency</u> will learn to walk very easily at this age, but may need a heavy push-along toy to give some extra support. It is helpful if the child and parents are referred to a physiotherapist so the child is encouraged to have a good gait pattern. These children may walk more slowly than their peers and children with a prosthetic knee joint are unable to run. They often find adjusting to new sockets difficult when they grow.

Children with <u>multiple limb deficiencies</u> will move out of the baby phase at this age. They now have some independent balance and are beginning to explore their environment without help. Children without arms but with fully developed legs will require some encouragement to walk. They think of their feet as hands and their feet are for manipulating toys not walking on! Use of a toddler trike can give the idea of foot mobility. They have no arms to help them balance or to break the fall when it does come. Teaching the child and parents safe ways of falling can build up their confidence. The child may require a helmet in the early stages of learning to walk to protect the head. The parents may want to use a crotch strap on a harness when walking outside because they have no hand to hold. It is helpful if the concept of independence can be started early, with the child beginning to undress him- or herself with loose fitting clothes. The child will be able to eat biscuits held in the toes when sitting on the floor, moving their head down to their feet. Feet should remain bare as much as possible and the child's joint flexibility maintained because this is essential to achieve independence later in life.

A child without legs may be fitted with prostheses, or wheelchair mobility may be considered. Independent mobility is important at this age. When a child has one upper and one lower limb affected, it is usual to fit the lower limb prosthesis first.

These children are more dependent than their peers, and are eligible to apply for the Disability Living Allowance. They should continue to have regular physiotherapy to maintain and increase the mobility of all their remaining joints.

Children who become <u>amputees</u> in this age group will probably adapt very well, but the parents have considerable difficulty. It is important that this is overcome so the child can progress. The child has minimal language to express his or her needs and anxieties at this stage, so great awareness is required by those treating and caring for the child. The child should be encouraged to use the residual limb as soon as possible and to maintain the full range of movement of the remaining joints. Prosthetic fitting will commence when the residual limb is sufficiently healed. Treatment will be required as for the child with limb deficiency.

Children of primary school age (5–11 years)

The child is now beginning to find his place in society. It is helpful when the child can move into school with children he or she knows either through nursery or through an older sibling. The transition into school varies with each parent, child and school. Some parents prefer to speak to the teacher and make sure that their child and his special needs are known, whereas others feel that their child does not have special needs and would rather he was not treated differently. It is a situation that needs to be dealt with sensitively. Some parents find the transition into school very stressful and the child is likely to be aware of this and may become anxious himself. Parents are sometimes concerned that their child may be teased. If this does occur it is important to discuss it with the child and the teacher, because strategies are required to respond to it appropriately. Parents find it very helpful to discuss the problem with other families.

The child with a single upper limb deficiency will probably be established as a prosthetic user or as a non-user at this age. It is helpful if options are kept open and they retain a fitting prosthesis which they are encouraged to use at times. Some children use the prosthesis naturally and spontaneously as if it were their own hand. The prosthetic choice at this stage is the body-powered or myoelectric prosthesis (Figures 13.5, 13.8 and 13.9), although some children prefer the lighter, cosmetic prosthesis.

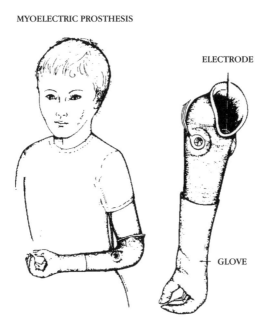

Figure 13.8: Drawing of a myoelectric prosthesis.

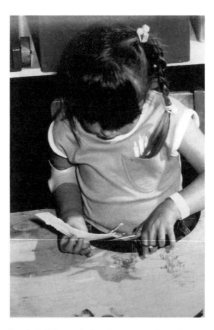

Figure 13.9: Photograph of child aged 6 using myoelectric prosthesis.

These children need to be good problem-solvers, because most tasks are possible with one hand, with or without a prosthesis. It is helpful if children are encouraged to try different tasks from an early age. Some children have established their hand dominance at this age. A child with one hand will have to write with this hand. Some of these children have great difficulty learning to write and use scissors, etc., particularly children who would have been strongly right-hand dominant but have been born without their right hand. This is further complicated by tools being designed for right-hand use. Special care should be given when teaching these children, using appropriate equipment. A number of children have difficulty managing construction tasks; some find a prosthesis helpful whereas others manage better without. When doing PE, some children prefer to remove their prosthesis; others prefer to wear it. They should be encouraged to participate as fully as possible. The first classroom task all one-handed children are unable to achieve is to play the recorder. They can manage a few notes but without an adapted instrument they cannot keep up with their peers. Reach, Association for Children with Hand or Arm Deficiency, has a scheme for hiring out one-handed recorders to members when they are 7 or 8 years old.

Outside the classroom the following are activities to consider:

- Skipping, which can be done by holding either the handle in the prosthesis or in the crook of the elbow, by tying the rope to the forearm or by using a tight sweat band into which the handle is fitted.
- Riding a bicycle: holding the handle bars can be difficult. If wearing a prosthesis the child's reach is correct; if not an extension on the handle bar may need to be fitted. Many children manage to ride using one hand. This is not a satisfactory long-term solution, as a result of poor posture and concern about safety. Braking can be achieved by using a tandem brake lever; both brake cables go into one brake lever.

The following is a personal ADL (activities of daily living) skill to consider:

- Dressing: this should become easier during this period; a child at primary school should manage to put clothes on. Problem areas are buttons, tights, socks and shoe laces. Buttons can be achieved with practice. Tights and socks are easiest when they are clean and dry and the child's foot is dry, i.e. it is difficult to put these on after PE. It is possible to tie shoe laces with one hand either using an alternative method of threading the lace or by using the residual limb, the prosthesis or a foot to hold the lace while the remaining hand does the tying. If a child does not learn to tie laces, he or she will be restricted later in the choice of footwear, and will have difficulty participating in sport, e.g. football.

A child at this age should be managing to cut up food, using a prosthesis, strap or holding the fork down with their residual limb. Use of the toilet is possible but reaching the toilet paper and managing their clothes may be difficult.

The child with a <u>lower limb deficiency</u> has a less obvious functional disability and can manage most tasks in the classroom. Most children will choose to wear a prosthesis. Some children with higher levels of loss may find sitting for long periods uncomfortable and may need attention paid to their seating. Some children find PE and sports difficult; ways of dealing with this should be discussed by the parents and teacher. Children often benefit from seeing a physiotherapist at this stage to encourage a good gait pattern and to discuss their mobility needs. Sometimes riding a bicycle is a problem because of the fit of the prosthesis. Several bicycles should be tried and if the problem continues it should be discussed with the child's prosthetist.

Children with <u>multiple limb deficiency</u> may require a Statement of Educational Need because they are likely to need help in the classroom.

The children should be encouraged to do as many tasks for themselves as possible in whatever way they can. Many of these children are very resourceful and this should be encouraged. Special scissors, sloping boards and use of easy writing tools should be considered, and early exposure to information technology should be encouraged. Some children may have difficulty participating in PE but should be encouraged to do as much as they can. They may need to have alternative exercise, e.g. swimming.

Toileting at home and at school may be a problem. This will be related to managing clothes and cleaning. In the early years of schooling help will be required, but this problem should be addressed as soon as the child is ready, with independence hopefully achieved before moving up to secondary school. This may involve a hook being attached to the wall, or the use of a dressing stick held in the child's fingers, or mouth. Cleansing is a difficult task, achieved by toilet paper on the toilet seat or in an appliance. Some are unable to do this and continue to need help. At home it is then necessary to consider a toilet that cleans and dries the child. The child should be managing more of his or her own dressing, and be encouraged to wear easy clothes with few fastenings. Extra loops, dressing sticks or hooks on the wall may help the child to learn independence.

A child using the feet should be feeding him- or herself with a spoon or fork in the toes, lifting food up to the mouth. Children with short upper limbs may benefit from adapted cutlery.

A child who becomes <u>an amputee</u> during this time will miss periods of schooling. This is not detrimental academically, but may be difficult for them socially, their friends having formed other social groups. Children of this age group are generally very accepting of others' misfortune and will support and help the child when he or she returns. It is important that the classmates have an understanding of what has happened and the way the return to school is planned is critical.

The child should be encouraged to look at, and handle, the residual limb as soon as possible. Movement of the remaining joints and muscle strength should be maintained and increased. The child will need to be encouraged to talk about the loss, possibly through play. Phantom sensation should be talked about so the child is assured of his or her sanity. Functional tasks should be addressed at an age-appropriate level. The parents and siblings will require support and help.

Some children do not like participating in sport and PE. This may be because of anxieties about the activity, the difficulties getting dressed and undressed, or concern about being seen without their prosthesis on. This should be dealt with as quickly as possible so self-consciousness does not become an issue. Aspects discussed in the limb deficiency sections also apply.

Secondary school children aged 11–18 years

This is when the child makes the transition through adolescence/puberty to adulthood. Progress for the child with limb deficiency may be smooth or difficult as with any child. The first transition is to a considerably larger school, with much more autonomy and more personal demands. It is helpful if the child can move school with friends so that there is some continuity of peer support. It is a stressful time for both parents and children. It is the time for decision-making – decisions that make a difference to the rest of their life, courses chosen, hobbies pursued, friendships formed. Children become more aware of their body image, and are very concerned about how they are accepted by their peers.

The child with a <u>single upper limb deficiency</u> may want to consider using a different prosthesis or, if they have lapsed, reconsider prosthetic use. All prostheses, or none, are appropriate for this age group. For a child who is very aware of body image the cosmetic prosthesis may be most appropriate. Others require more function and will consider the body-powered prosthesis with all its versatility, using the split hook, other activity specific terminal devices, or cosmetic or mechanical hand. Others will need the combination of cosmesis and function, so they will use the myoelectric prosthesis (Weaver et al., 1988). It is very important at this age that the children are aware of all available options and the advantages and disadvantages of each system. Children at this age should be encouraged to make decisions based on their own needs, rather than those of their parents.

Children with a partial hand or a longitudinal deficiency will sometimes consider a cosmetic or functional prosthesis at this stage.

In secondary school, the amount of writing increases considerably and some children find it difficult to keep up, especially if they are depending on their non-dominant hand. Some need greater exposure to information technology; others require extra time in examinations. If a child's hand becomes painful it should be rested to prevent repetitive strain injury. Some children have problems with tasks requiring dexterity, e.g. science, design and technology and art, whereas others achieve great success. There is a need to be able to carry books and equipment around the school, which can be difficult. These children should be achieving all personal care, and be participating in domestic tasks as appropriate in the family. They may require information about special equipment and techniques to make tasks easier. Children sometimes want to pursue sports and hobbies that may require some adaptation or special tools. The Amputee and les Autres Sports Association can be helpful, or activity-specific groups, e.g. Swimming for the Disabled, or activity and amputee specific, e.g. the One Armed Golfer's Association. During adolescence some children become aware that their limb-deficient side is less developed than their full arm, and some benefit from referral to physiotherapy for advice and guidance about suitable exercises to perform to build up the limb-deficient side.

Driving is of importance to 17 year olds. A child with a single upper limb deficiency should have no difficulty driving (Verral and Kulkani, 1995). Those with a right arm absence will be able to drive a geared car, those with a left arm absence will find driving an automatic car easiest, but it may be possible for them to drive a geared vehicle. Both will benefit from a steering ball either held in a prosthesis or in their hand.

The child with a lower limb deficiency will be facing greater distances to walk within a large school, and the need to change classrooms quickly. They may need special arrangements, e.g. leaving class a few minutes early. Some children will actively pursue sport, whereas others would rather not! Some will be needing specialised sports prostheses to enable them to participate in sport safely and satisfactorily.

Children with multiple limb deficiency will have the same struggles regarding the size of the new school and managing to get around it. Children with bilateral lower limb absence may choose to wear their prostheses rarely and will need to consider use of wheelchairs for the distances and speed. Children with upper limb absences are expected to be independent in personal care, using their feet and assistive equipment, e.g. wall hooks, dressing sticks. They should be encouraged to participate in domestic tasks as appropriate in the family. Sometimes these children look ungainly using their feet for a period, regaining grace once through adolescence.

Children with upper and lower limbs affected should be encouraged to participate in as many areas as possible. Information technology should be used to its greatest benefit. Use of prostheses or devices should be considered and the child involved at all times in problem-solving. Environmental controls can be advantageous for controlling television, radio, curtains, etc. It is very important that these children remain slim; all activity is more difficult when they are overweight.

They will still need a Statement of Educational Needs and may require use of a lap-top or voice-activated computer so they are able to communicate their level of knowledge. Mobility and functional ability must be regularly addressed.

A child who becomes an amputee during this period may have great difficulty making the inevitable adjustments. They may have long periods off school which is disruptive at this time, and the child's friends may have difficulty knowing how to respond to them, so the child may become isolated. The child requires physiotherapy in the early stages to be sure that he or she maintains range of movement in the remaining joints. Some children have very strong phantom limb sensations and these may be painful. Prosthetic rehabilitation will begin when the residual limb is healed. The child should be actively involved in the prescription decisions. A lower limb amputee will require physiotherapy to achieve a good gait pattern. An upper limb amputee will require training with the prosthesis to realise its full potential. They will also need to learn to do tasks with their remaining hand, especially if the dominant hand has been amputated.

Sometimes the amputation can have positive results, giving the child an unforeseen opportunity to re-evaluate where they are heading. This could be a good time to redirect and reconsider their personal goals. It is important that the parents and child get the support that they need together or separately. Aspects discussed in the limb deficiency sections also apply.

Children with limb deficiencies, congenital or acquired, are able to live full and fulfilling lives. The aim of the occupational therapist is to enable them to grow up to reach their greatest potential.

Case study 1

Kay is the eldest of four children; her parents did not know that she had a limb deficiency before she was born. Her deficiencies are: bilateral terminal transverse arrest at mid-humeral level and longitudinal deficiency of her right leg (femur partial, fibula total, rays 4 and 5 total). Later it became evident that she had an unstable left hip and knee, and that she suffered from sensory defensiveness.

Her first independent mobility was bottom shuffling, and a buggy was used for longer distances. She used her feet to explore her environment, play, and later to feed herself and write. At 4 years she was fitted with a right extension prosthesis and a KAFO (knee–ankle–foot orthosis) for her left leg. She could stand, progressing slowly to walking with her 'hands' held, to using a rollator with arm sockets attached. She walked independently at 7 years of age. She was fitted with arm prostheses, but these were too bulky and complex for her to use effectively. She now has arm sockets which are tools to use for typing, writing and carrying toys. She loves to walk but she is more independent when not wearing her extension prosthesis.

Now, aged 8 years, she can undress, put on some clothes, transfer on and off chairs, bed and toilet, and feed herself. Until now she has attended a school for children with physical disabilities and is progressing well. It is hoped that she will gradually transfer into mainstream school. She requires input from the occupational therapists within school and at home

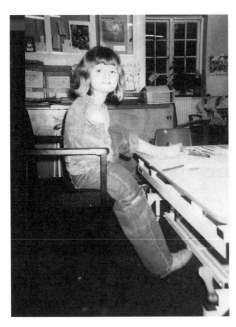

Figure 13.10: Kay aged 8, with bilateral transverse arrest at mid humerous level, wearing a right extension. She is writing with her left foot.

to increase her independence through provision of adaptations and equipment. This involvement is likely to continue throughout her life as her needs and circumstances change.

The multidisciplinary team involved in her care is very large: several different occupational therapy specialists, paediatrician, surgeons, rehabilitation consultant, prosthetist, orthotist, physiotherapists, school teachers, and most importantly, herself, her parents and siblings. Good communication between these people is essential if Kay is to reach her full potential.

Case study 2

Nicholas was 16 when he was diagnosed with meningitis. He developed meningococcal septicaemia and required amputation of both legs: left transfemoral, right transtibial; he also had a left partial hand, consisting of two metacarpal bones divided to act as two fingers, and his right hand had median nerve damage. He was in a critical condition, but became medically stable and was transferred to a rehabilitation environment.

He had been an easy-going, music-loving boy, who played the organ, and enjoyed dancing. He was not very keen on study but had been persuaded to go to college. All this suddenly changed with no period of preparation. He had great difficulty being in a rehabilitation environment with demands being made on him. He regressed to childhood, needing his mother to be with him and to help him with all tasks. His mother needed a lot of support and Nicholas required gentle, firm handling to help him towards recovery. He was encouraged to take some responsibility by being involved in his treatment planning. He started by using an electric wheelchair, with right hand controls and forward/backward transfers, and he fed himself with adapted cutlery. He had a full physiotherapy and occupational therapy programme, the occupational therapist addressing hand function and ADL issues, as well as psychological adjustment.

All his limbs took a long time to heal because of the nature of septicaemia. Once healed he was fitted with a PTB (patellar tendon-bearing) prosthesis for his left leg, and an ischial weight-bearing socket for his right leg. He always wore a mitten to cover his partial hand because he was very concerned about its appearance. This was a problem but it was decided not to force him to take the mitten off. Before he was discharged home, he began to remove it himself; once he felt confident at home he did not wear it at all.

When his prostheses were fitting well, standing activities were commenced to encourage good standing tolerance and enable functional tasks to be carried out. Donning and doffing the prostheses, managing transfers, dressing and toileting were practised. Planning for discharge included walking outside, managing steps and slopes, communicating closely with social service occupational therapists and with his family. Discussion was also required with Nicholas and college staff regarding the timing of his return to college.

Nicholas has grown into a confident young man of 21. He misses playing the organ but continues to enjoy listening to music; he is very fashion conscious and can spend many hours walking around the shops. He is learning to drive and is now living independently in a ground floor flat a short distance from his parents.

Resources

CIGOPW–COT Specialist Section: the Clinical Interest Group in Orthotics Prosthetics and Wheelchairs. College of Occupational Therapy.
Reach: The Association for Children with Hand or Arm Deficiency.
STEPS: The National Association for Children with Lower Limbs Abnormalities.
Thalidomide Society: for children and adults with multiple limb deficiency.
International Society for Prosthetics and Orthotics, Borgerraenget 5, 2100, Copenhagen, Denmark.

Chapter 14
Children with juvenile idiopathic arthritis

JANINE HACKETT

Arthritis characterised by joint swelling, pain and stiffness was first recognised as a distinct illness in childhood from that in adults by Sir George Frederick Still in 1897.

The most recent proposal from the International League of Associations for Rheumatology (ILAR) is to refer to chronic arthritis in children as 'juvenile idiopathic arthritis'. It is hoped that this umbrella term to classify all chronic arthritis of unknown cause will provide an internationally agreed classification of the disease, which will enable greater communication and facilitate research:

- 'Juvenile' refers to the onset of arthritis before the age of 16.
- 'Idiopathic' refers to the disease being of unknown cause.
- 'Arthritis' refers to inflammation of the joint.

Although rheumatic symptoms are common in childhood, juvenile idiopathic arthritis (JIA) is a relatively uncommon disease with approximately 1 in every 1000 children affected at any one time (Southwood and Malleson, 1993).

For a diagnosis of JIA to be made symptoms must have been present for at least 6 weeks. It is a disease of exclusion which often necessitates a variety of blood tests, radiographs and scans, and involves careful examination on the part of the physician to detect often subtle joint swelling and reduced range of movement. In some cases the diagnosis is made in the presence of systemic rather than articular features.

There are six major categories of juvenile idiopathic arthritis. These represent the major clinical patterns of the disease. The number of affected joints plays a major part in determining classification (Table 14.1, pages 310–11). Other factors including family medical history and laboratory markers also play a part in the specific diagnosis. Not only does the classification of the disease prove helpful in predicting the outcome of the disease; it is also useful in the prescription of particular treatment regimens, as well as for providing education and support.

Oligoarthritis

This is the most common form of idiopathic arthritis, which usually presents asymmetrically and affects between one and four joints. Onset is usually in early childhood and affects girls more than boys. One serious but asymptomatic complication of this disease is chronic uveitis (inflammation of the eye) which when left untreated can cause permanent blindness. Regular screening with a slit lamp by an ophthalmologist is therefore essential for this patient group.

For most of these children the prognosis is good. However, approximately a third will go on to develop extended oligoarthritis which affects more than four joints.

Polyarthritis

Polyarthritis affects five or more joints and is usually symmetrical in its presentation. Girls are affected more than boys and, although the most common age of onset is between 3 and 6 years, it can present throughout childhood.

Polyarthritis usually has a poorer prognosis than oligoarthritis, with a third of children having persistent disease into adulthood.

Systemic arthritis

Systemic arthritis may be diagnosed in the presence or absence of articular symptoms if the characteristic intermittent salmon-pink rash and quotidian fever (spikes in temperature) are present. Other systemic features, e.g. inflammation of the liver, heart, spleen and lymph nodes, etc., may also be present.

Although this is the least common type of arthritis, it is potentially the most serious because of its effects on the organs, particularly the heart (pericarditis) and amyloidosis. It affects boys and girls equally. Onset may be at any age throughout childhood and any number of joints can be affected.

Psoriatic arthritis

Psoriatic arthritis may be diagnosed in the presence or absence of psoriasis if the child has a dactylitis, changes in the nails or if there is a family history of the disease in parents or siblings.

Table 14.1: Summary of ILAR classification of JIA (1998)

Classification	Oligoarthritis	Polyarthritis	Systemic arthritis	Psoriatic arthritis	Enthesitis-related arthritis
Main characteristics	Asymmetrical presentation affecting one to four joints	Symmetrical presentation affecting five or more joints	Quotidian fever Rash Systemic features ± arthritis	Psoriasis ± or family history Arthritis Nail changes associated with psoriasis	Inflammation of attachments of ligaments/ tendons/fascia
Sex ratio	F > m E > r 5:1	F > m E > r 3:1	E = r F = m	Slightly more F E than r M 1.5:1	m > F E > r 7:1
Age of onset	Early childhood Peak age 2–4 years	Throughout childhood	Throughout childhood	Later childhood Peak age 10–11 years	Onset 8 years +
Complications	Chronic uveitis Growth disturbance	Joint erosion Generalized growth disturbance	Systemic illness Anaemia Amyloidosis		Acute uveitis Inflammatory bowel disease
Prognosis	Usually good A third may go on to develop extended oligoarthritis	Moderately good. A third will persist into adulthood	Poorer for those with polyarticular disease	Variable	Two-thirds will go on to develop ankylosing spondylitis

(contd)

Table 14.1: (contd)

Classification	Oligoarthritis	Polyarthritis	Systemic arthritis	Psoriatic arthritis	Enthesitis-related arthritis
Treatment	Non-steroidal anti-inflammatory drugs Joint injections	Non-steroidal anti-inflammatory drugs Joint injections Intravenous pulse steroids Second-line drugs, e.g. methotrexate, sulphasalazine	Non-steroidal anti-inflammatory drugs Joint injections Intravenous pulse steroids Oral corticosteroids Second-line drugs, e.g. methotrexate, sulphasalazine and cyclosporin	Non-steroidal anti-inflammatory drugs Joint injections Second line drugs	Non-steroidals Joint injections Sulphasalazine Methotrexate

Onset is usually later in childhood around the ages of 10 or 11 and affects only slightly more girls than boys. Prognosis is variable for this group.

Enthesitis-related arthritis

Enthesitis-related arthritis is diagnosed in the presence of inflammation around the attachments of tendons, ligaments or fascia, i.e. the entheses. It is more common in boys in later childhood or adolescence. Other presentations can include back pain, sacroiliac tenderness or the presence of the genetic marker HLA-B27. Acute uveitis, unlike chronic uveitis, is not clinically silent and may also be present.

There is often a family history of ankylosing spondylitis and in fact about two-thirds of these children will go on to develop this condition.

Other arthritis

This category refers to those children who have arthritis for a duration of at least 6 weeks but who, however, fall into either none or more than one of the above categories.

Juvenile idiopathic arthritis characteristics

Juvenile idiopathic arthritis is an autoimmune disease characterised by persistent joint swelling. Inflammation begins in the synovial membrane of the joint capsule and, as increased synovial fluid is produced, the intra-articular pressure in the joint also increases. This is often very painful and a position of flexion is often adopted in order to reduce this. This flexed position will lead to a shortening in the muscles, tendons and ligaments. Uncontrolled swelling can also lead to the destruction of these tissues and, if left untreated, destruction of cartilage can begin. Later, with continued destruction, joints can become eroded or ankylosed, i.e. bony fusion of the joints.

Growth disturbances

Juvenile idiopathic arthritis can affect growth in children, particularly those with oligoarthritis. Increased blood supply at the site of an inflamed joint can lead to asymmetrical increased growth. Leg-length discrepancies are therefore not uncommon in this group and may require a shoe raise. On the other hand, prolonged arthritis at a particular site may also have the reverse effect, where growth is stunted as a result of premature closure of the epiphyses. Generalised growth suppression can also occur with the long-term use of steroids or as a consequence of severe systemic polyarthritis.

Occupational therapy in JIA

A team approach in the management of the child with JIA is essential to maximise function and quality of life. Good communication skills are, therefore, essential in order to facilitate the exchange of information and to participate in shared treatment planning with other team members.

The occupational therapist's role is challenging and varied, and offers an excellent opportunity for therapists to work in a truly holistic way, which considers the child's physical, emotional and psychosocial needs. The occupational therapist's unique core skill of assessment of functional performance and her or his ability to determine a child's interests, analyse activities and plan treatment accordingly can be of great benefit in helping a child with a chronic illness bring about a positive adaptive response.

Assessment

Thorough assessment of a child with JIA is essential in order to establish the impact of the disease on their general health status. Assessment broadly uses a biomechanical approach to assess joint range of movement and strength accurately, as well as a developmental approach to ensure that the child has acquired age-appropriate skills, which will equip them for daily life. The following assessment outline offers a structure that may prove useful to other therapists. It is not intended as a checklist or cookbook approach; rather it is hoped that it will provide colleagues with a loose framework on which to build in order to complete a comprehensive and child-centred assessment.

Information gathering

A comprehensive assessment will include information from a number of sources. Medical records can provide details on past medical history, drug therapies and interventions by other professionals. Current radiographs, magnetic resonance imaging (MRI) and blood tests should also be considered, because they may have a bearing on treatment interventions. Information from the child and parent is valuable in providing details about the individual disease experience and severity, e.g. presence and duration of early morning stiffness, pain, fatigue and psychological adjustment, as well as the impact on the child's activities of daily living (ADL).

Observation

Good observation skills are necessary, not only during formal assessments, but also informally. By observing the child either in a waiting area or rising from a chair and walking into a clinic room, the occupational therapist can gain useful information, e.g. at rest, is the child adopting patterns of flexion in order to reduce the pain in her joints and is she thus prone to developing flexion contractures? Alternatively, she may be avoiding use of a particular limb during play and is thus reducing her opportunity for exploration and normal development. Similarly, when a child rises from a chair does she weight bear on the small joints of the fingers to compensate for reduced range of movement at the wrist and is she in danger of further complications? By observing the child walking, we are able to evaluate posture and may be able to detect leg-length discrepancies caused by localised disturbances in growth. Observing the child's face for evidence of pain when walking may also provide clues as to the severity of the disease because children are often unable to express pain verbally. For this reason, visual analogue scales are often used in the assessment of pain.

Upper limb

For an accurate assessment of range of movement, it is useful to use a goniometer. This is a valid and reliable tool, which can provide information on disease severity and the effectiveness of drug therapy, as well as providing baseline measures for physiotherapy and occupational therapy treatment interventions. Muscle strength can be measured using the Oxford scale.

The hand requires detailed assessment because disease activity in the wrist and fingers will have a significant impact on functional status.

Hand screening

A quick screening test may prove useful because major abnormalities are unlikely if a child can press the palms together with wrists at 90° (and vice versa for flexion), make full fists and a distal interphalangeal joint (DIP) tuck, and demonstrate full thumb opposition. Figure 14.1 illustrates reduced range of movement in the right wrist and flexion contractures in the PIP joints of the right hand.

Appearance

A good indication of disease activity can be gained by feeling the child's hands for heat and sweatiness because inflamed joints will cause increased temperature. Red swollen joints may also be observed as well as tenderness on palpation. Muscle atrophy, particularly of the thenar and hypothenar eminences, can also provide evidence of reduced strength and impaired hand function.

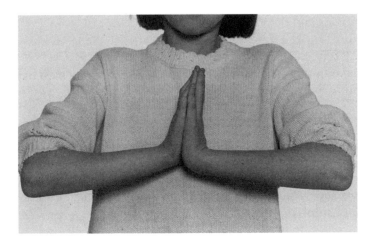

Figure 14.1: A quick and simple screening test will highlight any abnormalities.

Deformity

During assessment, careful note should be made of any flexion contractures. Joint integrity should also be considered along with any subluxations, joint instability or crepitations. Any deviations from the normal joint alignments should also be documented.

Common hand deformities

- Wrist:
    - loss of extension leading to flexion contracture
    - wrist subluxation/dinner fork deformity
    - ulnar deviation caused by growth disturbance and relative shortening of ulna
    - ankylosis (bony fusion of joint)
- Metacarpophalangeal (MCP) joints:
    - loss of extension → flexion contractures
    - radial deviations (if ulnar deviation of wrist present)
- Proximal interphalangeal (PIP) joints:
    - flexion contractures
    - Boutonnière's deformity, i.e. flexion at PIP with hyperextension of DIP caused by lengthening of the central slip as a result of chronic synovitis and the displacement of the lateral bands
    - swan neck deformity (less common), i.e. hyperextension of PIP joint with flexion at DIP joint
- DIP joints:
    - involvement more common in psoriatic arthritis

  – synovitis and flexion contractures
- Thumb:
  – MCP synovitis resulting in flexion contracture
  – weakening of tendons can result in a 'Z' deformity with hyperextension of interphalangeal joint.

Range of movement

Active and passive range of movement can be measured using a finger goniometer. A ruler may also be used to take linear measurements from the fingertips to the distal palmar crease. The rule of '9', which assigns a number to several key areas of the four digits, can be used to measure thumb opposition.

Muscle strength

A dynamometer or vigorometer can be used to measure gross grip strength as well as pinch and lateral pinch strength.

Hand function

Although the goniometer and dynamometer are useful in measuring joint range and strength, they provide little insight into the difficulties that a child may be experiencing with everyday activities. It is, therefore, important to include an activity-based hand function test, which includes the six major classifications of prehensile patterns (Light et al., 1999). A variety of assessments is commercially available. However, therapists may wish to include their own observation of particular tasks, e.g. pencil skills, peg moving, cone stacking, ball throwing and key turning, which incorporate these major patterns. Particular attention should be paid to manipulation, dexterity, coordination and strength.

Splints

Some children with arthritis are likely to have been prescribed splints. Continuous reassessment of these is necessary to ensure adequate fit, comfort and function. The precise reason for the prescription needs to be established in order to ensure that it is still effective in its purpose. The child's view of the splint is also important in determining whether or not the splint is actually worn. By negotiating the design of the splint, e.g. colour and material, the child may be more accepting of a light-weight splint, which is cooler and more cosmetically pleasing. Finally, if the child has a good understanding of the reasons behind splint wearing, she or he is more likely to comply with treatment.

Functional assessment

A number of functional assessments are available to therapists, including: the Juvenile Arthritis Functional Assessment Scale (JAFAS); the JAFAR-C, a self-assessment report; the JAFAR-P, a parental report on ability to perform activities over a week (Howe et al., 1991); and the Childhood Health Assessment Questionnaire (CHAQ). Designed to be more general than ADL assessments, functional assessments attempt to measure change in patients objectively; currently they are in vogue with physicians as a result of the move towards evidence-based medicine. The validated age range for the JAFAS is 7–16 years and consists of 10 timed activities, e.g. pulling on socks, buttoning a shirt, etc. Although the tool is considered valid and reliable, it does require a degree of training and standardised equipment. The Childhood HAQ, on the other hand, is a questionnaire, that measures function in eight areas, the scores of which are then averaged to calculate a disability index. It can also be used on those children aged under 7 because it can be administered by parents. This tool has been found to be valid and reliable and sensitive to change (Singh et al., 1994).

Activities of daily living

A more detailed assessment of ADLs is required to ensure that the child is performing at his or her optimal functional level. An assessment of self-care skills, mobility, transfers, safety, productivity and leisure, as well as consideration of any environmental barriers that may be hindering independence, can provide information for effective occupational therapy treatment planning.

Assistive devices

In some instances, a piece of ADL equipment will help to facilitate function. However, in the first instance an alternative technique of doing a particular activity is usually more appropriate. Before prescribing any piece of equipment, consideration should be given to whether or not it will be cosmetically acceptable to the child, and whether or not it will increase feelings of disability or actually hinder performance. If a device is indicated, teaching should be provided and a willingness to practise on the part of the child should be forthcoming. In some circumstances, an occupational therapist may have to adapt a particular piece of equipment because most ADL equipment is designed for adults.

School

School visits are useful, not only to assess the particular demands placed on a child but also to liaise with teachers and help them to gain more understanding of the disease. Areas for particular consideration include the following:

- School environment, e.g. stairs
- Demands placed upon mobility, e.g. regular classroom changes
- Hand-writing difficulties
- Posture and seating
- PE
- Lunch-time/break-time provision
- Carrying books and other equipment
- Pain/fatigue levels
- Requirements for technology classes.

A helpful checklist has been designed by Wetherbee and Neil (1989).

Development

Lack of mobility, pain, stiffness and reduced range of movement can all lead to a lack of exploration or experimentation with new skills. A lack of self-confidence, poor self-esteem and assertion, or a lack of opportunity to practise normal developmental activities, can also lead to a delay in acquiring new skills in a variety of areas. It is the occupational therapist's unique ability to analyse activities and plan treatment accordingly to promote development along a normal developmental sequence, which is of the utmost importance here (Figure 14.2).

Disease education

An evaluation of the child's level of understanding of the disease is important as is that of their parents. This will have a major impact on how they perceive their illness, their sense of control, their ability to cope and their willingness to cooperate with therapy regimens.

Occupational therapy treatment interventions

The main aim of occupational therapy in JIA is to ensure a positive adaptive response to this chronic illness. This involves preventing deformity, maximising function and facilitating independence.

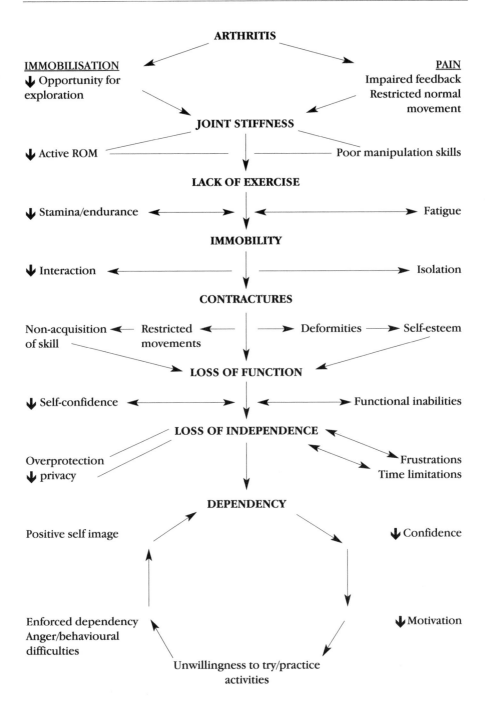

Figure 14.2: Development of juvenile idiopathic arthritis. (Adapted from Cycle of Inflammation – Helen Emery, 1987.)

Splinting

Splinting plays a major part in the role of the occupational therapist working with children with idiopathic arthritis. However, evidence for the effectiveness of splinting remains largely anecdotal. At present the main consensus surrounding the benefits of hand splint wearing in adults is that of pain relief (Adams, 1996). Other reasons for splinting include the following:

- Rest a joint and thus reduce pain and inflammation
- Support a joint and provide joint stability
- Mobilise a joint, e.g. by using dynamic splinting
- Prevent/correct a deformity
- Facilitate function.

Occupational therapists may find themselves involved in the fabrication of a variety of splints, including elbow, wrist, finger, ankle and knee splints, as well as neck collars. Responsibility for splint manufacture may vary from centre to centre and may involve joint working with physiotherapists and orthotists. Other centres may use prefabricated splints. The pros and cons of each are outlined below (Table 14.2).

Table 14.2: A comparison between prefabricated and custom-made splints

	Prefabricated splints	Custom made splints
Pros	Labour saving Soft materials are often comfortable and light weight Choice of colours usually available Range from relatively cheap May be cosmetically more acceptable	Custom made, conforms well Variety of thermoplastics available, e.g. light, breathable Choice of colours Rigidity facilitates good positioning and alignment Durable Adjustable memory of material allows remoulding
Cons	Some designs can be expensive Universal sizes, therefore often a poor fit Function of thumbs and fingers may be impeded as a result of poor fit Often difficult to achieve desired optimum position	Materials often expensive Shape can be altered inadvertently Equipment required, e.g. splint bath, heat gun. Some complaints of sweatiness Slight changes in swelling can make splint unwearable

Adapted from a comparison of splinting materials used at five paediatric rheumatology centres (Hackett et al., 1996).

Considerations

Occupational therapists should always consider the following basic rules before providing any splints:

- Splinting should never be provided in the absence of any active exercises or therapeutic activity regimen because muscles need to remain strong and eventually take over from the splint.
- Always control joints using three-point pressure.
- Give careful consideration to the position of any strapping because careless positioning can result in subluxation of a joint.
- Ascertain joint priorities.
- Always splint proximal joints before distal ones.
- Ensure even pressure and accurate fit, maintaining natural arches, and allowing room for any bony prominences, e.g. ulnar styloid.
- Only restrict joints that are to be splinted.
- Use corrective moulding techniques.
- Use strong and adjustable materials.
- Ensure that the child has had some active participation in the splinting process.

Adapted from Lawton (1994).

Regular follow-up visits to review the splint are of the utmost importance to ensure that the splint remains comfortable and functional, and continues to meet the aims of therapy. Occupational therapists should ensure that the following happen:

- The child and carer understand the reasons for wearing the splint (provide written information if necessary).
- The correct method of fitting the splint is understood.
- The splinting regimen is established, e.g. at night only/during functional tasks.
- Washing and after-care instructions are provided, because cleaning with hot water and leaving to dry on a radiator can alter the shape of the splint.
- The requirement to use an activity/exercise regimen is established.

Hand splints

There are two main types of hand splints worn by children with idiopathic arthritis: night resting splints and working splints.

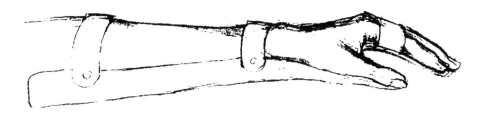

Figure 14.3: Night resting splint.

Night resting splints (Figure 14.3)

Indications for use

- Pain during sleep
- Early morning stiffness resulting in poor hand use first thing in the morning
- Disease activity in wrist and fingers
- Prophylactic measure.

Choice of material ranges from centre to centre depending on therapist preferences and budget limitations. However, the commonly accepted positioning for wrist night resting splints is as follows.

Positioning

- Splint covers approximately two-thirds of the forearm length
- Wrist is positioned in approximately 15° extension
- Slight flexion of all finger joints to prevent shortening of collateral ligaments
- Thumb supported on lateral and palmar aspects in slightly opposed and abducted position
- Transverse and longitudinal arches of the hand are maintained
- Straps sighted at lower end of radius/ulnar top of splint and proximal phalanx of fingers and thumb.

Regimen

It is usually considered unreasonable to expect a child to wear two splints at once, because this is likely to disturb sleep patterns. Alternating the left and right splint each night is therefore the preferred option.

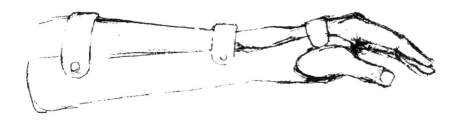

Figure 14.4: Wrist work splint.

Wrist work splints (Figure 14.4)

Wrist work splints are usually indicated in the following instances.

Indications

- Pain during function
- Impaired function resulting from reduced wrist extension
- Active wrist disease with reduced range of movement or deformity
- Inevitable ankylosis of a joint.

Again choices of materials vary and leather is a common alternative in North America. Generally accepted principles of work splints include:

- Wrists positioned in approximately 15° extension/neutral if inevitable ankylosis
- Splint should not impede thumb opposition and MCP flexion and thus impede hand function
- Splint should conform precisely to the anatomy of the hand and avoid bony prominences
- Splint should extend to at least the midpoint of the forearm
- Gauntlet-style splints are indicated for those with more deformed wrists
- Strapping at top of splint and at lower end of radius/ulna
- Dorsal splints should be avoided to prevent risk of subluxation.

Adapted from Hackett et al. (1996).

Regimen

Splints to be worn during functional tasks, e.g. writing, PE and craft activities. Twice daily exercises are recommended.

Collar

Collars may be indicated for children with neck pain. Flexion deformity or torticollis, i.e. neck lateral flexion and rotation, may be prevalent in some children with JIA with cervical spine involvement. Off-the-shelf collars are available, but it may be better to use Plastazote, which can be moulded into the required position. Joint working with a physiotherapist, who can provide hot packs and manual traction, if indicated, is helpful in achieving the optimal functional position. Collars are always provided with an active exercise programme. Where there are signs that a neck may be ankylosing, a more permanent collar is needed to ensure a functional fusion.

Leg splints

Joint working with a physiotherapist is also recommended when making leg splints because they possess specialist knowledge of foot anatomy and can apply treatment modalities. Heat therapy and passive stretching can ensure the best outcome. Care should be taken when extending the knee because careless handling techniques can cause tibial subluxation.

Knee splints

Indications

- Early morning stiffness causing poor mobility first thing
- Flexion contractures
- Knee pain and active arthritis.

Positioning

- Optimum degree of extension – beware of hyperextension
- Ensure hip is not internally/externally rotated
- Splint extends from above malleoli to three-quarters of the way up the outer thigh (slightly lower on medial side)
- Bandaging a knee splint allows best positioning because it is often difficult to strap comfortably. It can be worn over pyjamas or stockinette.

Regimen

- Alternate splints each night.

Ankle splint

Indication

- Ankle and foot involvement, i.e. active disease or deformity.

Positioning

- Splint extends from below head of fibula and includes the ankle and extends to the toes
- Correct any valgus/varus hind foot deformity
- Neutral forefoot
- Ankle at 90°
- Beware of pressure around malleolus and tibia
- Strapping is fixed at the top of the splint; a figure-of-eight strap around the ankle and a strap over the toes will ensure a good position. Alternatively the splint can be bandaged on.

Regimen

- Alternate splints each night.

Finger splints

A variety of splints is available to treat finger flexion contractures. These include commercially available silver ringer splints and dynamic spring-loaded devices. Therapists can also manufacture their own using gutter-style splints and securing strapping along the phalanges. Three point-pressure designs are also relatively easy to make from light-weight thermoplastic materials.

Serial splinting

When splinting, it may not always be possible for occupational therapists to achieve the desired outcome in one treatment session. Joints should never be splinted in a position that causes pain, and deformities should never be forced. Serial splinting where the joint is gently and gradually stretched over a period of time may therefore prove useful in treating joint contractures. Thermoplastics are ideal when serial splinting because these materials can be remoulded and reused, thus ensuring a cost-effective treatment intervention.

Serial casting

For long-standing contractures that may have been unresponsive to other treatment, serial casting can be used to increase range of movement. This is more permanent than serial splinting and may therefore be useful for those children with poor compliance with splint wearing. Serial casting involves encasing a joint in either plaster of Paris or other casting material for a period of up to 72 hours. Before casting, careful consideration of joint integrity needs to be given. Radiographs should always be reviewed to ensure adequate joint space, and those with ankylosed joints or osteoporosis should not be considered for this procedure.

It is often useful to work with physiotherapy colleagues who may be able to use massage or heat therapy before casting to ease joint stiffness and reduce muscle spasm.

Procedure

A layer of stockinette followed by a generous wrapping of padding is applied to the affected limb and then the child is carefully positioned while another therapist applies the casting material. The desired position is held for 3–5 min until the cast hardens. The cast is then worn for 48 h before being removed and another applied. As progress begins to slow down casts can be left on for slightly longer, i.e. 72 h. Treatment is discontinued if no gains have been made during two consecutive casts.

Precautions

- All bony prominences should be well padded to avoid pressure areas.
- Patients should be advised of emergency procedures if swelling or discomfort arises.
- The correct method of stretching should be ensured to avoid the risk of subluxation; this involves holding immediately proximal and distal to the affected joint.
- Particular attention should be given to the wrist when positioning. If the joint appears to be subluxing, upward pressure should be applied to the carpal bones before extending.
- In between casts, active exercise should be carried out to reduce muscle wasting and the minimisation of flexion loss, which may be vital for functional tasks.

Dynamic splinting

For those children who cannot tolerate a cast, commercially available, dynamic, spring-loaded, hinged splints may prove beneficial. These supply a constant gentle extension force to the joint, but allow active flexion and may therefore be more comfortable to wear. Unfortunately, these splints often prove difficult to fit correctly; considerable teaching and practice are therefore required before prescribing such a splint.

Compliance

Compliance with splinting regimens is variable. To improve compliance rates, it is helpful to look at the results of a recent telephone survey, which considered why children do not wear splints (Hebdon, 1998):

- Uncomfortable
- Difficult to put on and take off
- Lack of understanding of the need for wearing splints

- Too hot
- Appearance
- Need to be altered
- Impractical.

Regular follow-up reviews are therefore vital for ensuring comfort and fit. Involvement of the child during fabrication allows consideration of practical issues, and splints can be designed to facilitate taking them on and off. Finally, the importance of disease education in helping the child to understand their disease and the importance of therapy cannot be understated.

Remedial activities (Table 14.3)

Children with JIA are often given twice daily exercise regimens in order to promote good range of motion and normal movement, with an overall aim of reducing flexion deformities and improving muscle strength, stamina and cardiovascular fitness. As for splinting, compliance with exercise regimens is questionable because JIA is a very time-consuming disease with an estimated 22 hours per week being lost to treatment regimens (Southwood and Malleson, 1993). Occupational therapists, therefore, have a vital role to play in determining a child's particular interests in order to plan appropriate treatment programmes, which will be regarded as enjoyable as well as therapeutic. All activity suggestions should be age appropriate and tailor made to meet the child's physical, social and emotional needs.

Activities of daily living

The occupational therapist plays an important role in maximising function and facilitating independence. In most circumstances, children are taught an alternative compensatory method to complete a task that serves to promote independence and increase levels of self-esteem. Environmental barriers, which may be causing a particular handicap for the child, are also considered and adapted accordingly. In some instances, however, assistive devices may be prescribed for children but perhaps more commonly in teenagers with idiopathic arthritis. Generally, however, this is done less frequently than with adults with arthritis.

Manipulation difficulties

Some children may experience difficulty opening jars, bottles and doors, turning on taps, as well as opening packets and cleaning teeth. This is often the result of poor grip strength. Therapists should, therefore, initially provide a comprehensive treatment programme, which includes

Table 14.3: Activity suggestions

	Young children	Children	Teenagers
Shoulder	Throwing and catching beach ball Painting at an easel Parachute games Bubble popping	Bellow ball Swimming Working at a chalk board Plastic ball and bat games	Badminton Basket ball Kite flying Sketching/painting at an easel
Elbow	Pushing a toy pram Rolling a small ball Play dough Drawing on a wipe board	Pegging out toys on washing line Skittles Plasticine Air hockey	Clay work – rolling for slab pots Juggling Golf
Wrist	Push along toys Stacking games Hand printing Puppets	Catch ball Block printing Jenga Pick-up-stix	Bread making Salt dough moulding Table tennis Yo Yo
Fingers	Finger painting Finger puppets Pop up toys Water play	Subuteo football Cat's cradle Adapted finger draughts Paper weaving	Friendship bracelets Paper quilling Solitaire peg game Badge making Fimo fridge magnet
Strengthening	Popoids Sticklebricks Squeezing toys	Theraputty Water pistols Cutting different paper thickness	Clay work, squeezing for coil pots Ripping paper for papier mâché work Macramé

strengthening the wrist extensors and deviators, the interossei and lumbricals, as well as the muscles of the thumb. Small devices, including tap turners, toothpaste dispensers, large-handled utensils and jar openers, may also be indicated.

Decreased mobility

A bike or tricycle is a great method for improving mobility and encouraging social interaction and independence. However, a major buggy or wheelchair may be indicated. Children are encouraged to maintain a balance between walking and rest.

Bathing and toileting

It is extremely important for children and young people to be as independent as possible in these areas and thus ensure some degree of privacy. It may, therefore, be helpful to install grab bars, and small platforms for those of short stature. Hydraulic bath aids are the preferred option for those children experiencing difficulty getting in or out of the bath. This device allows children to become fully immersed in the warm water and thus enables them to carry out daily hydrotherapy exercises and reduce the duration of early morning stiffness. It also has the added advantage of assisting those children with reduced wrist extension to rise without adopting the often seen compensatory technique of weight bearing on the small joints of the fingers.

Non-slip mats are always useful for ensuring safety with transfers, and long-handled sponges can facilitate independence with washing.

Dressing

Children and parents should be advised that loose fitting clothing is always easier to put on. Difficulty with buttons and laces can always be overcome by the covert use of Velcro. Dressing sticks, long-handled shoehorns and combs may also prove useful in facilitating independence. Socks often pose a particular difficulty for children with hip and knee involvement. Commercially available sock aids are designed for adults; however, they can be cut down to shape and, for those with poor grip, small toggles can be tied to the strings to allow children to grip the strings and pull up.

Kitchen tasks

For older children wishing to participate in household chores, a number of assistive devices may be beneficial. These include perching stools, kettle tipper, Stirex scissors and cook baskets, which reduce the need to lift heavy pans. Independent living skills training may also be useful to help with meal planning, preparation, budgeting, etc.

Feeding

Some children with temporomandibular joint involvement may experience difficulty with chewing. Extra time to eat should therefore be allowed and the re-heating of food may be necessary midway through a meal.

Joint protection

As a general rule children are not instructed to avoid particular activities except in extreme cases, e.g. horse riding in the presence of hip disease or trampolining in the presence of neck involvement.

Children are encouraged to participate in all desired activities because they are usually likely to restrict their own participation. Some general advice is offered, however:

- Avoid long sedentary periods
- Avoid positions that involve the child being in a flexed position for any length of time
- Protect the joints that have arthritis, e.g. do not weight bear through the small joints of the fingers
- Use strongest joints available to perform everyday tasks, e.g. use of backpack rather than school bag
- Recognise limits and rest if necessary.

School

Most children with JIA attend mainstream schools. As children spend a major part of their waking life in school, it is important that occupational therapists appreciate the variety of physical, social and emotional demands placed on them and plan treatment accordingly. A school visit is often necessary to educate the teachers about the disease and the effect that it may have on their pupil: to offer advice on posture and seating, the provision of equipment, the environment, as well as advice about school activities.

Common problems may include the following.

Early morning stiffness

Early morning stiffness, which is a characteristic symptom of JIA, can last a matter of minutes or hours. Although night resting splints can assist function first thing in the morning, an early morning soak in the bath may be required to get joints mobile. It may, therefore, be necessary to arrange for the child to come into school a little later to allow for this regimen.

Gelling

Sitting still for a prolonged period can lead to 'gelling', where the joints become very stiff and lead to discomfort and reduced mobility. Regular stretches throughout the day are therefore important to keep joints mobile. This can be done surreptitiously by positioning the child at the back of the class or by asking him or her to act as a regular monitor, e.g. handing out papers, etc.

Mobility difficulties

In some instances therapists may be involved in arranging special transport to school if it proves difficult with conventional transport.

Mobility around the school may also prove difficult if children are required to walk to different classes, at different ends of the school or on different floors throughout the day. With negotiation it may be possible for all classes to be arranged on the ground floor or to confine them to a particular area of school.

Permission for the child to leave class 5 min early to avoid the crush in the corridors, or have access to restricted areas, e.g. lifts, staff areas, to allow short cuts, can also be requested.

In junior and infant schools children may be allowed to use tricycles to mobilise around schools. For older children, a wheelchair may be necessary. It is important not to become too reliant on wheelchairs, because weight bearing during mobility will facilitate normal growth and development.

Pain/Fatigue

Medications are important for relieving pain. It is, therefore, important for teachers to recognise this and provide an environment where the child feels comfortable in taking his or her drugs. In some instances a child may need to take a rest during the day and so a comfortable room should be available for this purpose. Those children complaining of fatigue should not be forced to go out at break and lunch times. However, they should not be penalised by spending the period alone or doing extra work; rather, by allowing them to stay in with one or two friends, they can enjoy the benefits of peer interaction.

Ensuring a good work posture can also reduce fatigue. This may involve adapting seating to facilitate hips, knee and ankles at 90°; a small wooden plinth under the feet can also help. An angled desktop surface can also ensure good positioning of the neck and back (Figures 14.5 and 14.6).

Carrying difficulties

It is always advisable for students to use a backpack because this will help spread weight evenly and reduce pressure on the small joints of the hand. It may also be possible to duplicate books for home and school purposes, thus reducing the need to carry them back and forth. School lockers are also helpful in storing books and equipment that are not required.

Writing

Children often complain of difficulties writing, especially as the volume of written work increases as they progress through the school system. Splints may reduce wrist pain and fatigue, but dictated answers or extra time is often required to complete examinations and assignments. The volume of work can be reduced by asking for copies of the teacher's notes or by

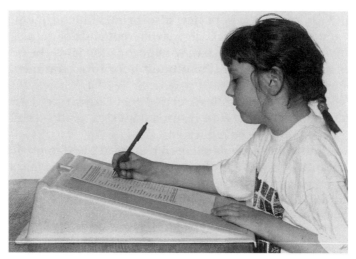

Figure 14.5: Angled desktop surfaces can facilitate good postures and provide a comfortable position from which to work.

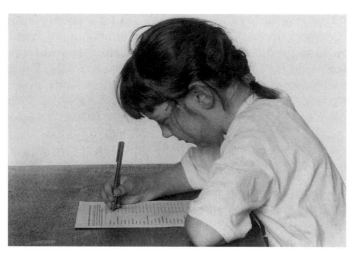

Figure 14.6: Children spending long periods in a flexed position are in danger of developing flexion contractures of the neck.

writing the answers only, rather than the question and answer that is usually required. Larger or rollerball felt pens can reduce the grip required to grasp a pen; however, for some children a compact word processor or PC may be required. These should be used alongside a wrist guard to reduce repetitive strain injuries and regular hand exercises to stretch fingers should be encouraged.

Technology classes

The use of adaptive equipment is often indicated in order to maximise independence in these areas. Seating is of major concern in these classes because high stool seating is usually the norm. Stools with arm and backrests may therefore be necessary or, in some instances, a hydraulic chair that can be adjusted to any height may prove useful for all classroom activities.

Physical education

It is important that children with JIA gain some cardiovascular fitness. Swimming and cycling are therefore excellent activities because they do not require weight bearing. Children should not be barred from PE classes; in fact it is often helpful to consult them about their feelings. If they feel unable to participate, they may wish to be involved with keeping score or refereeing. etc,, rather than having extra schoolwork or sitting on the sidelines.

Very often children can join in and activities can be adapted to meet individual needs, e.g. lightweight balls and bats, having a runner. As a general rule gymnastics, e.g. somersaults and headstands, is not suitable for those with neck involvement, nor is jumping for those with painful lower limb involvement. Contact sports, especially at secondary level, should be avoided for those with more severe or active arthritis for fear of damaging the joints.

Peer relationships

A study carried out by Arthritis Care in 1992 reported that many children with arthritis experience teasing. This may be as a result of their appearance, e.g. cushingoid face as a result of steroid use, deformed joints, splint wearing or waddling gait, or by a perceived notion that they are receiving special attention. It is therefore important for the occupational therapist to help increase the understanding of arthritis in other students. This can be done by providing information, e.g. booklets or a video, or may involve a visit to school to give a talk subject to the child's agreement. Treatment may also be focused on building self-esteem and helping the child deal with unwelcome teasing.

Although in many instances occupational therapists may be able to arrange for the provision of specialist equipment without too much difficulty, in some instances it may be necessary for the child to be statemented (Education Act 1981) to ensure that their needs are being adequately met. Occupational therapists will play a major role in the statementing process.

Pain control

Children may regularly experience pain but may have difficulty expressing it. Using a visual analogue scale, or asking the child to represent pain diagrammatically, may provide the therapist with a good insight into their pain experience (Figure 14.7). This is important because it may be having an impact on the child's affect, motivation levels and ability to perform functional tasks, as well as their learning capacity.

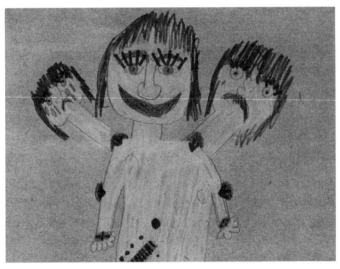

Figure 14.7: This picture shows the personal emotional and pain experience of an 8-year-old child with JIA.

A relaxation technique may prove useful in pain management and a variety of methods should be used in order to meet the child's needs fully. One method that should perhaps be avoided is the Jacobsen progressive muscular technique, which involves tensing and relaxing particular muscle groups, because they may cause muscle spasm in some children and therefore increase pain levels.

Methods of pain control include:

- Teaching deep breathing exercises
- Guided imagery where the child is taught to visualise a calm and tranquil environment in which she feels relaxed and calm
- Simple relaxation which focuses on drawing attention to relaxed postures and positions
- Internal diversion techniques where children can divert their attention to a favourite song, rhyme or poem

- External diversion techniques where attention is focused towards an object in the environment, e.g. a plant or picture
- Creative activities in a calming environment may also have a part to play in reducing pain levels in children with JIA.

Disease education

Children with a chronic illness have a lot to learn about their disease and its treatment. It is therefore important that information is developmentally appropriate for their level of comprehension in order for them to understand it and make use of it in daily life (Engvall, 1996). An understanding of Piaget's stages of cognitive development will therefore serve occupational therapists well. As improved compliance with treatment regimens is the desired outcome of patient education, therapists will find themselves spending a considerable amount of time teaching children if their interventions are to be successful.

Each session should be tailor-made to suit the child's individual needs. Special consideration should be given, not only to their developmental level, but also to their emotional and psychological state. Practical issues should also be considered because time of day, venue, pain, anxiety, fear and denial can all be barriers to effective learning. Teaching should always be interactive and should provide an opportunity for children to take increased responsibility for their disease and facilitate a good adaptive response. Methods of education commonly employed by occupational therapists include the following:

- Informal discussions, e.g. during treatment sessions
- Formal education sessions, e.g. running a group
- Treatment activities including quizzes, adapting commercially available games, e.g. trivial pursuits, making a video/newsletter, etc.
- Role models – inviting young adults who have successfully coped with their disease to events can be helpful in promoting good self-esteem and healthy outlook.

Video

A disease education video for children with arthritis entitled *Kids Like Us*, made by the Birmingham Childhood Arthritis Unit and produced by Yorkshire TV, is commercially available. It stars children's TV reporters and youngsters with the disease, and aims to teach children about arthritis and its management. The advantage of this method of education is that it can be watched repeatedly in the comfort of their own home.

Computer

Interactive computer games have been used to teach children with other diseases including diabetes. A recently developed interactive computer game for children with JIA is currently being evaluated at Birmingham and Coventry Universities.

Various teaching materials are useful in helping children to understand their disease. Interventions should be provided on a regular basis because needs will change. Booklets (ARC), videos and computers are a useful adjunct to interaction with professionals; however, they can never replace them because education needs to be individualised and interactive, and understanding needs to be reviewed.

Adolescence

This stage of development may be a particularly difficult time for those with a chronic illness, who may have to deal with a variety of issues including restricted mobility and dependence on others, deformities, growth disturbance and changes in physical appearance as a result of drug therapy, as well as the normal difficulties of growing up.

Occupational therapists can play a key role in facilitating teenagers to achieve autonomy and functional independence. Group sessions can often prove beneficial for these youngsters because they are able to strike up friendships with 'like others' and provide support for one another. Sessions can include teenage hydrotherapy groups, recreation groups or remedial activity sessions. Life skills training can also be useful. The opportunity to go on trips away from home and participate in activities from which they have previously been excluded is also helpful. Such events may not only be fun but can also encourage taking control of their disease and weighing up the pros and cons of certain actions, e.g. staying up all night versus having a good night's sleep. Creative activities, which encourage self-expression and facilitate positive self-esteem, can be of enormous benefit to this group.

Support agencies

Juvenile idiopathic arthritis affects not only the child with the disease, but the whole family, because they have to adjust to a new way of life which can incorporate regular hospital visits, hydrotherapy, daily medication, exercises and splint wearing. Finances may become stretched and relationships strained. Family outings may become less frequent or dramatically changed to accommodate the child's restricted mobility. Siblings can often be left feeling neglected and it is also not uncommon for parents to report an impact on their own health status.

For this reason, occupational therapists often find themselves providing support for the whole family. However, this can sometimes prove difficult in a busy hospital environment. Other professionals can be called in or advice can be provided about other relevant organisations that may be able to offer badly needed practical, emotional and social support in coping with the disease.

Lady Hoare Trust
87 Worship Street
London EC2A 2BE

Children's Chronic Arthritis Association (CCAA)
Caroline Cox
Ground Floor Office
Amber Gate
City Walls Road
Worcester WR2 2AH

Arthritis Care
18 Stephenson Way
London NW1 2HD

Conclusion

Juvenile idiopathic arthritis is a chronic disease that impacts on many aspects of the child's life. It is the occupational therapist's role to ensure a good adaptive response, which facilitates maximum function and improved quality of life. Although intensive treatment is sometimes indicated, emphasis should be placed on disease management and monitoring, to ensure that the child is empowered to manage her own disease and that her daily life is not regularly disrupted by hospital visits.

Case study

Two brief case studies follow to highlight the occupational therapist's role in JIA. Assessment and interventions are not exhaustive but aim to illustrate some occupational therapy practice when working with this client group.

Katie

Katie is an 8-year-old girl with systemic onset JIA which mainly affects her right (R) knee, left (L) elbow, both hips, R wrist and neck.

She lives with her mother and three sisters in a two-storey council house and attends a special school because of minor learning difficulties. She is independent in toileting, washing and dressing using assistive devices, but is experiencing difficulty getting in and out of the bath.

Katie is presently experiencing some problems at school, and is complaining of difficulty writing and discomfort in her wrist and neck. Mobility is also proving problematic, and she is unable to walk over long distances.

Assessment

Katie is left hand dominant, and has 75 degrees of active wrist range of motion (ROM) and full finger ROM.

She has weak wrist extensors, which are observed when making a fist. She displays a mature tripod grasp but is unable to write for long periods before complaining of fatigue and discomfort.

Right wrist has a flexion deformity with 0 degrees of active extension, and only a few degrees of flexion. On a radiograph there is early evidence of subluxation and minor joint destruction. Functionally, she is compensating for her reduced wrist extension by hyperextending her MCP to 90 degrees when weight bearing. She is unable to register any measurement on a vigorometer for grip strength.

There is pain on all neck movements; however, there is full ROM and poor posture is evident during classroom tasks.

Katie is able to walk with a rollator approximately 25 metres; however, she fatigues easily as a result of quadriceps wasting, and hip pain and stiffness. She is currently being lifted up stairs and in and out of the bath, and has difficulty entering and exiting the house independently.

Aims

1. Increase ROM at R wrist
2. Increase grip strength in R hand
3. Improve knowledge of joint protection techniques
4. Facilitate independent mobility and enable full participation in family activities
5. Facilitate bath transfer
6. Improve access in/out/throughout the house
7. Maximise performance in a class setting.

Treatment

1. Using the technique of serial casting to her R wrist, as outlined previously in this chapter, 15° of active extension was achieved after four

successful casts. These gains were maintained and indeed increased over the following year.

2. Provide active and passive ROM exercises and remedial activities to improve movement. Fabricate thermoplastic wrist working splint after casting to maintain gains.
3. Provide Theraputty and other functional hand activities to increase strength.
4. Advise Katie to weight bear through large joints, ensure good postures and conserve energy.
5. Provide trike for independent mobility around school; prescribe attendant propelled wheelchair for family and community activities.
6. Assess and provide hydraulic bath aid to allow independent transfer and full immersion in the water to carry out daily hydrotherapy exercises.
7. Liaise with city council to provide ramped access and stair lift to facilitate safety and independence.
8. Trial angled desktop surface to avoid prolonged periods of neck flexion and improve overall posture by ensuring good supportive seating and a small plinth to rest feet on, ensuring hips, knees and ankles at 90 degrees.
9. Consider collar for class use only if desktop proves unsuccessful at relieving neck pain. Provide L wrist work splint for use when writing only along with exercise/activity programme. A pencil grip may also prove useful in reducing the amount of pencil pressure.

Eleanor

Eleanor is a 13-year-old girl with extended oligo-JIA which mainly affects her L knee, R ankle, R wrist and index finger MCP, and PIP joints.

She complains of occasional wrist pain; however, her main difficulty is keeping up with her peers when writing. She also experiences difficulty with opening jars, bottles and packages.

Her mother reports some difficulty accepting the disease and an avoidance of particular activities.

Assessment

Eleanor is right hand dominant. She has full active and passive ROM in her right and left wrists. In her fingers she has full ROM in her L, but has only a 90 per cent DIP tuck and reduced grip strength.

In her left knee she has a small effusion. More swelling is also reported at the end of the day. She has a few minutes of early morning stiffness.

She is independent in all self-care tasks, but Eleanor tends to avoid household chores because of some difficulty with manipulation and an over-protectiveness by her parents. Difficulty keeping up with her peers at school is giving rise to some anxiety about examinations and she is complaining of gelling when she rises from her chair. She avoids all PE lessons.

Eleanor is a bright girl and appears to have a good understanding of her disease; however, she has not made a good adaptive response.

Aims

1. Maintain range of movement and increase strength at the wrist
2. Increase grip strength and range of movement in the fingers
3. Increase independence in ADLs
4. Maximise performance in a class setting
5. Provide emotional/social support to promote good adaptive response.

Treatment

1. Provide active and passive exercise regimen for wrist to be carried out before activities of interest, e.g. bread making, sketching at an easel, clay work, etc.
2. Teach passive stretching to encourage full PIP flexion, encourage activities to increase strength, e.g. macramé, clay work, etc.
3. Provide assistive devices if acceptable, e.g. tap turners, jar openers, etc. Emphasise importance of active strengthening. Educate parents as to the importance of encouraging age-appropriate activities, e.g. household chores.
4. Provide general advice to school about the disease. Suggest regular stretches, and a trial of a pencil grip and a wrist splint to increase written output; allow extra time for examinations and assignments. Encourage gradual return to PE classes; adapt activities if necessary.
5. Provide an opportunity for Eleanor to mix with other children with arthritis, e.g. group therapy sessions, teenage holiday camps or independence training schemes. This will provide a network of informal support and will increase self-confidence levels.

An illustration of the benefits of such a training scheme are highlighted in the following written comments from Eleanor's parents:

> Her attitude towards arthritis is now very different. Before the holiday she had not known anyone else with the disease and often asked 'why me', and was very angry about her predicament. After the trip Eleanor felt very lucky, in the sense that her disease was well under control compared to some of her new friends who were suffering more. She has never complained about the disease to me again. She has taken an active role in school sports and has played hockey and netball. I feel that much of her change in attitude is due to the trip.

Acknowledgements

I would like to thank my physiotherapy colleague, Bernadette Johnson, for her helpful suggestions. Thanks also to Jenny Abraham and Carolyn Bardsley, rheumatology secretaries, for typing this work and Mark Shattock for his illustrations.

Chapter 15
Children with acquired brain injury

SUE MIDDLETON AND JO LLOYD

Children with acquired brain injury (ABI) are an enormously challenging and rewarding client group. They demand an extremely flexible and resourceful approach from their occupational therapist.

The paediatric occupational therapist may encounter children with ABI at different stages in their recovery and in a variety of environments. This could be in intensive care, acute wards, rehabilitation centres, special schools, mainstream schools, child and family psychiatric services or in the home. The length of intervention may be short as in intensive care or over many years in the community as the child develops and meets different challenges.

Acquired brain injury accounts for at least 20 000 admissions a year for children aged from 0 to 18, with the majority being boys between 0 and 15. Causes of ABI include accidents (falls, road accidents), non-accidental injury, infections (such as meningitis) or anoxia.

Many of these admissions will be for mild or moderate head injury. Mild injury can be defined as a loss of consciousness between zero up to 15 min with post-traumatic amnesia (PTA) of up to 1 hour. Moderate injuries can be defined as being unconscious for less than 6 h with PTA of up to 24 h. Most of these cases will recover with little or no medical intervention and no significant consequences. This should not be taken for granted, however, and there is evidence to suggest that even mild injuries can impact on cognitive function. It is therefore important that a thorough past medical history is taken of any child referred to an occupational therapist with cognitive or perceptual difficulties.

Severe head injury, which can be defined as being in a coma for longer than 6 h and PTA of over 24 h, usually results in more complex presentations and is the main emphasis of this chapter. This will be referred to as ABI.

After a severe ABI, the child can be expected to move through several stages of recovery. Stage 1 can be said to start with admission to hospital. Most children will be unconscious, unable to breathe for themselves and requiring a tracheostomy and ventilation. They are likely to have other injuries such as fractures or lacerations or to have serious medical problems, as well as increased intracranial pressure. The child will be transferred to an intensive care or high dependency unit and the medical team will be most active at this stage. Neurosurgery and other aggressive interventions and investigations may be necessary.

As the child becomes more medically stable, he or she may emerge from the coma with PTA, and often agitated, sometimes bizarre, behaviour.

Stage 2 is a state of stable consciousness when children are better able to cope with more dynamic rehabilitation. Children in this state usually go through a consistent period of recovery. The medical team will become less involved because the multi- or interdisciplinary team plays a bigger part. The child may continue to be treated on a hospital ward or be transferred to a specialised rehabilitation centre.

Recovery, which initially may be rapid, will start to plateau and the child will move into stage 3 as longer-term residual effects become apparent. At this stage, the child may be resettled into his or her own community. It is important at this stage that the child's residual abilities are integrated into his or her home and daily living situation. Evaluation of the amount of support and suitable educational placement will also be needed.

These stages are defined to help the therapist classify the client, and to aim treatment appropriately – there are no fixed divisions or clear distinctions between stages. Some children will pass rapidly through them all whereas others may take longer or may not progress so far.

As a result of the diversity and complexity of the problems caused by ABI, the occupational therapist needs to take a holistic view, and use of a model is considered advantageous. A model favoured by the authors is the Conceptual Model of Occupational Performance (American Occupational Therapy Association, 1994), which considers clients in terms of performance contexts, performance components and performance skills (Figure 15.1).

Presentation

Each child with an ABI presents differently, with a unique set of strengths and weaknesses. They can have minor difficulties with balance or memory to severe physical, cognitive or communication problems.

Common presentations of ABI are examined below using the Conceptual Model of Occupational Performance.

PERFORMANCE CONTEXTS

Temporal Aspects   **Environment**
Chronological   Physical
Developmental   Social
Life cycle   Cultural
Disability status   Spiritual

PERFORMANCE COMPONENTS		PERFORMANCE AREAS
Sensorimotor components		**Activities of daily living**
Sensory processing		
Perceptual processing	→	**Work/school and**
Neuromusculoskeletal		**productive activities**
Motor	←	
Cognitive integration		**Play or leisure activities**
and cognitive components		
Psychosocial skills and		
psychological components		

Figure 15.1: Conceptual model of occupational performance.

Sensorimotor components

Sensory processing

One teenager described feeling as if a CD was spinning in her head as a way of expressing her confusing sensory information. Some of the sensory processing impairments a child with an ABI can experience are listed below:

- Reduced awareness of light touch, deep pressure and temperature discrimination
- Hypersensitivity
- Altered autonomic control, including increased sweating, hair and nail growth and poor temperature regulation
- Visual impairments including visual field loss, visual acuity, difficulties in binocular vision, blurred vision, paralysis of nerve x, nystagmus, abnormal eye movements and cortical damage
- Auditory impairments include hearing loss and tinnitus
- Gustatory and olfactory senses damaged.

Perceptual processing

Perceptual problems are often noted in a child's difficulties in learning, completing puzzles and playing games. They result from poor awareness of body scheme or body image and visual–perception problems, including reduced spatial awareness.

Neuromusculoskeletal and motor problems refer to a child's changed patterns of movement after an ABI. They can include combinations of the list below:

- Little or no control of one to four limbs, the head or the trunk
- Bilateral involvement caused by the contre-coup effect of trauma (damage to opposite sides of the brain as it is thrown around within the skull), the secondary effects of brain injury, damage to the midbrain or brain stem
- Tone may be high or low; a mixed pattern is common, and tone is often high in the limbs
- Flexor patterning of their upper limbs and extensor patterning of lower limbs
- Strong spasms
- Ataxia
- Primitive reflexes
- Associated reactions
- Fine motor integration difficulties
- Dysphagia (being unable to swallow safely)
- Dysarthria (finding it difficult to speak clearly).

Cognitive components

Cognitive components are a common problem following ABI. Difficulties include:

- Poor awareness of the environment
- Poor awareness of cause and effect
- Information processing difficulties
- Attention deficit
- Memory loss
- Dysexecutive function (problems with planning, problem-solving and monitoring performance)
- Visual–perceptual processing skills difficulties.

Psychosocial skills and psychological components

- Communication problems
- Expressive communication

- Receptive communication
- Written language
- Emotional expression.

Psychological and social skills

Initially the child may show bizarre behaviours such as pulling out the tubes or being physically and verbally aggressive towards the people around them. Difficulties with behaviour may become apparent only as the child regains physical skills and increased independence. Disturbed behaviour can result from frustration in dealing with cognitive or dysexecutive impairments. Depression and grieving often follow as a child comes to terms with any disability and loss.

Common behaviours include the following:

- Agitation
- Increased competitiveness
- Emotional lability
- Socially or sexually inappropriate behaviours
- Passivity
- Impulsiveness
- Lack of initiative
- Low self-esteem
- Post-traumatic stress
- Anger towards others seen as responsible.

Impact on the child's occupation

The effects of an ABI on a child's occupational performance can be multiple, far-reaching and almost impossible to predict. Studies show statistical generalities, but for every generalisation another child will respond with startling differences.

Performance contexts

Age

Until recently, it was widely thought that the younger a child sustained a brain injury, the greater the chance of making a good recovery as a result of neuroplasticity. It seems, however, that children younger than 6 years have worse outcomes than older children. The younger the child, the less acquired knowledge they have on which to build and the more new material they need to learn, often in the presence of cognitive, perceptual and other learning difficulties. Neuroplastic changes may allow transfer of existing functions to other areas of the brain, initially to take over from the damaged area. However, areas in the brain used up in this way may not be available for when they are needed later on in a child's development (known as the crowding effect).

Damage to the young brain may disrupt the acquisition of skills. This is particularly noticeable in children with frontal lobe damage because many frontal lobe functions develop later on in the child's development, causing further difficulties as they grow and develop. A child may respond well to therapy, regain independence in mobility and personal care, but be less able to become socially skilled as he or she grows up. This delay in presentation is referred to as 'growing into their disability'.

Family life

Clinical experience indicates that a strong family unit and family involvement in rehabilitation are indicators of a good outcome for children with ABI; however, the disruption to family life and relationships when a child suffers a severe brain injury cannot be underestimated. Once discharged from a formal rehabilitation environment, performance falls away unless the family has been integrated into the rehabilitation programme.

It is now recognised that a family trying to come to terms with a child after an ABI go through the grieving process. The child they had previously bonded with is now very different, possibly with a changed, sometimes difficult, personality. The family dynamics will be affected if another member of the family is seen to be responsible for the accident.

Sadly, further difficulties for the child can be added if other family members are killed or severely injured in the same accident. The child will have to come to terms with his or her own disability as well as with losing a loved one and possibly having to be placed with part of his or her extended family or with a foster family.

Changes to living arrangements to accommodate the needs of a disabled child may add to disruption and stress for the child and his or her family. The family with a newly disabled child will also suddenly have to cope with an influx of outside agencies and people involved in their life. This will inevitably bring frustrations and resentments and a cold awakening to the limitations of a welfare state that they had had no reason to doubt before.

Many accidents that result in ABI end up with compensation claims going through the courts. This involves revisiting and reopening painful wounds for many years. The effect on siblings should not be underestimated because the sibling they used to play or fight with has changed and now receives all their parents' attention.

It can be seen that the family context of which the child is a part will change in many ways after an ABI, and it is important to acknowledge the influence of this in the approach to the child with ABI.

Performance areas

Activities of daily living

Cognitive, perceptual and physical consequences will impact on the child's ability to perform activities of daily living (ADL). In the medically acute stage, the child will be dependent on others for all personal care needs and in many cases the family will involve themselves in this. As consciousness and control over movement return the child can participate in his or her own care.

A child may demonstrate independence with activities that are familiar and routine, involving automatic and habitual patterns in a structured environment. When this environment is changed, e.g. dressing in the school changing room instead of an uncluttered, organised and familiar bedroom, he or she may not be so independent. Although adaptive equipment may be necessary because of motor limitations, his or her ability to use the equipment may be influenced by cognitive and perceptual dysfunction.

Sequencing difficulties and apraxia will affect the child's ability to complete a task. Swallowing difficulties may influence the child's feeding status and the child may be gastrostomy or tube fed.

Play and leisure

It is recognised that play is fundamental to how a child learns and develops. Leisure activities form an important area of occupation for children and adults. The child with ABI will have impaired access to both play and leisure activities, as a result of cognitive, physical, communicative or social limitations. Furthermore, more especially for the younger child, an inability to play will limit learning and compound any cognitive, perceptual and language difficulties present as a direct result of the brain injury.

Access to community and leisure activities may be difficult as a result of physical limitations or cognitive or organisational problems, such as remembering where and when to go and how to use public transport. Behavioural and social skill difficulties may also affect their ability to pursue leisure activities. Difficulties in attention, learning and memory will result in the child with ABI being more tired and exhausted after trying to overcome these at school. The child may therefore be less able to play or less willing to socialise when the school day is over. He or she is more likely to choose less demanding solitary and passive activities, such as watching TV, flipping through magazines or resting. This becomes a vicious cycle because this behaviour leads to losing contact with peers and further isolation.

School and productive activities

The cognitive, behavioural and emotional sequelae, not to mention any residual physical disability, have a profound effect on a child's school performance, academically and socially. Children with ABI may return to their own school or be placed in a special school or, if placement at home is too difficult as a result of medical and care demands, placement in a residential school may be considered. It is the author's experience that there are few places that are equipped for the special, dynamic and unique needs of the child with ABI.

Studies of ABI have uniformly reported significantly lower IQ scores in children who sustain severe brain injuries than in those with mild and moderate injuries. Memory, perception and cognitive skills facilitate learning, all areas often affected in severe brain injury. These skills enable a child to remember outcomes of behaviours, to learn from imitation and to predict that, if he behaves in a certain way, he will achieve certain consequences. Information processing and problem-solving are therefore affected. This may be observed in a variety of school tasks from reading to just following a timetable.

Attention, an essential component of learning, may be impaired, affecting the ability to learn and build on skills. Pupils may be disruptive because they show difficulties in focusing and sustaining attention, controlling distractibility and generally thinking at a normal pace in the classroom.

Residual physical disabilities will add further to difficulties getting around school, and access to facilities and manipulation and organisation of tools may be affected. Sensory problems will also affect their ability to learn and attend.

The child with ABI will have to expend greater effort to perform cognitive tasks than his or her peers; this again will have an impact or effect on his or her ability to learn.

Interpersonal relationships with peers will be influenced by the child's abilities to compete and play at a high level. Expressive and receptive language difficulties will affect communication. To the child returning to his or her old school, friends may have difficulties understanding or relating to any personality changes that may be evident. Also many children will have had a long period of absence, which not only means they will have lost valuable learning time but that relationships with old friends may have moved on and be difficult to re-establish.

Assessments

A variety of techniques and tools are used by occupational therapists to assess the children referred to them, including functional assessment, interviews, observation and standardised assessment batteries. Identifying appropriate assessment methods for children with ABI can seem daunting because the presentation is often diverse.

Assessment of performance components and performance areas is recommended, using a variety of tools and if possible in a variety of settings, to ensure a holistic picture of the child.

There is limited published information on standardised assessments in use clinically in this field (Rodger, 1994). Age-appropriate tests tend to be designed to assess developmental levels and most require a combination of motor, cognitive and communication skills. Many of the tests designed to assess neurologically impaired clients have few or no normative data for children.

Care must be taken when interpreting standardised assessments completed by children with ABI, e.g. the results of a formal motor ability assessment may suggest significant difficulties with motor planning, which are not reflected in the child's day-to-day life. His or her poor performance may, however, result from another problem such as poor verbal comprehension.

The following standardised assessments are considered to be valuable:

- The Glasgow Coma Scale (GCS) (Jennet et al., 1979)
- Test of Visual Perceptual Skills – Non Motor (TVPS) (Gardner, 1982)
- Developmental Test of Visual Motor Integration (VMI) (Beery and Buktenica, 1989)
- Motor-free Visual Perceptual Test (MVPT) (Colarusso and Hammill, 1995a)
- Test of Visual Motor Skills (TVMS) (Gardner, 1986)
- Bruininks–Oseretsky Movement Assessment Battery (Bruininks, 1978)
- MOVEMENT ABC (Henderson and Sugden, 1992)
- Rivermead Perceptual Assessment Battery (RPAB) (Whiting et al., 1984)
- Rivermead Behavioural Memory Test (RBMT) (some normative data for children available) (Wilson et al., 1985)
- Chessington Occupational Therapy Neurological Assessment Battery (COTNAB) (Tyerman et al., 1986)

Many other assessments are available on the market. When selecting and administering assessments for children with ABI, liaison with speech and language therapists, psychologists and physiotherapists is considered essential.

As children improve, functional assessments become appropriate; assessment of feeding ability, washing and dressing, transferring and mobility, handwriting and playing games will provide the occupational therapist with detailed information about their functional ability, as well as highlighting specific difficulties.

A particularly challenging area is the assessment of problems with executive function. Usually, in assessments, the therapist will provide the activity and the goals, and will control the environment to secure objective and specific results. By its very nature, executive function involves the child's ability to interpret a possibly confusing situation and make appropriate plans for action. A child's performance may vary greatly from one setting to another, and this area in particular requires assessment in a variety of settings.

Use of an appropriate outcome measure is also necessary if we are to justify the cost of our intervention for this client group, particularly as intervention may continue to be required over a number of years and in a variety of settings. The FIM (Byrnes and Powers, 1989), FAM (Granger et al., 1995) and WeeFIM (UDS, 1991) are used by the authors because they are considered an appropriate tool in a strongly interdisciplinary environment, with some comparative data for ABI (Corrigan et al., 1997). The Paediatric Evaluation Disability Index (PEDI) and Barthel Index are also thought to be of value.

It is not always easy to establish maladaptive or non-adaptive occupational performance in the absence of an accurate baseline against which functional changes can be assessed. Anecdotal evidence from parents and school can help.

Ongoing assessment and more formal periods of review are desirable in all occupational therapy intervention, but are of particular importance with this client group where change can be slow or rapid, and will also be affected by the child's development and growth. Ideally assessment should continue periodically after the child has plateaued, even if they are no longer receiving therapy because progress can continue, but also because new problems may become apparent as the child develops and 'grows into' their disability.

Therapeutic approaches

The occupational therapist's role is to enable the child to achieve his or her optimum level of independence in daily living activities. For the purpose of describing intervention, therapy can be divided into two areas: that targeting performance components, and that which targets performance areas. As a result of the complex nature of the problems resulting from ABI, occupational therapy intervention will frequently target performance components and performance areas at the same time, and consideration of performance contexts is essential all the time.

Team working

Whether working in a multidisciplinary team in a hospital or the community, in a rehabilitation setting, school or home situation, liaison and collaboration with an extensive team are considered essential. Each area will have its own local arrangements to suit the resources but, where children are being seen away from a specialist centre, every effort should be made to coordinate intervention from the whole team. Clinical evidence suggests that a child's progress will be most successful if there is true collaboration among health professionals, the child, family and education services.

Where possible, an interdisciplinary team approach is considered beneficial, as a result of the complex needs of the child covering many domains (Figure 15.2).

Good communication between disciplines can ensure continuity of care and extend the therapy day, giving the child the best possible chance of a good recovery.

Treatment planning

Throughout all stages of recovery, treatment planning needs to be holistic. After assessment, discussion with the child and family and liaison with other professionals, the occupational therapist will identify goals. Intervention strategies will depend on the problems identified in assessment, the priorities of the child and the family, the therapy environment, and the theoretical frame of reference employed by the therapist and team. A variety of treatment techniques will almost certainly be required as a result of the complexity of the brain and the impact that problems in one area have on other skills.

The environment in which a child is referred and the anticipated time available for intervention will also impact on the planning of occupational therapy treatment, and the choice of approach. In an acute, short-stay or community environment, the therapist's role is more of an assessor of the child and educator of the family and carers; recommendations have to be straightforward and practical. In an intensive rehabilitation setting, it is more realistic to use approaches that demand a higher level of input to be effective.

Treatment continuum

As the child moves through different stages of recovery it is helpful to describe how the occupational therapist's therapeutic intervention will

PREADMISSION ASSESSMENT Including discussion with child and family and assessment of current abilities	NO → Referral to alternative resources

ADMISSION

ALLOCATION OF KEY WORKER Nurse to liase with family, child and interdisciplinary team	MOVING AND HANDLING ASSESSMENT OF RISK by trained assessors *Usually a nurse and therapist*
INITIAL INTERDISCIPLINARY ASSESSMENT	ONGOING INTERDISCIPLINARY AND PROFESSION-SPECIFIC ASSESSMENT over 2 weeks
INTERDISCIPLINARY TEAM MEETING To identify: ◆ strengths and weaknesses ◆ overall aims of admission ◆ long-term goals ◆ short-term goals *Includes discussion with parents and child*	INTERDISCIPLINARY THERAPY PROGRAMME Programmes for positioning and ADL are set up, carers attend sessions and many sessions involve two or more disciplines to promote continuity of care

INTERDISCIPLINARY TEAM MEETING to discuss progress	Weekly
INTERDISCIPLINARY REVIEW of team goals	Fortnightly
REFERRAL TO / LIAISION WITH community therapists; teachers; carers; family	
REVIEW OF THERAPY PRIORITIES AND TIMETABLE PROGRAMME	Monthly
INTERDISCIPLINARY TEAM REPORT on progress and current problems. Team recommendations	3-monthly
CASE REVIEW includes parents; referring team; community therapists; local teachers; child *as appropriate*	3-monthly

PREPARATIONS FOR PLACEMENT OR SCHOOL REINTEGRATION Co-ordinated by educational psychologist; occupational therapist; teachers; family

DISCHARGE

Figure 15.2: Flow chart to demonstrate interdisciplinary working.

reflect these changes. In stage 1, the occupational therapist, in conjunction with the multi- or interdisciplinary team, is concerned with assessing and treating the performance components, i.e. prerequisites for function such as the sensory and motor areas. In stage 2, the occupational therapist will still be concerned with the assessment and treatment of performance components, especially those that become more apparent as motor and sensory recovery occurs, such as the areas of cognition and perception. Increasing emphasis will be on performance skills involving active practice of such skills, e.g. dressing, washing, eating. In stage 3, as the child's progress slows, therapy focuses more on teaching strategies for adaptive equipment, and techniques to increase independence in performance skills and to compensate for residual inabilities. Treatment emphasis will be more clearly based on community skills, independence at home and integration into an appropriate school. Ongoing assessment is required, and intervention for performance components and performance skills may be needed at any time as the child develops.

Therapeutic intervention

A number of therapeutic approaches have been proposed for effective intervention with many of the difficulties observed in ABI, and it is beyond our remit to discuss these here. We have attempted to summarise the role of the occupational therapist working with these problems, and to highlight the areas of particular relevance to children with ABI.

Treatment of sensorimotor components

The occupational therapist working with children in stage 1 will often be working to increase the child's level of responsiveness and overall arousal through sensory stimulation. This involves exposing the child to a variety of stimuli that target a specific sense, e.g. listening to music, looking at photographs, smelling pleasant and unpleasant smells, etc. There is conflicting evidence to prove that this has an effect on raising arousal. It is, however, often something that the family can be involved in at an early stage.

Certain principles should be observed when carrying out a sensory stimulation programme. Initial observation of behaviour at rest such as involuntary movements, facial movements, etc. will enable the therapist to be more objective in recording responses and emergence from coma. Coma stimulation, where possible, should be carried out after a time of complete rest and quiet to avoid overloading the sensory systems, and to enable optimum responses.

The therapist should see her role as that of sensory regulation not just stimulation because minimising and structuring the stimulation of the environment will also be of benefit. For similar reasons, not all modalities should be worked on in each session. Stimulation should be carried out regularly but for short periods, i.e. 10 min several times a day.

Coma stimulation is not recommended in the presence of raised intracranial pressure. If the child is not yet medically stable, medical opinion should be sought before starting a stimulation programme, and careful monitoring of vital signs should be observed.

Sensory stimulation sessions can be unimodal or multimodal (working on one or several modalities) and can use familiar or unfamiliar stimuli. It should be done in a graded manner, i.e. looking at bright objects or a mirror and getting positive responses before moving on to less distinctive stimuli such as photographs.

Normalising sensory input through kinaesthetic and labyrinth systems, e.g. sitting so that the child can visually perceive the environment appropriately, will also help.

For the children who are slow to recover or diagnosed as being in persistent vegetative state coma, stimulation will become a major focus of treatment. In the authors' experience, the SMART programme developed for adults by Helen Gill, occupational therapist at the Royal Hospital for Neuro-Disability, offers valuable guidelines for working with such children.

As the child becomes more responsive to his of her environment, therapy focuses on skills considered preliminary to function, e.g. visual fixing and tracking which may be in preparation for eye pointing as a form of communication or visual choice making.

Treatment of neuromusculoskeletal and motor components

An understanding of normal development and knowledge of the child's developmental milestones are essential if treatment is to be aimed at the right level. Children with ABI have, until their accident or illness, usually experienced a relatively normal development, and are considered to have the potential to re-learn this normal movement.

In the early stages, positioning and postural control are the key to effective intervention for neuromusculoskeletal and motor components. Along with other members of the team, the occupational therapist may be involved in maintaining range of movement and preventing contractures, particularly in stages 1 and 2. Splinting and positioning equipment is needed, e.g. elbow splints, foot-drop and knee extension splints to prevent contractures. Resting splints may be required to rest and protect low toned hands, or to prevent contracture and stiffness in high tone.

Occupational therapists need to advise on techniques for personal care incorporating passive range movements, and on appropriate positions for functional activity.

Assessment for and prescription of specialist equipment are vital in the early stages, particularly if the child is to be at home, where the level of care and support is limited. Provision of a postural sleep system, such as Symmetrisleep or Chailey lying board, will promote good positioning throughout the night, and may reduce the need for turning, so relieving some of the strain on the child's carers.

Specialist supportive seating is often required. It is essential to consider the child's anticipated progress after a brain injury, and it may be appropriate to use a short-term system before prescription of an expensive, custom-built seat is made. Seating systems need to be incorporated into an appropriate wheelchair, and should be adaptable to meet the changing needs of the child as they progress. Referral to the Regional Special Seating Clinic may be required.

It is also essential to consider the purpose of the chair – to provide mobility and adequate support to promote function, and to influence the child's position, enabling the child to experience and re-learn normal movements and positions. The occupational therapist may be required to give advice to other members of the team on appropriate positions for therapeutic activities, whether a child is more able to work in sitting, prone lying or standing. They may also ask that a specific position be used in play and treatment sessions to promote improvements in neuromuscular control.

As the child progresses, the occupational therapist will incorporate neuromusculoskeletal aims more directly into ADLs, e.g. asking the child to bridge at the hips when dressing the lower half on the bed, to improve control of the pelvic and shoulder girdles.

Treatment of the upper limb focuses on encouraging bilateral activities, re-establishing or changing hand dominance, developing functional grips, and practising handwriting or keyboard skills. Children may be encouraged to work with assistance such as facilitation from the therapist, or using arm rests to encourage the development of normal tone and normal patterns of movement. Splinting may be required at this stage to promote function, e.g. a wrist extension splint putting the hand into a functional position, and enabling the child to hold a pencil.

In stage 3, emphasis moves towards functional independence and compromise may be necessary. A child at this stage may need to use abnormal patterns, which would otherwise be discouraged, in order to achieve function. Teaching adaptive techniques, and providing assistive equipment, such as table-mounted scissors, non-slip mats and pen grips for use in school, becomes appropriate.

Treatment of cognitive components

Attention skills are needed for all cognitive activities, and its importance in intervention cannot be overestimated. Attention is considered to be made up of several different processes.

Levels of attention have been identified:

* Focused attention: our ability to perceive individual pieces of information
* Sustained attention: concentration
* Selective attention: our ability to filter irrelevant information and avoid distractions
* Divided attention: our ability to attend to two tasks simultaneously.

Children with ABI may have difficulty with all of these areas, and in the early stages limited concentration and distractibility are commonly seen in all activities. The ABI patient may need to expend more effort to attend to activities, which is reflected in higher levels of fatigue.

Attention must be improved to allow the brain to carry out more complex processes. Children are often unable to carry out a performance skill despite having the other performance components, e.g. a child may be able to walk well with a frame, or to talk fluently in therapy sessions, but be unable to walk and talk at the same time. In the early stages, intervention will be similar to that for sensory components, targeting visual and auditory attention with single stimuli such as a light or a favourite story. As the child moves into stage 2, intervention should include skills training, functional activities training and strategy training. Skills training is literally practising the skills that we need to use. To improve concentration span, choose an activity that the child enjoys such as a computer game or a favourite story, and work in a distraction-free environment. Gradually increase the time for which the child concentrates, and provide encouragement and positive feedback when they do well. As the child becomes able to concentrate for longer, start targeting other areas of attention – working on two tasks at the same time such as typing and looking at the computer screen – or start to introduce small distractions. Continue to increase the demands made on the child: move from individual sessions to working in small groups and working alone. Try to integrate realistic goals for attention into the child's school environment, e.g. asking the child to concentrate for a short period of time on a favourite subject at school.

There are several memory problems associated with ABI:

- PTA when short-term or everyday memory is not functioning, and the individual is disorientated and confused
- Retrograde amnesia when an individual is unable to remember the events and personal information leading up to the accident
- Explicit memory loss: the ability to remember facts and events, particularly associated with temporal lobe damage
- Prospective memory loss: an individual's ability to act in the future.

All these have a great impact on the child's ability to function independently.

To be most effective, the occupational therapist must introduce the child to suitable memory aids and strategies, and then help the child to learn to incorporate them into everyday life. Internal strategies include techniques such as rehearsal, practising something repeatedly, use of rhymes such as 'Richard of York Gave Battle In Vain' to help remember colours of the rainbow. Forming 'associations' between items to be remembered and more familiar or regular items or events can be helpful, as can creating visual images.

Orientation to the day, place and time should be carried out regularly as soon as the child shows awareness. This can be backed up by making an individual organizer file, which includes a timetable, map and photos of relevant people. External strategies include use of diaries, calendars, lists, notes, alarms and electronic organisers. A wide variety of organisers is available in high street shops, and research is required to choose one suitable for the child's needs and abilities. Electronic organisers tend to be popular among older children, who may otherwise be embarrassed by their need to use external aids. As a child progresses, he or she will require assistance to transfer external strategies into more everyday living situations.

Information processing is our ability to interpret the environment and the sensory information that we receive. The skill of information processing includes perception and sequencing, and our ability to relate what we have just learned to information already received from other experiences. Reduced speed of information processing is common after an ABI, and impacts on all other activities. When asking a child with an ABI to complete a timed formal test, you must consider the probable effects of slow processing on their overall score, while evaluating their abilities in the area being tested. It is thought that information processing improves with improvement in other cognitive skills.

Initially, all activities should be presented to the child in small stages, to promote success and increase self-esteem and motivation. Work should be carried out in a distraction-free environment. The child should be encouraged to use external organisation strategies such as headings, dividers, labels and lists.

As the child progresses, he or she can be taught to break tasks up into stages, to choose a suitable environment and to double check for mistakes.

Analysing the components of many activities will show that they are an appropriate tool for working on information processing, but care should be taken to choose activities that are age appropriate and suited to the child's physical abilities, interests and lifestyle. Following a recipe in cooking, following the instructions to construct a toy or model and using the index to find a place on the map are all examples of activities that can easily be graded to suit a child's current level of ability.

> Chris was a 14-year-old independent teenager used to looking after himself while his mother worked in the evenings, when he was beaten up on his way to school one day and sustained a head injury. Chris made a good physical recovery but had a lot of difficulty with cognitive activities, and was particularly slow at processing information. Chris enjoyed cooking, and wanted to be able to cook for himself when his mum was out. His occupational therapist set up a graded cookery programme, designed to teach Chris cookery skills, at the same time as targeting his ability to process information. In the first week, the occupational therapist bought a pizza, and wrote out detailed instructions for Chris to follow to cook the pizza. The following week, the exercise was repeated, with less detailed instructions and, a week later, Chris was encouraged to add another topping to the pre-prepared pizza. Sessions continued and Chris moved on to be able to construct his own pizza from a bought base and sauce. Towards the end of the programme, Chris was able to choose a pizza from a recipe book, write a shopping list, create a pizza from scratch and serve it to his mum with salad.

Executive function describes how memory, attention and perception work together. Children with dysexecutive syndrome are unlikely to participate effectively in their treatment and to learn the compensatory strategies they need, being unable to monitor their own performance.

Normal development of executive function is thought to be gradual rather than hierarchical; executive skills develop at a simple level, at the same time as attention and memory rather than afterwards, so it is important to consider executive function in all three stages of intervention.

In the early stages, while providing a quiet, uncluttered and structured environment to reduce confusion, children should be encouraged to participate in activities by making simple choices, e.g. being offered a choice of orange or lemonade to drink. In this way, they can re-learn that they can have a positive effect on their environment, practise decision-making, and start to re-develop executive skills. At the same time, children should be encouraged to act, with assistance as required, e.g. hand-over-hand assistance when washing the face. This approach – of encouraging a child to participate in routine and familiar activities – is thought to activate sensorimotor neural loops, to add to the effects of sensory stimulation.

Intervention should include modelling and explanation. Direct intervention from the occupational therapist may involve setting up any activity in which the child may be interested, at a level that will be challenging.

As the child progresses and starts to become aware of his or her difficulties, using interviews or self-rating questionnaires can be helpful. Asking the child to predict his or her ability to complete a task, and how much help he or she will need, can ensure that the child becomes more able to evaluate and monitor performance, and begin to adjust it as necessary. To compensate for a more automatic monitoring process, the child can be taught a list of questions to help him or her plan a course of action, and to problem solve if the actions are not successful. As with the strategies for the other areas of cognitive impairment described above, strategies for dysexecutive function should initially be applied to fun and meaningful activities, before asking the child to apply them to more routine daily living skills.

As children 'grow into' their executive function disability, and fail to develop more mature executive function skills, the need for ongoing monitoring assessment of this client group is important. Some children may experience difficulties in school or social activities several years after their ABI, and may benefit from skills training in executive function at this time.

Psychosocial skills and psychological components

Emotional

It is important, when developing rehabilitation strategies, to address emotional and behavioural problems to asses and identify those that are a result of cognitive, physical or social effects caused by the ABI and to address these in treatment.

Performance areas

Activities of daily living

Most children who regain good motor function will resume independence in basic ADLs such as dressing, washing, continence, etc. More complex tasks of daily life involving problem-solving and planning, such as cooking a meal or making use of community resources, may cause more difficulty.

In the early stages, the occupational therapist can be involved in advising nursing staff on positioning, equipment, moving and handling, and procedures for simple ADL tasks. Incorporating even basic responses into some sort of function, e.g. sniffing the soap before application, eye pointing to which clothes they want to wear that day, etc. will have some value.

As the child begins to recover motor control, he or she can work on performance components as well as daily practice of skills relevant to the disability, age and lifestyle, e.g. a 3 year old would have a different type of dressing programme to a 10 year old. Following set routines, especially in the early stages, can be helpful for recovery of function in such skills as dressing and washing. This should be written down or put down in photographs, so that it can both cue the child and be followed by nursing staff and family in a consistent fashion.

As the child prepares for home, it is important to make the programmes more relevant for his or her home and school situation, and to encourage and practise more problem-solving techniques around personal care issues, e.g. 'if I can't find the soap I must ask where it is'.

The recommendation for the use of assistive devices must bear in mind the child's physical and cognitive abilities in using them. Regular practice of practical skills such as cooking is helpful in both developing executive skills and teaching independence. Planning the meal and analysing the activity with the child are important parts of this process. Community skills, such as shopping and using the library, are also tasks that involve many cognitive and executive functions and therefore need considerable planning and practice.

A referral to the social services occupational therapist should be made as early as possible if any physical disability or any adaptations or equipment needs are envisaged as a result of the length of the process of getting such things.

School skills

Most children who have suffered an ABI will need to return to an educational setting. If special needs are identified, the child should be statemented under the 1981 Education Act and the occupational therapist can make a valuable contribution to this. Recommendations the occupational therapist may advocate from her unique knowledge of the strengths and difficulties of the child could be:

• One-to-one classroom support: the learning and behavioural difficulties of the child who has made good motor and language recovery, especially if he or she is young, are not always recognised immediately. Therefore 1:1 support is not always a recognised need until later, when problems are becoming obvious and causing secondary problems such as behaviour difficulties caused by frustration. Evidence suggests that early 1:1 classroom support can be effective and withdrawn later on. It may need reinstating at certain periods such as transition to secondary school.

- Flexibility: it is important that a flexible approach is adopted where possible. Shorter days, rest periods, limited amounts of homework with more time to complete, smaller teaching groups and even learning strategies, such as more concrete approaches and the use of task analysis to help problem solve, may all be valid recommendations.
- Equipment, ramps, rails and other devices may be necessary to enable the child to access the school curriculum. Positioning the child will be dependent on motor, visual and auditory limitations, but may also have to take account of attention and how distractible the child is.
- Task modifications: this could include how material is presented, how much print is on the page, etc.

It is important to work on classroom competencies, as outlined above, as early as possible.

To write in school, hand dominance may need to be re-trained and specific perceptual problems may need to be remedied. In the author's experience, the 'Write from the Start' (LDA, 2000) programme has been found to have value.

Strategies to cope or low-tech assistive devices to accommodate difficulties can be given. When written recording will be too slow or difficult to be practical as a result of physical, cognitive or perceptual problems, the use of high-tech devices should be considered. The Switch Clicker Plus program has been found to be particularly helpful for children with severe physical difficulties. Referral to external agencies for advice such as the Advisory Centre for Education (ACE) is advised.

Strategies to help with effective reading can be taught in conjunction with speech and language therapists and teachers. The strategy SQRRR (Survey, Question, Read, Recall and Review) can be helpful where memory, language or speed of processing reduces a child's ability to read meaningfully for schoolwork.

The cognitive skills and strategies described above should be integrated into the skills needed for learning in the classroom and coping with the school day as soon as possible. The training and use of site maps of schools, etc. are effective in helping children get to where they are going. The monitored and well-planned use of friends to help cue where and when they should be at different places may also be useful.

Play and leisure

The ability to access play and leisure are important aspects of the child's life, aiding learning and enhancing quality of life; the occupational therapist will be involved in facilitating independence in these areas.

Adapting toys to enable access can be done in a high-tech or low-tech manner. The use of switches to access toys and computer use is well practised with a range of disabilities, including children with ABI. Switches can be attached to toys to enable simple 'cause-and-effect' play, as soon as some consistent voluntary motor movement is observed. Technical help may be needed to make a custom-made switch where voluntary movements are limited, e.g. raising an eyebrow, turning the head. Adapting favourite toys can be very rewarding.

Switches may be added to computers for children who lack the manipulative skills to use a keyboard and a mouse, along with the appropriate software such as Switch Clicker Plus.

Other toys may be adapted in more low-tech ways to enable children to access them, by making them easier to hold and stabilising them with non-slip mats or customising building blocks out of foam to make them lighter, e.g. according to the child's needs.

The effect of the ABI on the development of play should be considered. Developmental guidelines have been found to be helpful to follow when working with young children with ABI.

Older children need to develop skills in leisure pursuits and to learn strategies to use their time constructively. Children with significant residual problems may need to be introduced to new hobbies and interests, where their disability will have less impact on their ability to play and compete with peers. Often, favourite hobbies can be pursued, with a child taking part in a new capacity, such as score keeping. Children are often highly anxious and benefit from practising skills at home or in therapy sessions before trying them out in front of their friends. More complex activities will need to be broken down, with each part being practised to develop skills and increase confidence before the whole task is completed. For other children who have limited self-evaluation skills, practice and preparation in therapy may help them to establish more realistic goals, and avoid 'failing' in front of their friends.

Mark was a keen ice-skater before his accident, and enjoyed playing ice hockey for his local leisure centre. Having made a good physical recovery, Mark's main problems were balance and coordination, along with memory and dysexecutive function. Mark expected to be able to return to ice skating straight away, but his parents were anxious that he would fall and hit his head. Therapists were concerned that Mark would attempt too much too soon, and skate badly in front of his friends whose opinion Mark valued highly. Mark was persuaded to practise on roller skates, initially requiring two therapists to support him. With daily practice, his balance quickly improved. Ice-skating lessons were set up for Mark, who was then encouraged to teach his younger sister, reinforcing what he had learnt. The rules of ice hockey were introduced to sessions working on memory, and Mark was asked to describe games to improve his speed of processing. Mark regained the ability to ice skate well on his own, but continued to find the speed of ice hockey very hard. He now goes to his local club for practice sessions, and writes a review of the games for the newsletter instead of playing in competitive games.

Conclusion

Children with an ABI present with a unique set of problems that require an occupational therapist to use all the skills developed in training. The integrated nature of the strengths and weaknesses, problems and assets that present after a brain injury are challenging and exciting. Good communication with everyone involved, including the child and the family, as well as other professionals, is essential if the child is to reach his or her full potential. A wide range of therapeutic approaches may be helpful and possibilities for therapeutic activities are almost endless. Progress and improvements are hard to predict, but a holistic and integrated approach will provide a child with the best opportunity to regain independence, and enable occupational therapists to use their own skills to their full potential.

Chapter 16
Children with developmental dyspraxia

SIDNEY CHU

Developmental dyspraxia is a specific developmental disorder in which a child presents deficits in the conceptualisation and planning of motor acts. There is inconsistency in the use of this diagnostic term. Some professionals use it to describe a child with general motor impairment; others use it more specifically for children whose difficulties in motor execution are a result of poor praxis, especially in the processes of ideation and motor planning. Throughout the years, in various parts of the world, many terms have been used by medical, educational and psychological professionals to describe a child with specific problems in motor organisation, e.g. clumsy child syndrome, minimal brain dysfunction, perceptual–motor dysfunction, sensory integrative dysfunction, motor–learning difficulties, developmental coordination disorder and developmental dyspraxia.

Clumsiness in children is estimated to affect between 2 per cent and 15 per cent of the population and affects more males than females (Gubbay, 1975; Cratty, 1986; Henderson, 1993; DSM-IV – APA, 1994). In the UK, it is believed to affect around 10 per cent of the general population, with 4 per cent having significant difficulties. These ranges of prevalence reflect diverse theoretical positions and different interpretations that have characterised both the descriptive and empirical literature in the field (Missiuna and Polatajko, 1995).

Although there is agreement on what developmental dyspraxia is in general terms, consensus is difficult to find when it comes to specifics (Miller, 1986). Clinically, it is important to make an accurate diagnosis so that appropriate intervention can be provided to remediate the underlying causes of a child's difficulties in motor organisation. As there is a lack of consistency in the use of the term 'developmental dyspraxia', this chapter attempts to describe this childhood syndrome characterised by impaired conceptualisation and planning of skilled movement, and present current approaches to the assessment and treatment of these deficits.

Historical perspective

The description of subtle motor difficulties in children, not associated with frank neurological deficits, dates back to the early 1900s. Cermak (1985) suggested that the concept of developmental dyspraxia has been documented since that time. In the 1970s, the term 'developmental dyspraxia' was introduced in occupational therapy literature (Missiuna and Polatajko, 1995). Ayres (1972a), who originally used the term 'developmental apraxia', later expressed a preference for the term 'developmental dyspraxia' (Ayres, 1979, 1985) to describe the problems of children who are slow and inefficient when formulating a motor plan and executing skilled and non-habitual motor tasks. Gubbay (1975) defined the dyspraxic child as a clumsy child whose ability to perform skilled movement is impaired despite normal intelligence and normal findings in conventional neurological examination.

The Child Neurology Society (David et al., 1981) appears to have been the first group to attempt to distinguish developmental dyspraxia, a motor planning disorder, from a motor execution disorder that they labelled developmental maladroitness (cited in Missiuna and Polatajko, 1995). Cermak (1985) and Sugden and Keogh (1990) further reinforced this concept to differentiate different forms of motor dysfunction. They considered that any use of the term 'dyspraxia' should reflect observable difficulties in planning or conceptualising motor acts. In 1994, in the 4th edition of the *Diagnostic and Statistical Manual of Mental Disorders* (DSM-IV – APA, 1994), the term 'developmental coordination disorder' (DCD) is used to diagnose children with specific motor difficulties. In 'The London Consensus' Statement (Fox and Polatajko, 1994), a descriptive and clearer definition of DCD is provided, minimal requirements for assessment are outlined, and comments and suggestions on identification and intervention techniques are discussed. It recommends that the term 'DCD' should be used as a key word in all publications in order to facilitate interdisciplinary review and discussions.

However, it does not mean that the term 'DCD' should be used to label a child with either motor planning dysfunction or motor execution dysfunction. Missiuna and Polatajko (1995) examined different empirical literature and found that the four terms used most frequently to describe developmental motor problems in children – clumsy child syndrome, developmental dyspraxia, sensory integrative dysfunction and developmental coordination disorder – are not interchangeable. Miyahara and

Mobs (1995) proposed distinguishing developmental dyspraxia from DCD. Clinically, therapists have distinguished between the uncoordinated child and the dyspraxic child. The former appears to know how to approach a task, but seems to be clumsy in the execution, whereas the latter has difficulties in formulating the idea of what to do in planning a sequence of actions for a task (Cermak, 1985).

What is developmental dyspraxia?

The term dyspraxia is derived from the Greek word 'praxis' which means 'doing, acting, deed, and practice' (Safire, 1989). The word 'developmental' indicates that the problem begins early in the child's life and affects his development as he grows, and is not the result of a specific insult or injury (Ayres, 1979). Understanding of developmental dyspraxia could be enhanced by examining the concepts of praxis and the underlying processes involved.

What is praxis?

The concept of praxis is largely based on the knowledge derived from the studies of acquired apraxia in adults. As with many other developmental disorders, developmental dyspraxia has a presumed, but as yet unidentified, neuroanatomical substrate, which may reflect different anatomical and/or functional abnormalities from those associated with the identifiable lesion underlying acquired apraxia (Morris, 1997). Praxis is a uniquely human skill requiring conscious thought and 'enabling the brain to conceptualise, organise, and direct purposeful interaction with the physical world' (Ayres et al., 1987). It is the ability by which an individual figures out how to use his or her hands and body in skilled tasks such as playing with toys, using tools (including a pencil or fork), building a structure (whether a toy block tower or a house), tidying up a room or engaging in many occupations (Ayres, 1989).

Components of praxis

Ayres (1979, 1985, 1989) describes three components of praxis:

1. Ideation: the ability to grasp the idea or concept to allow purposeful interaction with the environment, i.e. knowing what to do.
2. Motor planning/programming: the ability to plan and structure a purposeful, adaptive response. It entails knowing how to move, sequence and predict the end result, i.e. knowing how to do it.
3. Execution: the ability to carry out the planned sequence of actions for a task in a smooth process, i.e. how to complete it successfully.

Ideation and motor planning distinguish praxis from other basic neuro-motor functions. Execution is not likely to be the major source of difficulty in children with dyspraxia, but it is only in the execution of a motor act that the quality of ideation and motor planning can be observed.

The concept of developmental dyspraxia

Cermak (1991) defined dyspraxia as difficulty in planning and carrying out skilled, non-habitual motor acts in the correct sequence. It is not a primary problem in motor coordination (motor execution), but rather the problem is hypothesised to result from difficulty in formulating a plan of action. Dewey (1995) proposed a neuropsychologically based definition that developmental dyspraxia is a disorder in gestural performance in children whose basic motor skills are intact, i.e. unable to imitate different postures or actions for a task.

Ayres (1972a) suggested that 'if the information which the body receives from its somatosensory receptors is not precise, the brain has a poor basis on which to build its scheme of the body'. She consistently hypothesised (Ayres, 1972a, 1979, 1985) that the body scheme is critical to the ability to motor plan, and that processing of tactile as well as proprioceptive information is of critical importance in the development of an adequate body scheme, which in turn forms the foundation for the development of praxis and perceptual functions. Ayres (1985) further suggested that the main problem of dyspraxia lies in the neural activity that takes place before motor execution is begun. Although dyspraxia is sometimes viewed as an output disorder because the motor component is more observable than the sensory component, it is actually a dysfunction of information integration and planning rather than of the motor system (Goodgold-Edwards and Cermak, 1990).

Although our understanding of normal praxis development is quite limited, it is appropriate to presume that it is contingent on the integrity of many other functions outside the motor domain, such as attention, perception, memory, and conceptual and linguistic abilities. Thus, deficits in other cognitive domains are more likely to be present in a developmental disorder (Morris, 1997). McConnell (1995) reviewed four distinct perspectives on the causes of clumsiness: neuropathological, visual perceptual, kinaesthetic processing and motor programming. He suggested that occupational therapists need to consider all these four perspectives when assessing children with coordination difficulties.

Cermak (1985) and Morris (1997) list different aetiological theories of practic dysfunctions proposed by different researchers between the 1930s and 1990s, e.g. dysfunction of the left parietal lobe (Orton, 1937), alternation of typical cerebral mechanisms (Reuben and Bakwin, 1968), under-stimulation of an otherwise intact network as a result of faulty input pathways (Gubbay, 1975), delay and/or incomplete development of cerebellar functions (Lesny, 1980), etc. In terms of neurological level of function, dyspraxia could be classified at two levels (Chu, 1998a) resulting from:

- a specific deficit at the higher cortical function, especially the concep-tual–organisational level of motor functions, or
- inefficient subcortical functions in integrating different sensory infor-mation to enhance the development of body scheme for motor planning, i.e. sensory integration.

Diagnosis of developmental dyspraxia

Diagnostic criteria

The condition 'developmental dyspraxia' has been used to represent a single and recognisable entity. Whether or not such a condition can be isolated is far from clear because there is still no universal set of diagnostic criteria that could be used. Most often, exclusionary criteria are used, e.g. in the absence of primary deficits in other sensory, motor or cognitive functions. For example, Gubbay (1975, p. 39) stated that:

> The clumsy child is to be regarded as one who is mentally normal, without bodily deformity, and whose physical strength, sensation, and co-ordination are virtually normal by the standards of routine conventional neurological assess-ment, but whose ability to perform skilled, purposive movement is impaired.

There have been ongoing arguments on the use of intelligence quotient (IQ) as one of the criteria for the diagnosis of developmental dyspraxia. Gubbay (1975) stated that the single most important diagnostic criterion of dyspraxia is a significantly lower Performance IQ than Verbal IQ score (usually considered to be a 15-point discrepancy) on the Wechsler Intelligence Scale for Children – Revised (WISC-R). However, clinical experience indicates that not all children with dyspraxia meet these criteria, e.g. a child with concomitant specific language disorders and dyspraxia might manifest lower Verbal IQ than Performance IQ scores. Dawdy (1981) stated that 'it is probably unrealistic and theoretically restrictive to assume normal or near normal intellectual capacity as a diagnostic criterion'.

Cermak (1991) makes the following comments:

Can we consider a child with mental retardation to be dyspraxic? The child with a learning disability is typically delayed in all areas. When the delays in motor planning are consistent with the child's cognitive and motor development, the child would not be considered to be dyspraxic. Furthermore, delays in motor performance are not necessarily indicative of poor motor planning. Therefore, a child is considered to be dyspraxic if (a) motor deficits are due to poor motor planning and not poor motor skills, *per se*, and (b) the motor planning deficits are significantly below his or her performance in other areas.

The following descriptions are the primary clinical features of developmental dyspraxia which could be used as the basis for making diagnosis:

- Poor praxis, especially in the process of ideation and motor planning which in turn leads to poor motor execution.
- Poor praxis may be related to deficits in the integration and discrimination of tactile and proprioceptive information, or could be related to a higher cortical dysfunction, especially in the left cerebral hemisphere.
- Average general intellectual capacity, with Performance IQ lower than Verbal IQ if there are no other concomitant conditions.
- Immaturity of body scheme and awareness.
- May have visual–perceptual and auditory–perceptual dysfunctions.
- Poor spatial skills in two-dimensional and three-dimensional orientation.
- Poor perceptual–motor integration, e.g. visual–motor skills, auditory–motor skills.
- Poor postural–motor functions, e.g. weak muscle tone, poor postural control.
- Poor functional motor skills, e.g. bilateral integration, sequencing, rhythm and temporal awareness.
- Delay in the development of laterality/dominance with inconsistent use of body parts, e.g. hand, foot, eye and ear.
- Poor fine motor skills, including poor in-hand manipulations.

The above underlying dysfunctions will cause different secondary clinical features described later in this chapter. As a result of the nature of co-morbidity with other conditions, a child with dyspraxia may have the following associated clinical features:

- Poor fundamental motor skills, e.g. hopping, skipping, riding a bicycle, ball skills, etc.
- Soft neurological signs, e.g. associated movements, poor diadochokinesia, etc.

- Minor neurological deficits, e.g. overt associated reactions, mild tightness of muscles/tendons, mild positive signs in eliciting stretch reflex by fast passive movement of elbow.
- Articulation deficits.
- Minimal delays in attainment of early developmental milestones.
- Behavioural patterns associated with other co-morbid conditions, e.g. attention deficit hyperactivity disorder (ADHD), high functioning autism/Asperger's syndrome, semantic–pragmatic disorders, etc.
- Hyperreactivity to sensory inputs, associated with sensory modulation disorders.

Differential diagnosis

Differential diagnosis is complicated by the increased prevalence of several other specific developmental disorders in children with dyspraxic features. Clinical experiences indicated that children with more severe dyspraxia tend to overlap with children who have ADHD, high functioning autism, Asperger's syndrome and tic disorders; children with mild-to-moderate dyspraxia may present concomitant specific language disorder and specific learning difficulties (dyslexia).

Studies of children with specific learning difficulties have demonstrated an increased incidence of dyspraxia (Cermak et al., 1980; Lennox et al., 1988; Deuel and Doar, 1992). However, attempts to link dyspraxia to a specific pattern of cognitive deficit have not been successful. Both verbally and non-verbally impaired, learning-disabled children exhibit problems with praxis, but these two groups could not be differentiated on a battery of tests specifically designed to assess several distinct mechanisms underlying praxis. However, a careful examination of this group of studies does provide some preliminary support for the notion that all dyspraxic children are not alike (Morris, 1997). Studies of children with speech and language disorders (Aram and Horwitz, 1983; Cermak et al., 1986; Archer and Witelson, 1988; Dewey et al., 1988; Thal et al., 1991) have found an increased incidence of limb dyspraxia. It is consistent with the findings in adults with left-hemispheric dysfunction, i.e. apraxia and aphasia. It also further reinforces the theory that the left hemisphere has an important role in the development of both auditory–language skills and motor planning function.

In the motor domain, it is difficult to draw a boundary between the child whose motor dysfunction falls at the mildest end of the neuromotor dysfunctions and the most severely affected dyspraxic child who may exhibit subtle motor findings on neurological examination (Denckla and Roeltgen, 1992). Although a neuromotor dysfunction, e.g. mild abnormality in muscle tone, interferes with precise execution of specific motor acts, practic dysfunction interferes with the organisation of functional behaviour in a broader sense. It impedes the person's conceptualisation of how to organise action effectively (Parham, 1986). Morris (1997) states that the number of empirical studies that have assessed praxis in a population of children selected for the presence of documented developmental motor deficits is quite small. Those studies identified have used diverse measures for selection, encompassing both gross and fine motor behaviours; they have often failed to describe adequately the specific selective criteria employed and have rarely provided data about the range of co-morbid diagnoses in their samples. These factors hinder efforts to replicate findings and to integrate information across studies.

Even though developmental dyspraxia may occur concomitantly with other handicapping conditions (e.g. cerebral palsy, learning disabilities, sensory impairment, emotional and behavioural dysfunctions), or environmental influences (e.g. cultural difference, insufficient/inappropriate instruction, psychogenic factors), it is not the direct result of those conditions or influences.

Effect of developmental dyspraxia on the development of learning and behaviour

Skilled motor behaviour is essential in many aspects of life. The development of motor functions influences intellectual, social and emotional development (Holt, 1975; Rosenbloom, 1975; Gelman, 1978). The link between motor and cognitive functioning seems to be an indirect one (Williams, 1983). Motor functioning, through its emphasis on and concern with the development of sensory and motor processes associated with active movement and physical exploration of the internal environment, probably provides the basic foundation for the development of a higher-order information-processing system upon which more sophisticated perceptual and cognitive processes can ultimately be built. Social and emotional development is facilitated by an interaction with others through the complex skills of gesturing, playing and speech. It plays an important role in the development of self-concept and self-confidence. Gallahue (1982) discussed that a child who moves with ease and performs motor tasks skilfully tends to have confidence in him- or herself and builds a positive self-image.

Developmental dyspraxia may pervade many aspects of a child's life, making it difficult for the child to perform adequately at home, in school and in social settings. Unfortunately, as these children generally do not look handicapped, the expectations placed on them by caregivers, teachers, peers and siblings may be unrealistic. The following descriptions of secondary clinical features result from the primary clinical features discussed before:

- Clumsy or awkward in movement, frequently bumping into things, dropping things, tripping and falling, sustaining more than his or her fair share of bumps and bruises.
- Constantly needs to think about planning movements, thus presents moments of hesitation in between tasks.
- Difficulties in organising approach to tasks, in solving problems and adapting behaviour to new or unexpected situational demands, in analysing task requirements and components, and preparing for actions and learning new and unfamiliar tasks. However, once they are learnt, he or she will be able to perform tasks, but be unable to generalise them into other similar situations.
- 'Talking' through the tasks, i.e. uses verbalisation to assist the planning of actions.
- 'Watching' others in order to formulate the ideas of what to do and model the plan of actions.
- Delays in acquiring skills in activities of daily living, especially those requiring motor planning, perceptual analysis and fine motor manipulation, e.g. tying shoe laces.
- Difficulties in developing mature and efficient manual handwriting skills.
- Low self-esteem and avoidant behaviour when faced with situations in which motor planning and skills are essential.
- Secondary emotional/behavioural difficulties as a result of repeated episodes of failure, teasing and social rejection by peers.
- Poor attention control, fidgety and overactive behaviour resulting from different primary deficits.

Evaluation of developmental dyspraxia

Evaluation is the planned process of gathering and interpreting objective/subjective and quantitative/qualitative data necessary for making a diagnosis, selecting appropriate treatment methods and planning treatment programmes with stated goals and objectives. Accurate diagnosis of the processes underlying dyspraxia depends on therapists selecting appropriate assessment tools and using informed clinical reasoning for interpretation (McConnell, 1995). The question must be asked 'Why assess?'. The answer, quite simply put, is 'to diagnose in order to remediate' (Thomson and Watkins, 1990). Early identification of this specific developmental disorder is important, to provide intervention and to prevent the development of subsequent difficulties. The evaluation process is also important to make a differential diagnosis in order to ascertain the child's condition and to choose the most appropriate treatment approach.

The recognition of signs and symptoms of dyspraxia also varies according to the child's age, because developmental dyspraxia manifests itself differently at different times in development, and according to the range of behaviour that different clinicians or educationalists are assessing. Typically, a child with developmental dyspraxia will be assessed by a paediatric neurologist or consultant paediatrician in order to ascertain the diagnosis, identify any co-morbid diagnoses, and eliminate any other medical conditions that may also contribute to the child's presenting clinical picture. Then the child should be referred to different professionals for further assessment and treatment. Occupational therapy is one of the primary services for children with developmental dyspraxia.

Preliminary assessment

The 'art' of assessment really focuses our attention as one looks at a number of attributes that contribute to the successful motor organisation of a child, e.g. when a child presents with problems in balance, coordination and a range of other motor organisational difficulties, the therapist may choose to review the events surrounding pregnancy, labour and delivery, and the acquisition of early developmental milestones. This type of history-taking endeavour may illuminate any number of potentially pathological events, which may have been responsible for the observed motor organisation difficulties. After this or coincidental with it, the therapist may observe the manner in which the child speaks and moves, and the posture that he or she adopts in an attempt to eliminate any presenting signs or symptoms of a particular form of neuromotor abnormality, e.g. mild cerebral palsy. Then, the therapist may perform an assessment of practic functions in which standardised tests could be used.

Use of standardised tests

Skilled motor behaviour can be assessed at two levels, either in terms of the different tasks or activities that constitute the motor repertoire (i.e. task-oriented approach), or in terms of the processes that underlie motor behaviour (i.e. process-oriented approach) (Laszlo and Bairstow, 1985). The process-oriented standardised tests are usually based on underlying models of motor function and on theories that causally link sensory, perceptual and cognitive deficits to motor dysfunctions. One of the most comprehensive process-oriented standardised tests designed to identify practic dysfunction is the Sensory Integration and Praxis Test (SIPT) which was developed by the late Dr A.J. Ayres, occupational therapist, in 1989. The SIPT is described in Chapter 7.

Besides the SIPT, there are many other standardised tests that focus on the assessment of motor skills, i.e. task-oriented approach, e.g. the Bruininks–Oseretsky Test of Motor Proficiency (Bruininks, 1978) and the Movement Assessment Battery for Children (Henderson and Sugden, 1992) are commonly used by paediatric occupational therapists and physiotherapists in the UK. It is important to note that these tests do not include measures of praxis. Thus, in order to use the results of these tests appropriately, therapists need to be able to make an observational assessment and to interpret the information with respect to the concepts of praxis and dyspraxia described previously.

Observational assessment

The three components of praxis – ideation, motor planning and execution – should be addressed during evaluation. Ayres (1985) distinguished between those children who have difficulty with the idea or conceptualisation of the action and those who have the idea but have difficulty planning the action. She suggested that the child with difficulty in ideation will also have difficulty with general organisation. Parham (1986) suggested that observation of motor activity is basic to evaluating all three processes. She provided the following suggestions:

- Ideation can be difficult to assess because there are no objective tests for evaluating this construct and it is highly inferential. One of the best ways to evaluate this ability is to observe the way that a child plays spontaneously with toys and therapeutic equipment. It is particularly revealing to observe what is done with novel equipment that the child has never seen before.
- Sometimes a child will have an idea of what to do and may be able to express verbally the desired action, but cannot organise body parts to execute the action effectively. The child may have a problem in motor planning.
- The child may be able to motor plan a specific task in one situation, but, when presented with a similar task in a different situation, the child is not able adequately to organise a response.

Ayres (1985) stated that, when problems of motor execution are observed, the therapist should analyse the possibility that difficulties are the result of either poor ideation or limited motor planning. Motor execution can also be impeded by a neuromotor involvement such as abnormal patterns of muscle tone, tremor, choreiform movements and primitive reflexes. If present, the impact of these should be assessed. More detailed evaluation of neuromotor problems can be initiated if necessary.

Treatment of developmental dyspraxia

Treatment planning

After determining the dyspraxic child's remedial needs, reasonable decisions can then be made pertaining to the intervention that would best fit this information. Intervention should be holistic, client centred, multifaceted and individualised to meet the unique needs of each child. The case therapist should set goals of treatment with parents, teachers, other professionals involved and possibly the child. Specific treatment objectives should be established as stepping stones in achieving the goals. The objectives selected should be achievable, observable, measurable and proven to be important from the child's perspective.

Example of goal

• To improve Peter's motor planning function in order to enhance his quality of movement and efficient organisation of self for effective participation in school and home activities.

Examples of objectives

• To demonstrate the ability to generate a sequence of ideas for action, Peter will physically or verbally communicate three ideas for play or work activities without cues.
• To demonstrate the improved ability to plan and carry out movement, Peter will assume two postures that involve movement of only one arm or leg, within 5 seconds of demonstration.

Treatment approaches

Therapeutic activities should be selected and integrated into the child's daily routine within different natural environments, e.g. school and home. A holistic treatment programme should incorporate a spectrum of treatment approaches (Mosey, 1993). No matter which approach the therapist adopts, the realistic remedial plan for the dyspraxic child may employ various treatment strategies, programme formats, and treatment style and techniques, depending on the nature of the child's motor impairment and other variables, e.g. the type of training of the therapists. The following approaches of treatment may be used concurrently and/or sequentially (Mosey, 1993; Chu, 1998b).

Remedial approaches

Remedial approaches emphasise facilitating the improvement of underlying processes, e.g. improving practic function in a child with dyspraxia. It is diagnostic–prescriptive in nature. Treatment planning is based on a diagnosis that results from the assessment of processes underlying motor skill performance. In essence, this approach assumes that adequate skill performance depends on the integrity and integration of the child's sensory, perceptual, cognitive and motor performance components. There are many different approaches employed by a therapist to overcome a child's motor organisation difficulties. Each approach has a basis for its theory and practice, and is usually targeted at a specific problem or to general sensorimotor integration. The most common remedial approaches are:

- Sensory Integrative Therapy (Ayres, 1972a, 1972b, 1972c, 1979; Fisher et al., 1991).
- Sensorimotor Therapy, i.e. the application of sensory integrative theory into a perceptual–motor programme (Fink, 1989; Scheerer, 1997).
- Neurodevelopmental Treatment on Postural–Motor Control (Magrun, 1989, 1990; Blanche et al., 1995).
- Perceptual–Motor (Kephart, 1960; Getman, 1965; Barsch, 1968).
- Movement Education such as Laban (Thornton, 1971); and (Frostig, 1982).
- Visual Perceptual Training (Frostig and Horne, 1973; Todd, 1993; Schneck, 1998).
- Fine Motor and Visual–Motor Skill Training (Levine, 1991; Berry, 1993).
- Cognitive–Behavioural Therapy (Reinecke et al., 1995; Graham, 1998).

Functional approaches

Functional approaches emphasise facilitating mastery of tasks, e.g. specific motor skills training, practice of handwriting skills, etc. Strategies to develop functional skills are particularly important for an 'older' child with dyspraxia because remedial work may not be available as a result of restricted criteria of service delivery in some occupational therapy departments. It is also important to equip the child with adequate skills to cope with the demand in different learning and daily activities. Recent research studies have demonstrated that training in specific functional skills is sometimes more appropriate for some children with developmental dyspraxia. For example, Polatajko et al. (1995) compared the effectiveness of a process-oriented treatment approach (i.e. increase the kinaesthetic performance) with a traditional or general motor approach and with no treatment in a randomised clinical trial of 75 children with developmental coordination disorder. The data suggest that these children do not improve spontaneously, and that their motor problems are very resistant to treatment. The data also suggest that an appropriate treatment strategy might be one that involves direct, repetitive training of a specific skill.

Examples of functional approaches are:

- Perceptual–motor programmes and movement education (emphasise developing specific motor skills) (Gilroy, 1985, 1989a, 1989b).
- Training on functional handwriting skills (Olsen, 1980; Alston and Taylor, 1988; Laufer, 1995).
- Self-care skills training, e.g. tying shoe laces (Klein, 1983; Christiansen, 1994).
- Social skills training (Cartledge and Milburn, 1980; Spence, 1980; Stephens, 1992).
- Task analysis and behavioural techniques in developing specific functional skills (Christiansen, 1994; Watson, 1997).

Compensatory approaches

Compensatory approaches emphasise minimising the effect of underlying deficits in areas of functional performance, e.g. using different colour codes to classify lesson files, using a checklist to help the child follow each step of a task, etc. Examples of compensatory strategies are to:

- teach coping strategies and study skills
- use IT equipment to compensate for weak functional skills, e.g. use computer for written work
- use specific strategies to compensate for perceptual dysfunctions, e.g. use colour code to indicate orientation or categorise materials
- set appropriate level of expectation
- allow more time to complete a task.

Adaptive approaches

Adaptive approaches emphasise changing the task, or aspects of the environment, to minimise the effect of underlying deficits, and/or related behaviours, in areas of functional performance, e.g. reducing the amount of written work. Examples of adaptive techniques are:

- modification of the National Curriculum
- modification of the environment, e.g. reduce unnecessary sensory stimulation from the environment
- use of adaptive devices or tools, e.g. adjustable furniture, pencil grip, etc.

- adaptation of a specific task, e.g. for a child with handwriting difficulties, teacher could reduce the amount of copying tasks or put main points or headings on a piece of paper.

Management approaches

Management approaches emphasise minimising distressing or disruptive feelings and behaviour so that the dyspraxic child is able to deal more directly with primary problems, e.g. psychological support, praise/reward, social skill training, etc. The therapist may provide considerable therapeutic benefit by providing an explanation for the child's presenting problems, helping to build up the child's self-esteem by providing appropriate physical, psychological, emotional and social support. Examples of management approaches are:

- promoting the understanding of the child's problems
- consultation with teachers, parents and others
- use of the motivational approach – intrinsic and extrinsic factors
- reinforcement programme, e.g. token economy, star chart, praise/ rewards
- direct intervention towards preventing secondary psychosocial– emotional complications.

Maintenance approaches

Maintenance approaches emphasise preserving and supporting the child's current level of function, in a protected environment, e.g. use of high-power IT equipment for a dyspraxic child who has extreme difficulty in manual handwriting skills. Clinically, maintenance approaches are not commonly applied to this care group. The therapist should devise an effective treatment programme by integrating relevant strategies for different service provision approaches described. Examples of maintenance approaches are to:

- recommend for participation in community-based recreational, fitness and social activities
- emphasise the child's strength and interests
- reassess and ongoing monitoring of changing needs.

Case study

Tom is an 8-year-old boy with problems in coordination and behavioural organisation. He was referred to occupational therapy by the school doctor because his teacher and parents expressed concerns about his development and also his performance in different learning tasks. He is described as being clumsy in movement. He has difficulty in catching and throwing a ball, and participating in different team games in the PE lessons. He has poor body balance and is described as accident prone. He also has difficulties with poor fine motor skills, including pencil control and handwriting.

Evaluation

An occupational therapy evaluation was carried out by using the following assessment procedures:

- Clinical Observations for the Evaluation of Sensory Integrative Functions (Chu, 1993)
- Sensory Integration and Praxis Tests (SIPT) (Ayres, 1989)
- Goodenough–Harris Drawing Test (Harris, 1963)
- Handwriting Checklist (Chu, 1999)
- Parent's questionnaire (non-standardised assessment developed in the Department)
- Teacher's questionnaire (non-standardised assessment developed in the Department).

Tom attended three 45-minute assessment sessions with his mother. He was friendly, cheerful and cooperative in all three sessions. He was able to maintain fair attention throughout all the assessment tasks. He presented difficulties in following a sequence of instructions. A school visit was carried out to observe his behaviours and performance within the classroom and during playground time. Results of all the assessment procedures indicated that he has the following underlying dysfunctions and performance difficulties:

- Poor somatosensory perception in discriminating different tactile and kinaesthetic information.
- Poor praxis functions with low scores in the Postural Praxis Test, Oral Praxis Test and Constructional Praxis Test of the SIPT.
- Mild deficits in his postural control (i.e. inadequate supine flexion posture), bilateral integration and sequencing functions.
- Immature performance in drawing a human figure, possibly indicating a poor body scheme or awareness.
- Problems in different gross and fine motor skills, including handwriting skills.
- Difficulties in acquiring certain self-care skills, e.g. using knife and fork, tying shoe laces, etc.

Information from both teacher's and parent's questionnaires, observation during assessment, within classroom and also during playground time provide the following additional information:

- Prefers 'talking' to 'doing', tends to talk to himself when doing different motor tasks.
- Often late and forgetful, needs a lot of help in organising himself in the morning.
- Described as having a disorganised approach to tasks.
- Has difficulty in learning new movement activities in PE lesson.
- Uses inefficient ways of doing things; tends to take excessive time for a task.
- Has difficulty in following a sequence of instructions.
- Problems in peer group interaction; unable to join in group activities in playground. Prefers to play with younger children.
- Low self-esteem and poor self-concept.
- Easily frustrated; avoids new situations.

The overall interpretation of the data suggested that Tom has somatodyspraxia, which affects his performance in different learning and daily activities, including interaction with peers within a social environment.

Intervention programme

An occupational therapy programme with stated goals and objectives was planned in conjunction with Tom's parents and teachers through a meeting in school. The programme consisted of the following components:

- Weekly individual sensory integrative therapy treatment sessions for 6 months. This aimed to enhance Tom's somatosensory processing functions and developed his postural–motor control, bilateral integrative functions, motor planning and sequencing functions by using different sensorimotor activities.
- Structured therapeutic programmes were prescribed to be integrated into classroom and home environment. These aimed to improve his gross motor skills, fine motor skills, handwriting skills, and those self-care skills that require motor planning and bilateral integrative functions.
- Therapeutic handling in developing his coping strategies, social interaction and also his organisational ability, e.g. organising himself in the morning.

- Participating in different extracurricular activities without a strong competition component, e.g. swimming, playing badminton with the family, etc.

Progress

After 6 months of intervention, Tom showed steady and good improvement in his underlying functions and performance in different learning and daily activities. His parents and teacher reported the following changes:

- Tom is much more confident with himself in doing different new activities. He is more readily participating in team games.
- He has established good relationships with several children in the class. They invited him to their birthday parties and involved him in different playground activities.
- He is able to tie shoe laces and can use a knife and fork competently during meal time.
- He also shows improvement in his handwriting skills though further training on his quality of writing is necessary.
- He can follow a structured daily routine and organise himself accordingly.

Further occupational therapy input will concentrate on generalising and extending his gains into different environments and situations of demand. Advice will be given to his teacher to improve Tom's quality of writing in the areas of directionality, spacing, levelling and relative size in letter formation.

Conclusion

It is important to note that the emergence and development of the concepts of developmental dyspraxia are seen in dynamic, gradually evolving terms. An attempt has been made to narrow down discussion of dyspraxia as a primary dysfunction in the process of ideation and motor planning. The contemporary concepts on the diagnostic criteria, evaluation procedures and intervention approaches are presented in order to provide therapists with a comprehensive view regarding this specific childhood condition. Therapists should use the information presented to make a differential diagnosis, identify any co-morbid conditions and devise a relevant treatment plan.

Unfortunately, valid and reliable data regarding the efficacy and efficiency of intervention techniques with dyspraxic children are almost non-existent. Serious faults have been identified in several poorly designed research studies carried out in the UK recently, e.g. inappropriate use of diagnostic and selection criteria, lack of appropriate knowledge in the subject matter, use of splinter skill training as treatment medium, lack of randomisation and a control group, and also invalid use of outcome measures. Unjustifiable claims made by these researchers have misled the general public and also raised concern within the professional field. Morris (1997) states that treatment efficacy research has been greatly hindered by the absence of clear diagnostic criteria for this disorder. Advances in understanding the causes of developmental dyspraxia and in knowing how to intervene effectively are contingent on our ability to address these diagnostic issues successfully. Therefore, professionals from different backgrounds should work together to come to a consensus on the diagnosis of developmental dyspraxia.

Chapter 17
Children who have been bereaved

SHONA COMBEN

Death is a universal experience which will affect everyone at some time in their life. This may be the death of a pet, friend or close relative. However, it is an experience that cannot be planned or prepared for, even if the death is preceded by a long illness. There is no way we can practise coping with feelings of loss and pain – feelings for which there is no easy explanation and seldom any speedy resolution.

As death is so unknown yet inevitable, it has become one of the last taboos in today's society. Many adults avoid discussing death with children because of their own anxiety about it and may substitute glib explanations in the hope of avoiding any distress to the child.

Children come home from school to find their hamster has subtly changed fur colour, which Mum and Dad insist is what happens to hamsters sometimes. If they are actually told that the hamster has died, they are immediately reassured that it is really very happy to have gone for a long sleep, or to live in the clouds with Jesus. It is understandable that parents wish to spare their children pain, but these explanations can cause confusion and some unusual responses in children who later experience the death of a close relative.

When we combine the taboo about death as it affects us directly with the endless images of real and fictionalised death portrayed on television, this leads to some unusual and idiosyncratic ideas about death in the minds of children.

A child's concept of death is subject to many variable external factors as well as to their own cognitive development and idiosyncratic understanding of events. Case studies, as in Krementz (1988) and in my own clinical experience, suggest that even very young children grieve, but this grief is different from that of adults in some aspects and may be hard for whoever is caring for a child at such a difficult time to understand. Boyd-

Webb (1993) suggests that there are four fundamental considerations that differentiate the grief of children from that of adults:

1. Their cognitive immaturity interferes with their understanding of the irreversibility, universality and inevitability of death.
2. They have a limited capacity to tolerate emotional pain.
3. They have a limited ability to verbalise their feelings.
4. They are sensitive about being 'different' from their peers.

It is worthwhile thinking about these differences and their possible effects on children at different stages of cognitive development.

Very young children between the ages of 2 and 7 years (Piaget's 'pre-operational' stage) are still egocentric and involved in magical thinking (Piaget, 1969). They are essentially unable to differentiate between thoughts and deeds and may wonder if their own anger was in some way responsible for the death. They are unable to understand that being dead means gone forever and may, although apparently accepting that Daddy has died, at the same time cheerfully expect him to come home for supper. Even if they are given the opportunity to view the body, they may wonder how the person will be able to breathe in the coffin and whether being buried will hurt.

Young children, by repeating the phrases used to explain the death to them, can sound as if they have a mature understanding of what has happened, only to reveal some time after the event that they have not really understood at all. One 3 year old surprised and distressed his mother 6 months after the death of his father by saying casually in the car on the way home from playgroup 'as it's such a nice sunny day, let's go and get Daddy back from Jesus this afternoon'.

Older children aged 7–10 years (Piaget's 'concrete operational' phase) have an improved capacity for reasoning and understanding. Their natural curiosity may lead to them asking questions in an attempt to clarify ideas that they have about death. They may wonder about ghosts and skeletons and struggle to relate these images to someone they love.

Understandably, some of their questions may be distressing for the adults to respond to and the predicament children find themselves in is how to gain accurate information about what has happened, without causing distress to the adults around them at the time. The reverse of this is that some adults, believing children should be told the truth, may not phrase their truth sensitively. The question 'what does cremation mean?' requires a kinder and more thoughtful response than 'it means burnt'. The loss of a body that once held and cuddled them lovingly can be acutely painful to some children and their developing understanding of the concept of the future makes the knowledge of their loss even greater.

Despite this, children at this stage of cognitive development may be able to put their grief aside for all or parts of every day and get on with the essential business of growing up. This too can lead to problems. I often encounter parents and teachers who tell me that they suspect a child is feigning sadness because they can run about and be happy at playtime and only start getting upset when given a page of maths to do. I can identify only too readily with someone who gets upset when given maths to do, but it seems possible to me that a bereaved child may welcome the release of running around as usual with their peers in the playground, but feel deeply upset 5 minutes later in class when faced with some work that may remind him that, for example, Mum is no longer at home waiting to help him with his homework.

Prepubertal children aged 9–12 and adolescents are more logical and capable of understanding complicated concepts such as being in the grave and in heaven simultaneously (Lonetto, 1980). They have an awareness of mortality and may be thinking about ideas to do with spirituality and life after death. Anger may be a more common feature of their bereavement process, coupled with fears about their own future development. They may be more aware of the practical implications of the death of a parent, such as financial restraints and other life changes. For this group of young people, the fear of being different from their peers may lead to them finding it hard to talk about what has happened outside the immediate family.

Client group

Not all children who experience bereavement require professional help to cope with it and most families find that in time they are able to adapt to a life without the loved one.

Increasingly, however, children are referred to child and adolescent mental health services after the death of a parent or sibling, especially if the death has been particularly traumatic or unexpected. I am not sure why this trend has arisen and wonder sometimes if it is symptomatic of a culture where there is a developing belief that all pain and suffering can be avoided if only the 'right expert' can be found.

In the clinic where I work, our advice on talking to children about illness and death was sought by the Macmillan nursing team, which has led to an increase in referrals of families who are coping with terminal illness. Not all of these families wish to attend the clinic either before or after the death, but find it helpful to be able to make telephone contact from time to time when they have particular anxieties about their children and want to talk things over with us. I think this is a sensible use of our service and it has the additional benefit of helping the remaining parent feel that he or she is still capable of resolving his or her own problems and difficulties.

Not all deaths are known about, and children who are referred for behavioural or mood disturbance may have underlying bereavement issues that come to light only during a routine initial assessment.

It is important to remember that loss impacts not only on the child, but on the entire family and this impact can compound the loss in a way that leaves the child feeling very vulnerable indeed. I have often been told by children that it was bad enough when Daddy died, but what makes it worse is that Mummy never laughs or smiles any more.

Sometimes referrals are made for teenagers whose behaviour is causing concern. Assessment reveals that the child's natural parent died many years before and the surviving parent has subsequently remarried and perhaps had more children with the new partner. Having lived happily as a new family for several years, it is particularly distressing for everyone to have to readdress the earlier loss that has surfaced in the adolescent's quest for his or her own adult identity.

It is generally accepted that the death of a parent or sibling can have serious consequences for children if they are unable to express and work through their grief at the time of the loss (Fox, 1985). However, everyone, young or old, grieves in their own way and in their own time and the difficulty for carers is to identify a normal grieving process in their children when they are themselves in a vulnerable emotional state. It is tempting for friends, teachers or health professionals seeing the remaining parent's bewilderment and distress to suggest that the child may benefit from therapy when what the child and the family actually need is support and loving understanding from those around them.

In making an assessment of the need for professional intervention, we must take account of the disabling effects of the bereavement and the degree to which it intrudes into the everyday life of the child.

Assessment

Before embarking on therapy it is important to make a detailed assessment of the identified child and the family to ensure that therapy is the most appropriate response to the referral.

Most families prefer to resolve their own problems and it can add to the remaining parent's distress if they feel that, in addition to everything else, they can no longer meet their children's needs. One young widowed mother who was referred to our service 3 months after her husband's death was particularly distressed because she and her husband had planned what to tell their children about his impending death and had even chosen his funeral hymns together, yet despite their careful and loving planning she had 'ended up in a place like this'. It felt like the ultimate betrayal of her husband's memory to have to seek outside help with one of her son's overwhelming anger at the loss of his father. It is important to hear and understand this sense of failure and reassure people that there is no way that feelings can be controlled by rehearsal or forward planning, however willing everyone is to cooperate with the idea that they might be.

The assessment should take place in a comfortable environment free from interruptions. A selection of age-appropriate toys, paper and crayons or felt pencils should be available, as well as an easily accessible box of paper tissues. I find it helpful to outline at the start how much time we have available and offer to give both parent and children time to talk alone if they would like it. I acknowledge that they have come to see me because something very upsetting has happened in their family and invite one of the family to tell me a bit about it if no one feels able to tell me what has happened. I go on to tell them that I have had a letter from their doctor/health visitor who says that they have all been feeling very sad because their mummy/daddy/gran died just before Christmas/during the school holidays (using a time reference which is meaningful to even the youngest child present). I then ask 'what happened?'.

This simple question nearly always prompts everyone to begin to tell me about the death, from their own perspective. Often the adult may interrupt to correct the child's apparent misconceptions and I try to reassure them that I am interested in what the children believe as much as in the true facts. Being invited to tell their story and being quietly listened to is an important part of the process of building a therapeutic relationship with the family. Many of their friends and family find listening to their sadness too hard to bear and rush in with platitudes and unwelcome advice, unwittingly adding to the burden for the family of 'being different'.

In the course of listening carefully, much of the information you need can be gathered.

- What is the cultural/belief system about life and death in this family?
- Do they have a religious belief?
- How did the family hear about the death and how were the children told?
- Is the story straightforward or are there concealed secrets and anomalies?
- Did everyone have an opportunity to say goodbye, either before or after the death?

- What sort of funeral service was there and were the children involved in planning it?
- Were they allowed to attend/not attend the funeral and what did they make of the experience?
- Does anyone have any ideas about why the death happened, e.g. 'those doctors were no good', or 'if I hadn't insisted on having a lift to football club the accident would never have happened'?
- How is what has happened affecting each family member now, e.g. disturbance of sleep, mood, appetite or relationships?
- How do people cope? What has been particularly helpful/difficult?
- How do they remember the person who has died?
- Extended family members or friends may become more intimately involved with the family after the death. How helpful/irritating is this? For example, a widowed father told me how supportive his parents had been after the death of his wife during the birth of their second child. He really valued and needed their help, but felt guilty because he knew how much his wife had disliked their old-fashioned approach to child rearing, and how angry she would be about some of the restraints they placed on his 4-year-old son.
- How supportive and understanding are other agencies, e.g. school, church?

For many families, the opportunity to sit down together and talk about what has happened and how everyone is feeling about it can be a great relief and they may feel that no further intervention is necessary. When this happens, I usually offer to keep the file open for a further 3 months or offer a review appointment some time in the future so that they will not feel too disappointed if difficulties recur and they have to seek another referral. I also explain that sometimes children need further help as they mature and their understanding of events develops.

Treatment

There are a variety of treatment options for working with bereaved children. The choice of the most appropriate must be based on a careful assessment of the presenting problems, the family's current situation, and an awareness of the child's cognitive and emotional development and present needs. In urban areas, group work may be an appropriate and viable therapeutic option, but in smaller communities it may lead to an unacceptably long wait for help.

Bearing in mind children's limited capacity to verbalise their feelings, I have found play therapy the most helpful approach with under-10s. Older children and adolescents are more likely to benefit from talking therapy. For all age groups, it is important to meet regularly with their carers to review progress and avoid them feeling shut out of the therapeutic process. It is often helpful to provide a therapist for the adult as well, both to help with their own needs and to advise on the effective management of the child's behaviour. Many people find it difficult to retain the usual boundaries and constraints around children's behaviour after a bereavement (S Comben, 2000, personal observations). They are aware of the child's upset feelings and they feel sorry for them, but it can be frightening and disorienting for a child to lose a parent and in addition feel uncontained by the adults around. This can be compounded if the adult who has died was usually the one who disciplined the child.

With parental permission, it is helpful to make contact with the child's school. Teachers often handle a bereavement for one of their pupils very well and are sensitive to the child's needs at a difficult time. However, they sometimes need reassurance that they are doing the right thing, and usually welcome advice and discussion about the child's identified needs. Attending therapy sessions may well interrupt the child's school day and the staff may feel that the school is left unsupported to deal with further upset after each session. Sometimes teachers are reluctant to tell the parent when a child is upset in school because they don't want to add to their burden. It is common for a child's school performance to deteriorate after a bereavement and it can be hard for teachers to decide when and how to do anything about this. Consultation with the family, school and therapist can help everyone feel involved and committed to providing the right sort of support at this difficult time.

Whatever the presenting symptoms, it is important to recognise that the underlying cause is likely to be issues to do with the bereavement and to reassure the child and their family that these are the sort of symptoms that occur when children are feeling upset, e.g. anger is one of the most common presenting symptoms and can be very distressing for everyone, especially if the child has previously been even tempered. It can also be one of the hardest symptoms to treat – after all, any child deprived of a parent by death has a right to feel very angry indeed! It is usually helpful to acknowledge this and make a few suggestions for externalising anger in a way that will not cause hurt to either the child or anyone else. However, it is important to recognise that the anger is only a symptom and try to find ways of helping the child express the thoughts, fears and anxieties that are troubling him or her.

Play therapy is an established treatment for children and one that I have found particularly helpful with bereaved children. It is hard for young children to express themselves verbally and it can be even harder for them to talk about something that raises such powerful emotions in everyone. Play therapy is a way of helping children express some of the thoughts and ideas that may be troubling them. As with counselling for adults, being listened to and feeling that one is understood often helps clients to resolve problems themselves. Children express themselves in words and actions. Often they will unconsciously play out their worries and fears, and a trained play therapist can help them to think about the problems they uncover and work on some solutions.

Although it is important that the parents do not feel excluded from the process, it is often easier for the children to share their concerns with someone who will not get upset by the things they want to explore, or be shocked by the sort of questions to which they need answers.

Lowenfeld (1979), who pioneered sandplay with children, said 'children have many ideas and experiences in their heads which won't go into words and even if they did, they seem to be the sort of ideas that people don't talk about'. Death is certainly the 'sort of idea that people don't talk about' and I have found the use of Lowenfeld's techniques of immense value in my work with young children.

The playroom should be equipped with all the usual essential equipment for play therapy – paper, crayons and paints, toys, dolls and puppets, dressing up clothes, clay or playdough, sand and water, as well as a home corner or doll's house. Interestingly, I find children often begin to explore ideas about death by burying objects and then figures in the sand. This can lead to discussions about some of the confused and painful ideas they have been holding on to – examples of this are illustrated in the following case studies.

Many children, like adults, fear that they will forget their loved one and need help to do their remembering. Towards the end of therapy, I encourage children to create a 'memory book' which they can take away with them and keep for ever. Memories can be stimulated by direct questions about bedtime routines or funny things that happened and also by family photographs. It seems to be particularly helpful for children to be reminded that their memories can always be accessed and that these memories, though sometimes painful, can also be very comforting.

It is important to remember that there is no cure for bereavement and the powerful feelings it arouses. It is probably not wise to engage in long-term therapy because a bereaved child has already suffered enough disruption to his or her normal life and needs to get on with that life as soon as the worst of the symptoms that led to referral have abated. Nevertheless, ending therapy is another loss that must be dealt with sensitively. I try to maintain contact on a regular but increasingly less frequent basis, until the child and the carer feel that they are once again able to cope.

It is not uncommon for children who have received therapy after bereavement to return later in their childhood when they have reached a new level of cognitive understanding.

Case studies

James

James was brought to our service by his distraught mother only a few weeks after the death of her husband. At the time of his father's death, James was aged 2 years 3 months. The presenting difficulty was James's disturbed sleep pattern. His mother described how he would wake every night screaming 'hysterically' for his daddy, and lashing out with his fists in a way that made it impossible for her to get close to him to offer comfort. He would scream and thrash around in his bed for hours at a time before falling into an exhausted sleep, while she sat in a corner of his room feeling powerless, ineffectual and overwhelmed by her loss.

James had been born after his parents had been married for several years. At the time of his birth his father was 56 years old and had given up hope of ever being a parent. He took great delight in James, getting up early every morning to bathe and change him and taking charge of the bedtime routine when he returned from work. James's mother had found late parenthood more difficult than her husband. She was a career woman in her mid-30s when he was born, and she was grateful for her husband's enthusiasm and more than willing to let him do as much caring for James as he wanted. His sudden death in an accident at work left her with parenting tasks with which she had never been involved before and unsure how she would manage in the future. In addition to the screaming at night, James was determined not to let his mother out of his sight and clung to her every minute he was awake.

Our first task in helping James and his mum was to help mum feel more effective as a parent and try to ensure that they both got a little more sleep to help them cope with the days. We acknowledged mum's sense of helplessness, but pointed out how James clung to her all day because he needed her. We suggested that she ignore his struggling and lashing out at night and try to hold him firmly, perhaps rocking him and singing to him as she did so, until he fell asleep. Initially she was sceptical, but returned the following week to say that it had been very effective and had additionally been a great comfort to her. With James in a more settled sleeping pattern, our next task was to help him separate from mum for brief periods of time so that she could have some respite from his constant demands. She had a good friend with a child of a similar age living nearby who had offered to look after James, to allow mum to have some rest periods, but had so far been unable to accept this offer of help because James became so distressed by any attempt at separation. From James's point of view, it was perfectly reasonable that he held on to his mum, after all, dad had suddenly disappeared and he couldn't be sure that mum might not do the same.

I began by engaging James in play in the room where a colleague and I met with his mum. Over a short space of time, James gave up holding on to mum and began moving more freely around the room, inviting me to join in his play. Although he was too young to have any clear idea about what had happened to his father, he always chose to play with the rescue vehicles or to play hide and seek games with toys in the sand tray.

After only a few sessions, James agreed to let his mum go into the room next door with her therapist while he remained in the playroom with me. Initially he needed to check regularly that she was still there, but increasingly he became involved in his play and was able to separate from his mum. He was soon able to carry this experience over into his home life and spend some time with mum's friend, allowing her some much needed respite.

Within a few months, James and his mum were settling down to a new routine without dad. As James developed speech he asked questions about his father and where he had gone to and it was a great relief to his mother to know that James wouldn't grow up without some memories of his dad – James was the child I quoted earlier in this chapter who wanted to go and get his daddy back from Jesus. His mum told me this story when she telephoned to ask whether I thought it would be all right for her to show James holiday videos of his dad, because she found them such a comfort. Having said this, she paused and said that on reflection James might want to go and get daddy back from holiday too, so perhaps she would leave it for a few years. I felt that was a sensible decision.

I recently met James's mother in town and she stopped me to tell me that James was now a big, bold 6 year old who had settled well in school and was interested in 'all the usual boys' stuff'. She was not only coping, but relishing her role as his mum and had found a part-time job to fit in with his school hours.

Liam

Liam came to the Clinic accompanied by his mum, dad and maternal grandmother. The presenting problems were his difficult behaviour, sleep difficulties and fear of the dark. He had been seen by the behavioural therapist for the initial assessment, but referred on to me because his parents were sure that all Liam's problems stemmed from the death of his maternal great-grandmother 2 years previously. At the time of referral, Liam was 6 years 2 months old.

During my assessment, I observed that Liam was a generally non-compliant child, but none of the adults seemed to make much of an attempt to insist on compliance. Both mum and gran were still grieving for the great-grandmother and wept when they spoke about their sense of loss when she died 'so unexpectedly' of a chronic heart condition aged 87. Throughout this conversation, Liam looked anxious and dad said very little. Mum told me how very close Liam had been to his 'Nanna' and that she had been the only member of the family who could get him to do as he was told. The request for help had been prompted by a recent episode of misbehaviour which had resulted in Liam being sent to his room. While there, he had written 'I miss my Nanna' on a piece of paper and brought it down to give to his Mother. She had let Liam off his punishment and gone to her GP for advice. Dad felt that Liam would benefit from firmer handling, but was prepared to concede to mum's anxieties about bereavement issues. When seen alone, Liam was not very forthcoming. He had good memories of Nanna and worried about gran and mum being upset so much. He agreed to come and see me for some individual play therapy sessions and these were duly arranged.

At the first session, Liam chose to play in the sand tray. He moved vehicles around the tray and began to add trees. Having done this, he formed a mound in the sand and drew a cross on it. Next he removed the vehicles and began to stroke the mound gently, making sure it was smooth and tidy. As he did so, he began to talk about visits to Nanna's grave. He disliked these visits because, although it was nice to go and think about Nanna, mum and gran always cried and that made him feel upset. He added that he knew that Nanna wasn't really in the grave anyway. I asked him where he thought Nanna was and after a long pause he replied in a low voice that gran said she had gone to live in the light. I wondered aloud what that might mean and Liam rolled his eyes up towards the ceiling. It transpired that Liam had interpreted this adult remark in a literal sense. He believed that somehow his Nanna was living in the light and felt anxious about lights being turned off for fear of what that might do to her. He had attempted to resolve this conflict by insisting that a light was left on in his room at all times. Unfortunately, this caused further problems for him, because if the light was on then Nanna could see what he was doing and, as he was often naughty, he lived in fear of her descending from the light to tell him off. He had thought of asking mum about all of this, but every time he mentioned Nanna she began crying again and he couldn't bear that. Dad wasn't very helpful either because he was 'fed up with people going on about Nanna'. I suggested that it might be helpful for me to have a talk to mum and dad and, if they agreed that it was all right, he could ask me questions about dying.

I met again with mum and dad on their own and we talked about the dilemma. They were astonished by the ideas that Liam had expressed and mum hadn't been aware that her own grief was having such a powerful effect on her son. She agreed to seek referral to the counsellor at her GP's surgery and gave me permission to tell Liam 'anything he wanted to know'. Liam and I spent the next two sessions trying to work out the answers to some very interesting questions, such as 'what do dead people look like?', 'what happens at a funeral?' and 'if dead people can't feel things, why do they have padding inside coffins?'.

At a follow-up session a few weeks later, mum and dad came without gran. They were happy to report an improvement in Liam's mood and behaviour, and had decided to be firmer with him and not let him use Nanna as an excuse to get out of trouble. Mum was receiving help with her own bereavement issues and dad had taken up my suggestion that Liam was now at an age when he would benefit from spending a bit more time with his dad. They had got involved with the school football team and the local Saturday football league and were having a good time together.

Jack

Jack was 8 years 1 month old when he was referred to the clinic after the death of his father 3 months previously. The presenting problem was Jack's overwhelming anger, which was upsetting his mother at home and beginning to get him into a lot of trouble at school. Jack's father had died of cancer and Jack and his little sister had been gradually introduced to the idea that he was ill, that he was so ill he might die and that he might die quite soon, over a period of about 18 months. Mum was disappointed that Jack needed referral, because she felt that she and her husband had done everything they could to prepare for his death, even down to planning his funeral together with the children, and somehow Jack's subsequent angry behaviour was letting everyone down. She had told him he was coming to talk to a woman who would help him get over his anger.

Jack glared at me from beneath his fringe and demanded to know what there was to talk about – his dad was dead. Thereafter, he refused to utter another word in the session. Leaving his mum with my colleague, I took Jack to the playroom and showed him what was available there and he had a good look around, while I explained about his anger being very reasonable given what had happened to his family. We discussed how he could let his anger out in ways that didn't hurt him or others and he drew a picture of himself with a steam valve on his head! Jack agreed to attend for some individual sessions and very soon his anger was replaced by an almost overwhelming sadness, which was almost harder for everyone to bear. During this phase of his grieving, Jack became very interested in playing with an old wooden fort which he set up in the sand tray. Terrible battles were fought, but the people inside the fort were kept safe from harm and always had a supply of fresh water. Jack confided in me that he believed that dad had died of a bug that he caught from drinking 'bad water'. He also told me that some of his peers in school were teasing him and saying that he was so horrible his dad had probably died to get away from him.

As he progressed he remembered more and more about the things he and dad had done together before dad became so ill and he was able to construct a memory book. At his final planned session with me, he invited his mum in to see what he had been doing. As soon as she saw the fort, she smiled and told us that it was almost identical to one that Jack's dad had had. He and Jack had played with it together when Jack was a little boy, but it had got broken and thrown out before Jack was 3. He had no conscious memory of it, but it had obviously formed a powerful link between him and his memories of his dad and playing with it had brought him great comfort and stimulated other memories that he feared were forgotten.

Chapter 18
Young people with chronic fatigue syndrome

BECKY DURANT

This chapter describes the management of chronic fatigue syndrome in an outpatient child and family unit in Norfolk. The method emphasises the importance of a joint paediatric, psychiatric and educational approach. Within this model, there is the opportunity for everyone in the client's family to express his or her opinion, feel validated and for the young person to return to 'normal' life.

Introduction

Over the past few years several children with chronic fatigue syndrome (CFS) have been given the diagnosis myalgic encephalomyelitis (ME). This term is controversial and has generated discussion, because there is little evidence to suggest inflammation of the brain (Wessely, 1990). The illness is also known as postviral fatigue although, to be correctly diagnosed, the client should demonstrate clinical evidence of a virus.

For the purpose of this chapter, no distinction is made between these terms and for convenience the initials CFS are adopted.

In 1992, Margaret Vereker highlighted the importance of a joint paediatric–psychiatric approach in the treatment of children with chronic fatigue. Since then numerous papers have attributed possible causes to the illness and a few have focused on rehabilitation strategies for adults; now we see the emergence of papers that mention children and adolescents (Jordan et al., 1997; Dobbins et al., 1997).

The condition affects many areas of the child's life – physical, social, emotional, psychological and family. It would seem appropriate, therefore, that young people are referred to a child and family centre so that all these factors may be addressed, and the child can have a thorough assessment before embarking on treatment.

The present treatment approach at the child and family centre in Norwich emerged from a joint seminar in Norfolk in 1995, organised by the local paediatric department, an occupational therapist from the centre and the visiting teacher service from the Norfolk Education Service.

As the condition is unpredictable and displays many forms, the programme is flexible and adapts to the needs of the individual and the family. It has also developed as a result of our experience and reflection on working with so many young people. It is therefore dynamic and changes according to the needs of the individual, the family and current research.

A user-friendly service is crucial for families with a child who has CFS. Many families are suspicious of the centre mainly because they believe that their previous experiences with traditional medicine were unhelpful and in some instances very distressing.

Some people still hold the view that psychiatry has nothing to offer people with mental health difficulties. This belief is also reinforced in the literature available from the various self-help groups (*Perspectives* – the magazine of the ME association; *Interaction* – the magazine for action for ME and chronic fatigue). Clients and parents may assume that the centre will look for deep-rooted emotional or psychological reasons for the condition.

To overcome this rather poor image, the centre strives to create an atmosphere of total acceptance and encourages each family member to tell his or her story without criticism, doubt or the worry of pressure of time. Individual, parent-only or sibling-only sessions are available, depending on need and appropriateness.

Children are normally referred by GPs, paediatricians, school nurses (school health advisers) or educational welfare officers. The occupational therapist often works with a psychologist or a nurse from the centre, but is viewed as the key worker.

The child's diagnosis is made by either the paediatrician or the GP. Sometimes the family forms its own diagnosis based on information received from neighbours, newspapers or the TV. Although the centre does not diagnose CFS, it has a responsibility to ensure that other illnesses have not been overlooked – in particular, depression, which is often a feature of CFS, either as a result of chronic fatigue or a predisposing factor. Chronic anxiety is often present as well and may be shared by all the family members.

At the onset of our intervention programme, we noticed that several people failed to attend. When we changed our style to a more flexible approach, our attendance rate improved as clients felt more comfortable in the psychiatric setting. This was accomplished by the occupational therapist joining the paediatrician in the general hospital and having a shared session with the family. Thus the family would be able to meet the occupational therapist at the point of referral, which helps with the engagement process.

In this way the occupational therapist was able to explain to the family why the referral was seen as necessary and the family could ask questions and discuss anxieties at an early stage.

After this first meeting with the referrer present, the subsequent sessions are held at the Family Centre.

The family are greeted by the occupational therapist who has sole responsibility for the assessment, planning and implementation of treatment, although these are always negotiated with the family and other professionals if appropriate. In this centre, the occupational therapist is the prime instigator because she is a clinical specialist in CFS.

The first task is to assess the family by interviewing as many members as possible, normally at the centre. A full family history is taken with special consideration given to a detailed developmental history.

If it seems likely that a clinical psychiatric disorder is present, another opinion from a psychiatrist is sought. The therapist is normally present to facilitate the session and enable the young person to feel at ease.

If the initial referrer requests a psychiatric opinion, the family will have its first assessment with a psychiatrist and the occupational therapist.

Since 1991, 55 young people with CFS have been seen at the Child and Family Centre. Many more were referred but failed to attend. The average age at referral is 13, the youngest 8 and the oldest 17. There are more females than males, which is in keeping with national figures relating to sex of adolescents referred to psychiatric units.

In the early 1990s there was a trend to refer young people who had experienced the condition for a long period. This reflected the lack of facilities for treatment and the inability to diagnose the condition. With greater awareness through a well-developed education system, GPs and paediatricians, the children are now referred during the early stages of the condition, suggesting a better prognosis.

Criteria for referral

There appears to be different diagnostic tools used to identify the condition. In the absence of agreed clinical guidelines for children, each referrer modifies the Holmes et al. (1998) criteria.

Six months in a developing child's life is a very long period for a child to experience an illness and not be given a diagnosis or offer of help. Therefore, in most instances if children have had this condition with no identifiable cause for about a month, if they have been off school and after all clinical investigations have been tried, they may be referred to the Child and Family Centre.

The condition often causes major disruptions in the lives of these children and their families. As they become isolated, they become less confident and soon do not want to go out. Many parents are confused about managing the problem and the Centre offers support and guidance.

Clinical features

Most of the young people share the following characteristics and many referrers identify at least four of them in order to make a diagnosis:

- A characteristic history of generalised fatigue causing significant disruption to social, family and educational life.
- Chronic fatiguability.
- A history of a viral-type illness preceding the onset, possibly glandular fever.
- Further symptoms such as headache, aches and pains, nausea, dizziness and cognitive problems.
- Trauma after a significant life event such as a change of school, a house move, loss of a family member, close friend or pet.
- A high degree of anxiety or complete indifference to the situation.
- No abnormalities on physical examination.
- Negative investigations to exclude other chronic diseases.

The treatment approach

More than one assessment session may be needed before treatment begins. The Centre has a standardised assessment form that therapists use with all families.

The process of being listened to is very important for many families because they feel that no one has listened to them before. They have rarely been allowed the opportunity to relate their stories in a climate of acceptance. This opportunity validates them as an individual or as a family. Parry (1991) suggests that Freud's greatest discovery may not be the unconscious but:

> . . . the validation that a person receives simply in the act of telling her story to an attentive listener.

First, it is important to identify the family's beliefs about the cause, duration and prognosis of the illness. The treatment that follows is often influenced by these beliefs, depending on how much the family feels the illness has physical or psychological roots. There is little point focusing on significant life events with a child whose family has strong beliefs that emotions play no part in the illness.

There are instances when individual family members have harboured anxieties about the real nature of the condition. The absence of a diagnosis may give rise to fears of serious undetected problems, such as leukaemia. Once these worries are voiced and shared, the families often feel greatly relieved and children feel more able to talk about their fears once they feel safe.

For some young people, especially in the early stages of therapy, the fatigue factor becomes the focus of attention and the occupational therapist offers a treatment programme that is designed to meet the needs of the individual.

Importance of negotiation

The therapist negotiates with the client and if appropriate with the family. This validates the person by recognising the importance of listening to them, e.g. relaxation techniques are more likely to work if the therapist incorporates the ideas of the client when designing a programme.

One young girl was particularly interested in meditation and had used this in the past. So, with some adaptation, the occupational therapist and client decided to try it again.

All suggestions need to be considered in the light of the natural lifestyle of the individual and the family. In this way new ideas can more easily be incorporated into their lives with the minimum of disruption while avoiding further stress. It is important to recognise that these families are vulnerable to stress and so each technique must be carefully explained and modified at regular intervals.

Activity avoidance cycle

Many children have developed an 'activity avoidance' cycle reinforced by their parents. As a consequence, the severity of their symptoms may well increase. Muscle wastage occurs and pain is experienced when the young person tries to move. This leads to further avoidance of activity.

It is at this point that the therapist needs to decide whether to include the skills of a psychologist as well as the intervention of a physiotherapist. To break away from this negative cycle, the client has to change his or her perceptions and behaviour. A psychologist may advise the occupational therapist about using cognitive therapy techniques and a physiotherapist may also be consulted for advice regarding a graded exercise plan.

Cognitive–behavioural therapy

There are numerous publications exploring the above therapy but readers are directed to some of the articles written by Chalder, a psychologist (Butler et al., 1989, 1991).

The principle of cognitive–behavioural therapy (CBT) is to help the client consider other reasons for the pain after activity. After any period of inactivity muscle wastage occurs. Once the inactive person becomes active again, they may experience pain and tire easily. Pain and fatiguability are the most common symptoms of CFS. Thus the activity avoidance cycle is reinforced.

Role of physiotherapy

It is essential for the occupational therapist and physiotherapist to liaise with each other because this is crucial to effective outcomes. The physiotherapist is also aware of the importance of listening to the client's story.

Physiotherapy has helped many young people recover. Some young-sters, through pain and anxiety, develop an abnormal breathing style. The physiotherapist teaches breathing techniques while the occupational therapist explores the cause of the anxiety. Both therapists explain to the young person exactly what is happening, while encouraging continuous feedback from them.

Thus, the young person feels empowered to express concerns as well as satisfaction about progress.

Sleep patterns

Often, youngsters with CFS complain that it is difficult to get to sleep because they are frightened by their thoughts, such as what is wrong with me? Why do I feel so ill? Am I dying? How is it that no one can help me?

Their thoughts keep them awake until they can no longer cope with the idea of going to bed at night. Instead they devise methods to stay awake, such as watching TV, playing with their computer or writing stories. As a result of this nocturnal behaviour, they feel tired during the day and they start to sleep in the mornings, often through lunch times into the after-noon. Thus, a poor sleeping pattern emerges.

Other reasons may be important, e.g. some young people experience boredom and isolation. Day-time sleeping helps to pass the time until a brother or sister returns from school. As well as sleep deprivation, friend-ship deprivation may be a factor, so the young person with CFS may stay up late at night in the company of adults.

Gradual return to school

Although the illness may not have developed as a result of school phobia, this often becomes a consequence after many months away from class. The long period away from school, with the loss of peer support, leaves the young person with plenty of opportunity to think and become fearful. This may not be a problem if the referral is made before the pattern of school non-attendance emerges. The stress that these children may experience as they try to maintain a regular attendance pattern during their illness should be recognised.

If schools allow the young people to attend just when they like, this may add to their stress because each absence suggests failure to the child. This affects confidence, increases anxiety and may perpetuate the illness.

It is preferable for the child to attend three mornings a week every week than to attend two full days then take three weeks off. Most schools understand this and are very flexible. The visiting teacher service should work with children with CFS to develop suitable programmes in schools.

The occupational therapist may organise a meeting with all professionals and the family to develop strategies regarding school attendance. It is important to give permission to the children to enjoy themselves while they are not at school. If days away from school are legitimised, the young person begins to relax and make good use of this time instead of worrying about trying to get to school.

Alternative education

Many young people have benefited from the experience of home tutors, groups for children who have problems attending school and the teacher at the family centre.

The tutor will arrange some sessions in the home which are tailored to the needs and health of the child.

When the young person is ready and feels confident, the teacher arranges for a visit to a teaching group designed especially for those unable to attend school. Gradually, more and more time is spent in the group until the child no longer needs to be taught at home, but may have lessons in a Portakabin in the grounds of the high school or occasionally in one of the school's classrooms.

These groups have been very successful in providing peer support and the opportunity for the child to continue the journey from childhood to adolescence. Many have been deprived of this experience because of the onset of the illness at this crucial stage in their development. Thus, the group offers a chance to make friendships and experiment with some of the issues that emerge during this phase.

Changes in the adolescent often confuse parents. Some find this new image difficult to manage. It is important for the therapist to work closely with the teacher and liaise regularly, so the therapist keeps in touch with current family issues which may then become a focus of the family therapy sessions (Willson, 1996).

The advantages of the group experience can best be understood by this short extract from an essay written by a group member and patient at the family centre:

> Six months ago I spent most of my days lying around feeling ill and depending on other people. I had home tutoring two hours a week and found the sessions difficult because the teacher arrived at 10.00. So I had to get up at 9.15 which was a real struggle.
>
> Then one day my tutor told me about this group and all the people in it who were like me off school and unable to do very much.
>
> So eventually I came here and felt very nervous at first. I soon made friends with one girl I used to know from school.
>
> I was surprised and slightly relieved that she had the same illness too. Another girl started coming to the group and eventually we all got very friendly and started talking to each other about lots of different things. We suddenly felt very confident and began to express ourselves by wearing hats and psychedelic leggings. We did a lot of art work and helped each other become more confident and independent.
>
> I started doing tap dancing again which I did before I was ill and really enjoyed it. As I started to do more physical activities I felt a lot better and was more able to concentrate on my school work.
>
> I'm still improving now and love the group; it finished for the summer holidays today and already I am missing my friends. I have made so many good friends. I hope the group will be as good next term.

This girl made a partial return to school before the Christmas break and was back in full-time education by Easter.

Case study

The following is a brief description of the treatment offered to a young boy. It analyses the response of his parents and emphasises the importance of joint work.

Simon was 15 when he was referred to the centre. Six months before the referral he had been a healthy boy, keen on sport, who enjoyed school. He then developed glandular fever and became very ill.

His condition deteriorated quickly until he could no longer do anything for himself. He was able to stand and support his body, but he was unable to move his legs. Simon stopped speaking and for 3 months his parents coped alone with him, carrying out all activities of daily living for him.

After several clinical tests that proved negative, his GP referred him to the occupational therapist at the child and family centre.

His parents were very grateful for this referral because it gave them an opportunity to talk at great length about their fears. They were seen by the occupational therapist and a nurse therapist for their initial assessment.

In the first session the occupational therapist planned to gain an understanding of the history of the illness, and find out about Simon before he was ill. However, his parents were so pleased to have someone with whom they could discuss their problems that most of the first session was devoted to talking about and explaining chronic fatigue syndrome. In their understanding, someone with ME, as they called the illness, had a bleak future and would probably have to spend several years in bed before there were signs of recovery.

We were able to share with them our knowledge of the illness and explain how young people do get better and reassure them that the stories they had read need not necessarily apply to their son.

During the next session we discussed possible causes of the illness, both generally and in relation to Simon. Although at first he was not able to speak, he was aware of everything that was going on and communicated by nodding or blinking. His father was confused by his son's illness and wondered if there was some psychological cause. This gave us a lead into a usually rather difficult area. His mother, however, was convinced that her son was dying of leukaemia.

The family sessions included his two siblings. They were pleased to attend because it gave them an opportunity to express their fears. During the sessions several stress-related issues were discussed, such as worries about the future, fear of meeting friends, fear of criticism from family members and the amount of time Simon was having off school. Eventually a detailed profile was obtained.

The occupational therapist believes that it was because the family were able to accept that there were both psychological and physical implications that the sessions were successful.

In addition to the family sessions, the occupational therapist and nurse therapist offered Simon some individual sessions; the initial focus was on his inability to speak. A physiological explanation was offered that the muscles necessary for voice control had weakened as a result of the illness and that Simon needed exercises to strengthen them.

Starting with very simple facial exercises, he then progressed to sounds. Within 2 weeks Simon was able to say a few words and after another 3 weeks he regained full control of his voice. At the same time, the occupational therapist organised physiotherapy and he soon regained independent movements.

The next step was to consider his education. The visiting teacher service offered a few hours a week, and the occupational therapist visited his school to talk to his teachers and find out about his general school performance. This occurred with permission from Simon and his parents.

These visits were particularly insightful. He had in fact been the victim of bullying but had never told his family. He had always found lunch times difficult and usually went home to avoid this time, and often stayed there for the rest of the afternoon. This pattern had gradually developed over 3 or 4 months before his glandular fever. Further discussions also revealed that he was not such an able athlete as his father had described him; in fact he was average and appeared quite unenthusiastic about sports.

We were able to look at these factors in the session. Simon discussed some of these issues with me in confidence and I was guided by him over the amount of information he wanted to share with his parents. Gradually, other issues emerged and we were able to understand that, for a very long time, Simon had felt confused and then unhappy, mainly about school-related issues. In particular he was very afraid of letting his father down. His interest changed as he grew older; however, his father still believed that his son was a good athlete.

After 9 months of therapy Simon was physically well. His symptoms disappeared, he put on weight and looked healthy. He even started a paper round and found a few odd jobs on farms in the evenings and at weekends.

He continued his education with the visiting tutor and also had a weekly session with the teacher at the centre.

As he had only a few months of compulsory education left, it was decided that he should not go back to school. Instead he engaged in his own educational projects at home. He designed, dug out and created a fish pond. He is now a happy young man who has a permanent job on a farm, and is due to start a part-time course at an agricultural college soon.

On reflection, the occupational therapist believes that the glandular fever left Simon very weak and vulnerable, with a low tolerance to stress.

General observations

Although the condition produces different symptomatology, there are common characteristics that appear to be shared by many families who have children with CFS.

Levels of achievement are often important. Many parents describe their children as bright and often with a talent for sport. Some youngsters relate stories about their high levels of academic ability, sporting performances and popularity. Young people with CFS appear to share some of the same personality characteristics as those with an eating disorder, such as anorexia nervosa.

However, there is a significant difference. Stories of success and achievement appear to be slightly exaggerated with children with CFS. The reports given by the schools, describing the child as average or a real 'trier', do not match the child's perception of his or her ability.

A similar distortion of *perception* has been implicated in some of the studies with adults. Gibson et al. (1993) indicate that adults with CFS have both a distorted and a lower threshold of effort, but have higher aspirations than other people without the condition.

Absent fathers can be another feature. They rarely come to the appointments but this is often the case with other families who attend the centre, because of the father's work commitments.

From the experience of the occupational therapist, most children with CFS come from middle-class families where the father works long hours away from home, leaving the mother to care for the children. Consequently, the mother and child develop a close relationship, which Minuchin (1974) describes as 'enmeshed'.

There may be a parallel between these families and adults who have CFS, most of whom are from professional and middle-class backgrounds.

Conclusion

This chapter has highlighted the need for a joint approach as was originally suggested by Vereker in 1992. As with most illnesses, CFS is probably a combination of psychological and physical factors.

As the problem is complicated by family, educational, social and developmental factors, it seems very relevant to refer these young people to a child and family centre so that most of their needs can be addressed in one setting.

Part IV
Evaluation of Practice

Chapter 19
An exploration and examination of a child's response to intervention alongside the impact of diagnosis on her family and their early response to treatment

SUSAN HENDERSON

Before working in Essex, I was a member of a Child and Family Psychiatry Team working in rural Scotland between 1986 and 1990. My formative experiences within this setting were based around family centred care. Families were an integral part of the assessment and treatment approaches. There was a commonly held belief within the team that to help children successfully we must include their parents. We followed the proposal made by D.W. Winnicott in 1964: 'there is no such thing as a baby, only a baby and someone else.'

It was during my time as a member of this team that a collaborative approach for children with communication disorders, including autism, was developed by myself, a speech and language therapist and a clinical psychologist. The approach was based on the use of modelled play techniques. The programme framework was six sessions each of 60 minutes' duration. The play techniques were demonstrated by the thera-pist while parents observed (weeks 1 + 4). This was followed by the parent working alongside the therapist and the child (weeks 2 + 5). Then the parent worked alongside their child while the therapist observed (weeks 3 + 6). Although there were observable changes both in the play behaviour of the children and in the engagement states between parent and child, no detailed evaluative studies were undertaken.

When I moved south to Essex my involvement with pre-school children with social and communication difficulties continued and developed. I work as part of an interdisciplinary child development team based in Essex. My interest in the condition described as autistic spectrum

411

disorder/autism deepened in parallel with my increasing awareness of the need to demonstrate clinical effectiveness.

I continued to refine the non-directive treatment approach that I used with these very young children. I was strongly committed to early intervention and parental involvement and I wanted to introduce parents to 'a way of being with their child'. A way that would allow parents to 'grasp the moment' with their child, which was not dependent on a particular environment, or particular toys, but which could be used in any situation when they were with their child and there was opportunity for interaction and engagement.

This intervention approach moves away from traditional child-centred practice towards a family-centred or family-focused way of practising.

I was provided with the opportunity to undertake an in-depth study on my use of non-directive play techniques with autistic children as part of my Master's programme for Paediatric Occupational Therapists at the University of East London.

I hoped that the study which would allow me the opportunity to look critically at my practice would:

- demonstrate that this approach is a promising therapeutic strategy for promoting social interaction and play in pre-school children with autism
- enhance my clinical reasoning abilities as a therapist
- deepen my insight into a family's situation when faced with the knowledge that their child is autistic
- provide a forum for debate among other therapists working in this field
- add to the existing body of knowledge on the treatment of children with autism.

Throughout the narrative text that relates to the child and her family I have used the name Helen to identify the child. This is a pseudonym chosen by the parents.

Literature review

Before the research, I carried out an extensive review of the literature on the following themes: historical overview of autism, causes, prevalence and characteristics of children with autism, occupational therapy, play, social learning and autism and parental experience of having a child with autism. The following publications were used:

- Ainsworth (1978), Ayres and Mailloux (1981), Ayres and Tickle (1980), Bailey et al. (1995), Baron-Cohen (1989), Beckman and Kohl (1984),

Bettelheim (1967), Bloomer and Rose (1989b), Bolton and Rutter (1990), Bowlby (1969), Brown (1996), Case-Smith (1991), Coleman and Gillberg (1990), Cook (1996), Dawson and Adams (1984), Dawson and Galpert (1990), Drotar et al. (1975), Frith (1989), Goldstein et al. (1992), Happé (1994), Harris et al. (1986), Hobson (1987), Howlin (1981), Humphrey (1962), Jordan (1993), Jupp (1992), Kanner (1943), Kawar (1973), King and Grandin (1990), Kjerland and Kovach (1990), Knox (1996), Kubler-Ross (1969), Lewis and Boucher (1995), Lewy and Dawson (1992), Lovaas (1977, 1987), Lovaas et al. (1987), McEvoy et al. (1993), MacKeith (1973), Magrun et al. (1981), Ornitz (1985), Rydell and Mirenda (1994), Schopler and Olley (1982), Sheridan (1993), Sigman et al. (1986), Sloman (1991), Stahmer and Schreibman (1992), Tiegerman and Primavera (1984), Trevarthen (1986), Trevarthen et al. (1996), Turnbull and Turnbull (1991), Williams (1996), Wing (1988), Wolfberg and Schuler (1993).

Methodology

The following section briefly outlines the method of research undertaken. A narrative sketch of the child and her family is included.

This concurrent study aims to consider the child's response to intervention alongside the parents' response to the information that their child has autism and their early perceptions of therapy.

These responses are described from the time of initial diagnosis over a 20-week period when the child begins to assimilate and integrate the therapeutic experiences offered to her and the parents begin to assimilate and accommodate the diagnosis and treatment.

This study acts as an illustration of an evolving working practice moving towards family-focused interventions for children with autism. This evolution is represented by Figure 19.1.

Research design

A case study design was chosen because this method of research allows for investigation of a unique event or condition, and is particularly suited to working with heterogeneous individuals such as children with autism (Bloomer and Rose, 1989a,b). Employing a case study design enabled me to investigate my practice and the situation of the family over time; it is a flexible approach which allows new information to be incorporated into the study as it progresses.

Case study design is particularly appropriate when the aim is to consider the effectiveness of a treatment programme or when devel-

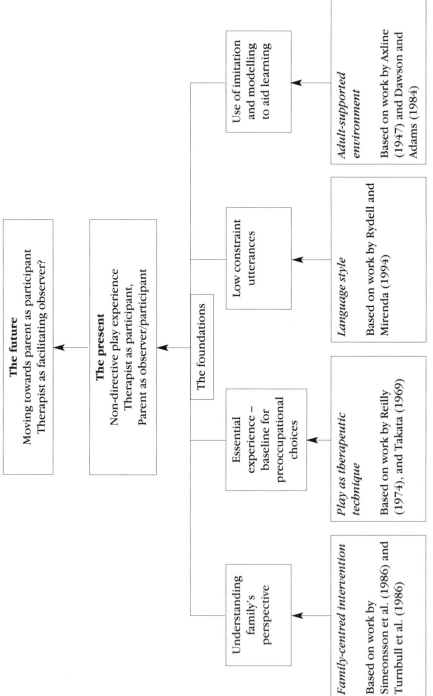

Figure 19.1: An illustration of the concepts underlying the development of a non-directive play approach as a family-centred interven-

oping theoretical concepts. I am attempting to re-conceptualise my practice and to develop a framework of intervention for therapists working with this client group and their families. At this stage it is too early to propose a fully developed working practice theory; more research is needed with other participants. Occupational therapists are traditionally involved in identifying needs; as Strupp and Bergin (1972) state, the therapist needs to know 'what' treatment by 'whom' is most effective for 'this' individual, with the specific problem under 'which' set of circumstances.

Within the context of this case study, I wished to consider change not only in the child with whom I was working but also within the family as a whole. The case, for the purpose of this study, therefore, is the family. It is a longitudinal study and considers change over a period of time.

The ultimate goals of this study were:

- To evaluate non-directive play techniques
- To gain an in depth insight into the family's journey between being told of the diagnosis and the end of the study
- To enhance my clinical reasoning abilities.

I wanted to consider not only my perspective with the intervention process but also that of the family, to allow them the opportunity to share their thoughts and feelings and to marry these separate experiences into an illuminating narrative to be considered together as a 'whole'. By examining the two aspects of this study as a whole and reflecting on these, my ongoing synthesis of this new way of working with children with autism and their families will be enriched.

Selection of the child/family

Inclusion criteria

The child will have been referred to the Child Development Centre for assessment. Following this assessment diagnosis of pervasive developmental disorder – autistic spectrum – will have been given by the consultant paediatrician according to the *Diagnostic Statistical Manual of the American Psychiatric Association*, 4th edn (DSM-IV; APA, 1994).

- The child will be aged between 2 and 4 years at time of diagnosis. The child can be either male or female.
- The child will be from a home using English as the first language.
- The child will be able to be accompanied for each treatment session by a parent.

- The child is not receiving regular intervention from another source.

Exclusion criteria

- A diagnosis of severe learning difficulties
- A child over 5 years
- A family where English is not the first language
- A family with parent(s) unable to accompany the child to the centre for treatment.

Procedures related to treatment

Treatment followed disclosure of disability to the family. For the purpose of this study, I focused on the first 10 intervention sessions.

Each session was a maximum of 60 min long, and took place in the Children's Centre in the same room, at the same time, on the same day, once a week over a 10-week period.

Within the room, I provided a selection of play equipment – totalling six items in all. Two of the items were constant – the sand tray and the platform swing. The other four items were systematically selected:

1. Large therapy ball
2. Crayons and paper
3. Playdoh and cutters
4. Large building bricks
5. Tactile mats
6. Doll's house
7. Scooter board
8. Musical instruments
9. Teaset/pretend food
10. Tunnel.

Use of a formula of 2 + 4 from 10 items over a 10-week period allowed each of the one to ten items to be used four times each. This is illustrated in Table 19.1.

The activities were chosen to offer the child a comprehensive play experience which encompassed exploratory, symbolic, constructive and creative opportunities – as related to Takata's taxonomy of play previously described.

The toys offered to the child were chosen to provide the full range of play experience and were all toys common to many homes, toddler groups and nurseries. They would therefore have a familiarity for the child.

Table 19.1: Choice of activities using formula described (2 + 4 from 10)

Treatment session	Items used			
Week	1	1	2	3	4
Week	2	2	3	4	5
Week	3	3	4	5	6
Week	4	4	5	6	7
Week	5	5	6	7	8
Week	6	6	7	8	9
Week	7	7	8	9	10
Week	8	8	9	10	1
Week	9	9	10	1	2
Week	10	10	1	2	3

I acted as participant during each session, i.e. I was involved in each of the sessions offering support and facilitation to the child employing the non-directive methods described below. The mother of the child was an observer in the room, joining activities when included by Helen.

The approach: non-directive play

The approach was developed initially by Axline in 1947. It has been used primarily within child psychiatry situations as an aid to resolving children's behavioural difficulties through self-expression and catharsis. Over the past 11 years, I have modified the application of the technique during my work with autistic children, because my objectives are not the resolution of emotional difficulties but are to develop connections with the child and enhance learning through play.

Non-directive play is essentially a child-led experience where the adult follows the lead of the child and reflects back to the child his or her own activity. This reflection is both visual – the adult imitates the play of the child – and auditory – the adult comments on the play of the child.

The commentary is contextual, contingent upon the child's activity. It is undertaken using the present tense and is factual. The commentary does not include interpretations, it does not question and it does not direct. The phrases are kept succinct, usually limited to single or two words, e.g. 'Billy drawing', 'round and round', 'up', 'down'.

The commentary can be accompanied by a mirroring of the child's activity if appropriate. The adult imitates the constructive play of the child. Inappropriate, destructive behaviours are ignored and the appropriate toy use reinforced by demonstration. If the child uses language or symbolic vocalisations appropriate to the situation, these are mirrored by the adult.

The adult adopts a position facing the child, at a similar height to the child and using an open posture – hands open, arms relaxed by their sides. The adult continually looks at the child to establish eye contact whenever possible. Facial expressions and body position/posture are used to reinforce the language commentary. The intonation patterns of the voice also reflect the activity, e.g. by raising the voice for the word 'up' and lowering it for the word 'down'.

There are two limits placed upon the approach:

- That the child is kept safe
- That the adult is kept safe.

No limits are placed beyond these on the activity of the child. If the child continually uses the toys presented in an inappropriate manner, then the adult models the constructive, appropriate use reinforcing the action with context specific language.

Within a treatment session the child is provided with a limited number of activities, the combination of which should provide opportunities for stimulation of the sensory modalities. These are:

- movement
- touch
- vision
- hearing.

The activities also allow for constructive exploration, development of symbolic understanding and problem-solving.

The non-directive approach starts where the child is now; it does not evaluate the child's activity or pressurise him or her to change and conform. The adult provides a secure accepting environment where the child can learn to develop relationships, make connections and enhance play skills.

The clinical reasoning underlying this approach is that constructive individual play is an essential occupational behaviour to be developed in any child.

Multiple sources of evidence were used to strengthen the validity of the data. In this study the sources of evidence were the following.

Observation

Observation is suitable for studying both verbal and non-verbal behaviours as well as the environment in which the behaviour occurs. It was particularly suited to this project because I was working directly with a child who was unable to take part in other more intellectually and socially demanding methods of data collection.

During each of the 10 treatment sessions, I acted as participant observer. At the close of each session, I completed a log of the treatment period. This log was part of my field journal.

Three of the ten treatment sessions were observed 'live' by a speech and language therapist not involved with the family after an observation schedule. The therapist/observer viewed the session via a video link. The camera was able to be moved by her via a remote control, thus ensuring that the complete session was observable.

The observation schedule was designed by myself. The semi-structured observation system was based on a category system and not a checklist. It followed the system derived by Weick (1968). It considered the following:

- Non-verbal behaviours (body movements)
- Spatial behaviours (the extent to which individuals move towards/away from each other)
- Extralinguistic behaviours (covers aspects of verbal behaviour other than words; includes volume, pitch and tone)
- Linguistic behaviours (the actual content of talking).

Notes were also taken regarding the physical, non-human environment. They considered three aspects of the intervention:

- the child
- the therapist
- the environment.

Field journal

Robson (1993) advised that records of participation should capture information unambiguously and as faithfully and fully as possible. The field journal was used throughout my study to record in detail each of the 10 individual treatment sessions.

It was also the 'safe' place for me to record my personal feelings and impressions. Those subjective reactions are often so important but are lost if not recorded. The journal was also used as an *aide-mémoire* for me. It allowed me to revisit and reflect on some of my earlier entries as the research process continued.

Semi-structured interviews

The three interviews were undertaken with Helen's parents. The first was before the start of the intervention, the second the week after the fifth treatment session and the third the week after the tenth treatment session.

In-depth interviewing was chosen as the way to capture the parents' understanding of the medical condition and how it related to their child, and also to attempt to gain insight into their perspectives as parents of a child with autism.

Each interview lasted 60–75 min. Three semi-structured questions were used as a framework to guide the course of the first two interviews, but did not restrict the conversational and narrative flow from the parents.

As the interviewer, I particularly wanted the parents to be free to express themselves openly; however, a certain amount of restriction was obviously placed on the parents by using a tape recorder to record their words because they were unused to this. To overcome some of this difficulty, the tape recorder was under the control of the parents at all times during the interview and could have been turned off if they had so desired.

Within this study, I was aware that the credibility could be compromised by the fact that I was Helen's therapist and also the researcher asking questions of the family, and that the family may have felt that they wanted to please me by providing me with 'what I wanted to hear'. In an effort to prevent this happening, I did not ask any 'value-laden' questions about Helen's therapy, or her involvement with me.

The third and final interview was conducted by the speech and language therapist who had observed the treatment sessions and completed the observation schedules. The questions she asked were directly related to the parents' understanding of the therapy and to their perceived changes in the child's behaviour in her home environment.

Parents' journal

I encouraged Helen's mother to consider keeping a personal journal and to see whether she felt that this would be a beneficial experience for her. I gave her my assurance that if, after the 10 weeks of the study, she did not wish me to read or use the content, I would not.

However, Helen's mother was able to keep a journal for the duration of the sessions and she allowed the content to be part of my gathered data.

Data analysis and interpretation

Use of multiple sources of evidence produces volumes of material, which I had to consider individually in order to gain control. These sources of evidence were:

- the observation schedules
- the field journal
- the parent journal
- the interview transcripts
- the video recordings.

Each of these sources of information was analysed as to content. The data were organised into categories and descriptive units, and patterns were developed and discussed with peers within my workplace. Developing patterns and themes laid the foundation for the subsequent analysis. Patterns allow networks of thoughts to develop and causal relationships to be examined. This constant comparative analysis allows these patterns and concepts to be refined and modified until a congruence emerges. In her paper on rigour in qualitative research, Krefting (1990) proposes that this intense participation and submersion in the data lends credibility to the information discovered. After considerable reflection and discussion, I decided to consider the clinical experience and the parents' experience separately.

Ethical considerations

When undertaking a research study, care must be taken to consider the relative importance and value of the costs to the participants and researcher fully, against the benefits of furthering knowledge, improving services and changing practices.

There are nationally accepted codes of conduct used by researchers when working with human subjects. I followed the principles designed by the British Psychological Society (1991).

Pen picture of Helen and her family

Helen lives with her parents, her older sister and two cats in a town in Essex. Mr and Mrs X are buying their own home, a semi-detached house in a quiet residential area of the town. The local primary school is within 200 yards of the home.

Mr X is in full-time employment working for a manufacturing industry on the outskirts of the town. He does not travel and is home each evening and at weekends. Mr X is a 'local' and has family and friends all around the district.

Mrs X is a full-time mum at home with her children. Before the birth of the children, Mrs X was a technician for the local university. Since the birth of her daughters, Mrs X has undertaken work that has enabled her to remain at home. Her current employment gives her the freedom to choose when she will undertake the tasks. Mr and Mrs X often work together in the evenings when the children are settled in bed. Mrs X also has close connections within the community, with family and friends close by.

Mr and Mrs X have provided their children with a wide range of play opportunities both in the garden and in the home. Toys are very much in evidence and the results of the children's efforts with paints, collage and crayons are displayed around the kitchen.

Carol, Helen's older sister, is 6 years old; she attends the primary school close to her home; she has settled well into school life and enjoys her days in the classroom. Carol is a diligent, caring child; she is keen to 'help' and enjoys being given small responsibilities.

The family support the school by attending organised fund-raising occasions and they attend Governors/Parents Annual General Meetings. Mrs X is a member of the committee for the Opportunity Playgroup. Helen is their second child; she will be 4 years old this summer – 1997. Helen attends the local 'Opportunity Playgroup' and a 'Mums and Toddlers' session each week.

Helen was born after an uneventful pregnancy at full term in the local maternity unit. She had no post-birth difficulties and mum and baby were discharged home within 48 hours.

Helen's early development was unremarkable; she made satisfactory progress and achieved all her early milestones as expected.

The first indication of a problem came when Helen was 7 months old and had difficulties with the routine hearing check. A 'wait and see' decision was taken and no immediate follow-up was undertaken. As Helen became increasingly physically able, she developed into a very active child; however, she was easily distressed and had many 'temper tantrums'. Helen was also failing to develop language. Throughout this period of her life, from 8 months to 2 years, Helen had many ear infections which were treated with antibiotics. At 2 years of age, Helen underwent a minor surgical procedure and had grommets fitted. This procedure did not improve Helen's ability to communicate and Mr and Mrs X sought further advice from their GP. Concerns about Helen had also been raised by the playgroup leader with Mrs X and a referral to the consultant paediatrician and the Child Assessment Centre followed. Helen was referred in October 1996; she was then 3 years and 3 months. An initial meeting took place in early November of that year and team assessment was undertaken in February 1997 when the diagnosis of autism was confirmed. Helen began attending the Children's Centre in March 1997 for therapy. I was her therapist.

Data interpretation

This section explores the common themes that emerged from the collected information.

It is divided into two discrete parts. The first section, the therapeutic experience, presents the conclusions reached from examining the clinically based data, i.e.

1. The field journal
2. The observation schedules of the external observer and of myself
3. The video recordings of sessions.

The second section details and explores the experience of the parents as they begin to deal with the diagnosis of autism.

In order to gain the valuable information about the parents' perceptions of the therapy, and in an effort to maintain credibility, the third interview was undertaken by a therapist not involved with the family. This allowed for truthful and genuine responses from the parents.

The therapeutic experience

The information that derived from the themes in the data has been organised into three classifications:

1. Creating a structure
2. Establishing connections
3. Learning through experience.

The categories emerged as descriptive of the actions of both therapist and child. Each will be considered in turn.

Creating a structure

This section illustrates how both physical and human resources were used to structure the experience and to influence the therapeutic relationship as the 10 sessions proceeded. It includes descriptions of how the space and time were organised and how the activities were chosen each time. Importantly, it includes the behaviours and interactions of myself and Helen. These formed the foundations upon which we built our relationships. As the sessions continued, the analysis of the findings illustrate the positive progression in engagement time that occurred.

Therapist behaviours that influenced the structure of the sessions

I had designed and arranged an environment that would offer Helen an opportunity to explore all her senses. It combined gross motor activities, tactile play opportunities and toys, which provided possibilities for 'let's pretend', play that is usual for a 4-year-old child. This play environment was provided for each of the 10 sessions. The time allowed for each session was 60 min. Initially, I adopted a position in the middle of the room, kneeling, facing the child to allow maximum opportunities for eye contact and use of gesture.

My language was reflexive, contingent upon the activity of the child. It comprised mainly simple one- or two-word comments. I used changes in pitch and tone to reinforce the meaning of words, e.g. I raised my voice for 'up' and lowered my voice for 'down'.

I did not ask questions or use tenses. I did not give instructions or directions. My actions would mirror those constructive, productive actions demonstrated by Helen. If she was unable to use toys adaptively, I would give a demonstration of a possible use but not a verbal direction.

The atmosphere within this environment was essentially permissive.

Child's behaviours that influenced the structure of the sessions

Helen is an active, lively, little girl. Her initial response on introduction to the therapy room was to move quickly between the activities offered, but her attention to each item was fleeting. Her initial exploration was to touch then discard; she did not remain still to play with any toy. Helen made several 'circuits' of the room before settling at the sand. Her activity in the sand tray was limited to fingering it; her attention to the swing was to climb on and immediately get off again. Helen communicated her need for the session to end by collecting her coat and pulling her mother to the door.

I accepted that I must respond to Helen's communicative overtures for the session to end. This acceptance reinforced Helen's understanding of the situation and gave her a degree of control and choice.

Helen's response to the intervention changed over the study period of 10 weeks. Table 19.2 illustrates how Helen's tolerance for each session improved. It is interesting to note that the improvements in engagement time were disrupted by a break in therapy of 3 weeks between weeks 5 and 6.

The structure of the sessions developed and changed over the intervention period. The initial framework, previously described, was moderated in response to Helen's behaviour. The structure was able to accommodate these changes. Initially, I had attempted to join Helen at her chosen activity but I realised I needed to adapt my structure when she

Table 19.2: Table to show improvements in Helen's ability to tolerate the full 60-min session

Week	1	2	3	4	5	6	7	8	9	10
Time	25 min	35 min	50 min	50 min	60 min	30 min	45 min	60 min	55 min	60 min

found this intrusive and disruptive to her exploratory play. At each session, I was able slowly to return to my original framework of imitation, demonstration and verbal reinforcement of actions by adopting a position closer to Helen's chosen activity. By week 4, Helen was tolerant of parallel play situations.

Helen had also adapted her initial structure of a 'circuit routine' to one of using her mother as her 'safe base' from which she could explore and return. Helen maintained this structure throughout the remaining intervention period.

Establishing connections

Making useful connections with our physical environment and the people within it is of integral importance to most people. It is the area that many children with autism find the most difficult to understand and develop.

For the purpose of this study, I considered 'connections' to be any communicative attempt, either verbal or non-verbal, any imitation of action or sound, any joint attention activities such as turn-taking and sharing, and any demonstration of symbolic pretend play.

Helen's social and play behaviours changed markedly over the study period. During session 1, Helen was only able to communicate her unwillingness to proceed with the session. Her other behaviours were exclusive. She was unable to include me in her activity or allow me to demonstrate possible toy use. Her attention to activity was short and she was unable purposefully to explore her environment. This is illustrated by the following entry from my field journal.

> Helen was very unsettled, her activity was high, rapidly moving between toys offered; her awareness of me was poor with no eye contact
> Session 1 (from my field journal)

The external observer's first record noted that Helen's use of jargon increased with activity and when approached by me.

> Social overtures, i.e. use of name precipitated movement away from chosen activity.

Subsequent observation records confirmed that jargon increased with periods of high activity and when my language usage became more socially based, e.g. use of child's name. Detailed notes taken in the journal identified the development of a definite pattern of behaviour.

Analysis of observation schedules, the field journal and the video tapes confirmed the emergence of a distinct pattern of social play behaviour. High activity levels showed a recognisable association with poor attention, decreased awareness of the therapist and increased use of non-functional expressive language, such as jargon.

Calm periods showed that an association with focused attention to task increased social play, e.g. sharing of activity and reduced use of jargon.

The positive changes in Helen's engagement behaviour are illustrated in Table 19.3.

The pattern of behaviour shown above was maintained throughout the 10 therapy sessions. The frequency of the high activity bursts decreased with a corresponding increase in settled behaviour.

Although Helen's ability to settle and play did show sequential improvement, entries from my field journal highlighted that, if there was a change to the accepted routine, then Helen's settled learning behaviours were adversely affected. This was demonstrated on two separate occasions, once when Helen and her mum were accompanied by an aunt and once when Helen had to attend after a paediatric outpatient appointment. The changes to Helen's expected structure produced deterioration in her periods of engagement and increased periods of high activity. However, it did not affect the total therapy time.

Analysis of the data also highlighted that over the intervention period Helen's initial response to the therapeutic environment changed. Between weeks 1 and 6, Helen's behaviours on entry into the playroom were of high activity, low attention type. Helen's initial period of high

Table 19.3: Different patterns of behaviour displayed by Helen within the sessions

	Periods of high activity signify:
	poor attention, increased non-functional (jargon) language, decreased awareness of therapist
Activity level	
	Periods of calm focused activity signify:
	increased attention to task, reduced jargon, increased awareness of therapist and social play behaviours
	Time in session

activity shortened each week until week 7 when her behaviour on entry into the playroom was calm and focused. She was immediately able to use the toys offered in a productive way (Figure 19.2).

Session 1

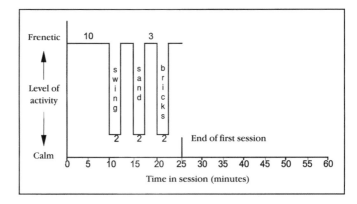

Session 5

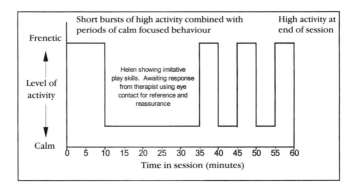

Session 10

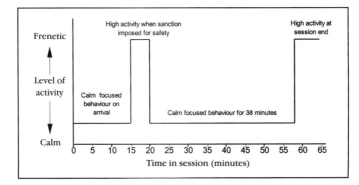

Figure 19.2: A pictorial representation to show Helen's difficulty in using the environment and how this changed over the 10-week intervention period.

It should be noted from these representations that changes in Helen's activity level were abrupt and immediate.

The periods of calm allowed me the opportunity to begin to build a relationship with Helen. Our developing relationship is illustrated by an extract from my field journal.

> Helen was able to imitate cutting playdoh with a knife, making round flat 'biscuits' and poking them with a fork. She was able to use several single words appropriately during this play – 'cut', 'thank you', 'knife'. She was able to include her mum in the play, passing her a plate and spoon. Helen used a toy salt cellar to 'season' her mum's 'food', then the 'food' on her plate, then on her dolly's. She fed teddy and accompanied this play with some lip smacking sounds.

Helen was using eye contact throughout this period of pretend play; she also used some natural gestures, pointing with eye contact to request an object.

My relationship with Helen was in many ways symbiotic – the one could not function well without the other. Helen's awareness of me and my response to her gradually synchronised over the intervention period.

By the end of the study period, Helen was able to take the initiative at times within the therapy sessions; she became confident of my role as her supporter.

The area of communication that showed least change during this timed therapy period was Helen's use of spontaneous appropriate verbal language. Helen had a single-word vocabulary of approximately 15–20 words at the start of the therapy. She did not always use them appropriately; she often used jargon and echoed speech on occasion. After the 10 sessions, Helen was making more useful non-verbal communicative overtures, but had not developed an increased vocabulary that she was able to demonstrate. However, the speech and language therapist noted that, by the tenth session, Helen was using this vocabulary of single whole words and some two-word phrases to comment on her own activity.

Learning through experience

This third and final section detailing the therapeutic experience considers how and what both the child and myself were learning.

Child

For the purpose of this study, I have considered Helen's learning as demonstrated by:

- using tools in constructive play
- creating play or let's pretend games
- adapting her behaviour to the environment
- communicating with others
- using her whole body to experience sensation.

I have used Takata's play epochs to illustrate Helen's gradual increase in play sophistication (Takata, 1969).

Initially, Helen's activity was limited to touching, e.g. she fingered the sand and had short bursts of movement stimulation – on swing, jumping on mats and knocking down bricks. She did not demonstrate constructive, creative or communicative play behaviours.

Over the intervention period, Helen showed an ability to learn from her environment. She was able to retain skills from week to week and build on them. Her purposeful exploration of her environment moved from a gross motor basis to a constructive and creative basis. This is summarised in Table 19.4. It illustrates Helen's ability to learn play skills within the therapeutic environment offered to her. The changes in play behaviours are shown by defining Helen's play in terms of Takata's Play Epochs. Only the first three epochs have been used because of Helen's age.

Learning through play (based on Takata's Play Epochs)

Therapist

For the purpose of this study, I have considered my learning experiences within the 'treatment context' as those demonstrated by my responses to the child.

It was necessary for me to moderate my physical approaches to Helen after she discarded the chosen items on my approach. My actions were reflexive. I reasoned that I must give Helen more space to explore and therefore maintained a still, central position within the room. I continued to give a verbal commentary using low constraint utterances and using facial expressions and eye contact to reinforce connection with Helen.

I recognised that I must respond to Helen's communicative overtures. One of the prime purposes of the therapy is to improve social understanding and the child's ability to communicate effectively. Therefore when Helen made definite indications of play choice, I needed to accept them. When Helen needed to finish the first session after only 20 minutes, my judgement was to accept her choice.

My learning throughout the whole period of intervention was led by Helen. I responded when she provided the opportunity; she indicated the pace of the development of understanding between us. I developed an

Table 19.4: Helen's ability to learn play skills within the therapeutic environment offered to her

	Sensorimotor epoch	Symbolic, constructive epoch	Dramatic, complex, constructive, pre-game epoch
Session 1	Rapid movement between activities Climbing on to swing Jumping on mats	Built tower of two bricks Poked fingers in sand	Not displayed
Session 5	Hiding and finding hands in sand Using 'rainmaker' for auditory stimulation Using swing for vestibular stimulation	Using bucket, spade, funnel and sieve in sand Using music-making toys appropriately – attempting to produce rhythms	Not displayed
Session 10	Using swing and large therapy ball for vestibular stimulation	Using shells/cups, hands as scoops in sand Using funnel to full bucket Using rolling pin and cutters with playdoh Scribbling on paper imitating circles, lines and dots	Using playdoh to make bracelets, rings and food Playing turn taking games on swing and large ball – demonstrating ability to wait her turn and share pleasure in cooperative game

awareness of her routine and that, after periods of concentrated attention and social interaction, she would need bursts of high activity when her overtures and responses to me would decrease. I provided her with the opportunity for this activity by ensuring that there was always a mix of creative/constructive toys and movement/touch toys.

Impact of diagnosis and early perceptions of therapy as described by the family

The second section within this chapter considers the impact of this diagnosis and the parents' early feelings about the therapy. It uses the information gathered from the three interviews and from the mother's diary. I have chosen to present the parents' stories separately and then have a combined conclusion.

To put this into a time perspective, Helen's family had been informed of the diagnosis only weeks before the therapy sessions began. I have explored their response to this information and their understanding of what it means for them at the beginning and the end of the intervention period. I looked for both attitudinal and behavioural change in this family.

The mother's story (considered from time of diagnosis until the end of therapy over a period of 20 weeks)

Until Helen reached the age of 2, there were few concerns about her development. Mrs X became concerned when Helen did not develop language abilities as her sister had done. She sought help from her local clinic and health visitor. Referrals to the ear, nose and throat department followed. Grommets were tried without success, so further investigations were needed.

This period of uncertainty was very difficult for Mrs X; she invested in hopes that proved fruitless and eventually, when the diagnosis came, it gave rise to many contradictory feelings: 'Half of it was relief in the sense of we always felt something was a little bit amiss with her, the other half was not my daughter, there can't be anything wrong.'

Mrs X felt partly to blame for the condition and also felt some shame as she tried to answer questions from her family and friends.

> I find it quite hard where people ask questions about it, sort of, having to, you know, admit it.
> Because you, you can't help but blame yourself, that was one of the hardest things, the pair of us said what did we do wrong? What have we done that's caused this?

Mrs X voiced great worries for the future of Helen. Se had a need to frame a possible future for Helen that could determine her role as parent.

Talking to various people, seeing programmes on television at least gives you some hope that she might be able to lead some sort of independent life, which is what I would like for her, you know, to find an independence that won't rely so much on us if, if something happens to us, I think that is my greatest fear.

Mrs X also felt bereft on occasion when faced with a difficult situation in a public place. She felt unable to cope with what she interpreted as condemnation of her position as mother.

When she's quite upset people come up and say things like – sounds like you're murdering that child – and I think, I think that's been the hardest thing, it's you know, it's always in a full shop it happens and you feel as if everybody stares at you.

Mrs X also had concerns about her mothering behaviours within the home. She felt under pressure to conform to the accepted child care routines of potty training and walking on reins instead of using the buggy, even though she recognised that Helen could not conform to these routines yet. Mrs X recorded her feelings in her diary.

I often feel I should be doing more normal things with her, potty training, walking with her, reading but it's always one step forward two steps back and you can't help feeling a failure for not doing these things.

These early responses from Mrs X typically demonstrate her general sadness and feelings of isolation, uncertainty and ignorance.

After diagnosis and over the treatment period, Mrs X was able to access a variety of information sources from the Children's Centre, the National Autistic Society and a local parent-run information and support group, to observe Helen within the treatment sessions and to develop her own coping strategies.

Over the weeks her early feelings of guilt and shame reduced. Mrs X was able to adopt a more constructive attitude when dealing with the public. She felt more ready to answer questions and was also prepared to discuss Helen with others. She was able to use the opportunities provided by her close community in the PTA and the Church Group to inform others and to develop their understanding of the condition. She herself gained support from this and so became more confident in her own abilities.

Having a child like Helen has also increased Mrs X's awareness of other people's situations; she is less judgemental and does not form an opinion as quickly as she used to. She is able to empathise more with each parent's individual situation. Mrs X also demonstrated behavioural changes both in her day-to-day management of her household duties and in the time spent with Helen. She adopted a pragmatic strategy when organising everyday tasks. She recognised that by changing routines the stresses could be reduced – she avoided certain shops that Helen found particularly distressing or she would leave Helen with her father while she went shopping alone.

Outings were considered in greater depth and contingencies were planned for, such as changes of clothes. Places that Helen enjoyed and were safe, such as those completely fenced with no water, were used again and again.

When playing with Helen, Mrs X was more able to enjoy the moment.

> I spend more time with her whenever I can, um, just doing silly things, not expecting her to, you know, say, start talking immediately or anything. It's just sort of playing with her now, you know, sort of looking for everything I've got.

This period of Mrs X's life has been very difficult; the process of change in her attitudes and behaviour is ongoing. It appears cyclical not sequential, but is forward moving.

It is apparent from Mrs X's journal that certain occasions have provoked a negative response in Helen, e.g. outpatient hospital visits, children's parties. When this happens, Mrs X is confronted again with feelings of fear and sadness; however, she is now able to reflect upon the situation and recognise what has provoked Helen's reaction. Her knowledge gives her a degree of control.

Mrs X has read widely on the topic of autism. She has joined the Autistic Research Council and the National Autistic Society and, although fears about the future remain, her attitude towards this unknown has changed. She is more able to deal with the 'next step' rather than the next 10 years.

> I do admit I do not look forward to sorting out her educational needs but I will do my best for her. A lot can happen in the next year and it's no good fretting over what has not happened yet.

The father's story

The initial reactions of Mr X on hearing the diagnosis were similar to those of his wife; he expressed disbelief and despair, and acknowledged his ignorance of autism. He also admitted that he, too, had invested hope in finding an alternative diagnosis, one that he felt offered a much more definite prognosis and treatment path.

> I think I would have found it easier to cope with had she been totally deaf, for which there is help and a cure.

Mr X also described his frustration at the slowness of the medical process from the time of initial concern through to diagnosis. He described a situation where he felt powerless to help his child as he did not know how. He did, however, view the diagnosis as positive, in that it gave a starting position from which to go forward. He also saw an opportunity in the early diagnosis for help to begin and so influence Helen's development. He also concentrated on Helen's physical prowess. He was proud of her agility and grasp of the workings of mechanical objects. He described her fleetness of foot and risk-taking in terms of achievement.

> She's a very adept child, physically adept, she's very good at running, jumping.

During the interviews, Mr X did not talk as readily or as openly as his wife about his emotional feelings. His contributions focused on the strengths that Helen had and the way forward for them as a family, and for Helen as child with special needs.

He developed his own coping strategies for dealing with difficult situations in public. These strategies were focused around protecting Helen.

> You are trying all the time to minimise the situation where she could get away from you, you try to be more aware for her, to help her not get into difficult situations.

During the second interview at the end of the sessions, Mr X acknowledged that he still found it difficult to talk to people about the condition. He described situations where, when faced with having to give explanations, he chose to avoid using the term 'autism' in favour of 'mentally handicapped'. Mr X felt that this term was more commonly understood and gained Helen and the family more understanding and sympathy. By the second interview, Mr X was able to share his positive feelings about his interactions with Helen; his words demonstrate his deepening insight into the condition.

> This is another thing I have learned with Helen, that what's good today might not be good tomorrow and we might have a nice walk today and tomorrow will be totally different, so the good moments with her are sort of heightened good moments [laughs] and you think, gosh that was brilliant.

Coming together and moving forward

Both parents were able to use words very effectively in describing this time of great transition for them as a family. Their stories were different, Mrs X focusing on the emotional demands and the changes that these have caused and Mr X focusing on the more concrete issues raised by the diagnosis – the way forward, how to manage the practicalities. But the stories also have many similarities: the focus on Helen's strengths, the investment of hope, the difficulties surrounding giving other people information and answering their questions, the acknowledgement of the need to restructure and reorganise the family life, and the deepening appreciation of special moments. The stories are complementary and demonstrate the evolving nature of growth of understanding. The need to understand was not confined to the issues surrounding diagnosis but also encompassed the therapy.

At the end of the 10-week intervention period the parents were able to voice their initial responses to the therapy that had been offered to them and their child. The parents' early reactions to the therapy were positive; however, they highlighted that assimilating the therapeutic objectives into their lives at the same time as accepting the diagnosis did place extra demands on them. These demands were intellectual, temporal and emotional.

> I didn't know how it would help her at the start, I must admit, I didn't quite see or understand. I think when it first started things were so negative, in lots of ways, it was an awful lot to take in and an awful lot to get on with and do. It was hard to see how we could cope, how we could change.

Mrs X, in particular, felt that the burden of responsibility for implementing change within the home was hers. Initially she was very apprehensive and became frustrated if the interaction with Helen did not reach her expectations. As the weeks progressed, Mrs X became more confident in her role as 'supporter' of Helen and the emphasis of the interaction began to change to one of recognising opportunities to develop play situations rather than attempting to lead them. The parents were also able to extend and develop certain aspects of the intervention themselves, e.g. they were able to recognise the positive benefits provided by using Makaton sign language. They purchased the video tape to expand their own and Helen's experiences.

Both parents described constructive changes in Helen's behaviour within the home environment since the start of the intervention; for the parents the most hopeful changes centred on Helen's ability to settle to play and to share and interact with other family members. Mrs X stressed the importance of them being able to play together as a family. Mr X expressed his happiness at being acknowledged and included by Helen.

> She came and sat on my lap facing me, she then shared my lunch of bread and ham, she fed me very precisely and gently and looked at me a lot until we finished. This made me feel very happy and pleased and I feel she and I are closer for the experience.

These stories give an illustration of the parental experience. They describe a process of accommodation that is dynamic, where the parents' reactions to the situation do change and apparently move forward, albeit cyclically. However, it is equally apparent that this is not a sequential ordering of events; it does involve reflection and re-examination of situations and it can involve revisiting and re-experiencing difficult times. They are honest and describe a painful time in this family's life. However, they are essentially hopeful; a quote from Mr X sums this up best:

> There are lots of shoots of green.

Discussion

This final section examines my study and reflects on my original aims. The relationship between the findings of my study and the literature is highlighted.

When I began this research, I believed that early intervention was very important if children and their families were to gain maximum benefit from a treatment programme. I also believed that such a programme should provide the child with as much cooperative, culturally relevant, social learning opportunity as possible.

I considered that to be most useful any intervention programme should include the parents because they hold the key position in a young child's life. I believed that, by involving the parent, they would also benefit, that their relationship with their child could be enriched.

One of my original aims was 'to consider to what extent does the use of non-directive play techniques promote social learning and communication skills in a pre-school child diagnosed as autistic?'.

The results from this study do indicate that the use of a non-confrontational child-led intervention strategy is a useful method of facilitating social learning, developing useful play and improving functional non-verbal communication.

Over the course of this intervention programme, Helen's appropriate play behaviours across all parameters used, i.e. sensorimotor, symbolic and constructive and dramatic/complex abilities, showed improvement.

Helen was able to demonstrate week-on-week learning and retention of skills. Her activity level moderated and her accommodation of the therapist increased. The results of this study would also indicate that Helen's learning through play was facilitated by the reinforcement, visual and auditory, provided by the therapist commenting on and imitating the play of the child.

This study builds on work previously undertaken by Dawson and Galpert (1990) and Tiegerman and Primavera (1984), which supported the use of imitation as a means of promoting eye gaze and toy play with autistic children. This study extends the use of imitation from an experimental, rigidly constrained context into a wider, less-structured, intervention programme. The beneficial effects of imitation are especially encouraging in the light of the fact that this was a flexible application of the imitative responses proposed by Dawson and Galpert (1990).

The results of this study also support the findings of previous research, indicating that language used by adults when working with children with autism has a direct effect on their behaviour. Previous work undertaken by Rydell and Mirenda (1994) found that, when autistic children were placed in highly controlled contexts, which typically included the use of numerous high constraint utterances, they resorted to inefficient communicative behaviours such as echolalia. This study confirms that an adult facilitative style, which typically uses low constraint utterances, such as comments, is more likely to result in increased communicative attempts, including non-verbal attempts and increased joint attention activities such as sharing and turn-taking. Indeed, my study indicated that the child's behaviour was altered negatively even by the limited use of socially demanding language such as the use of her name.

It is interesting to note that the area that showed least change during the study was Helen's vocabulary.

This study also supports previous work undertaken, which considers play as a useful treatment medium for occupational therapists working with children with developmental disorders. In their paper of 1994, Restall and Magill Evans suggested that the therapeutic use of play with children with autism should be considered as a means of developing skills for communication and social interaction.

A play environment was used as the basis of the intervention programme; the results from my study indicated that such an environment, which provides the child with a range of opportunities for exploration and learning, is very important.

The findings of this study suggest that, by providing a balanced but comprehensive play environment, the therapist can facilitate the autistic child's learning through play. The provision of an attractive play environment combined with an adult facilitating the child's performance within that environment appeared, from my study, to increase the child's competency to play.

This study also began to fill a gap in the published literature regarding the intervention regimen as perceived by the therapist. The study acknowledges the essential symbiosis that exists between therapist and client. It demonstrates that this relationship is dynamic and reflexive on both sides; it also suggests that, in this particular instance, the therapist acknowledged that the pace of change was dictated by the client, that her learning was led by the child's responses.

The second aim of my study was to consider the impact of diagnosis on a family and their early perceptions of therapy. The findings related to the experiences of the parents strongly echo those findings of previous researchers who have considered the impact of disability on a family.

The work of Jupp (1992) about the emotional confusion experienced by the parents has been confirmed by my study. It adds to the very limited literature that considers the responses of mothers and fathers separately. Many of the findings of this study almost directly replicate those of Cook (1996) in her paper, which considered the impact of having a child with autism on two families. This study is important because it is one of the first to consider a British family's experience of having an autistic child. It highlights the pressures and responsibilities that they have in coping with their child, but it also describes how they are developing their understanding of autism, and details insights into their developing understanding of their child and what she and they can achieve.

This study highlights the positive feelings that the parents have concerning the therapy and the constructive changes that they have experienced in the home environment. However, they also stress the challenges that faced them when attempting to understand and incorporate the therapy principles into their daily lives.

I have used this case study to illustrate a changing method of practice when working with pre-school children with autism. A move away from child-centred working towards a family-centred service. This is an emerging way of working; to be most effective in engaging with families, all the research emphasises the essential need to understand the structure, communication, concerns and strengths of the family with whom you are working (Simeonsson et al., 1986; Case-Smith, 1991; Turnbull and Turnbull, 1991). Early intervention that considers family variables and most importantly the family's perception of and relationship with their child is most likely to result in positive experiences of therapy for both child and parent (Kjerland and Kovach, 1990).

By considering all these family dynamics, I have developed a framework for a collaborative intervention activity that can effectively match the needs of the child, the family and the goals of therapy.

Undertaking this combined study within my clinical practice has enhanced my clinical reasoning skills. Not only have I developed my diagnostic and intervention skills, I have also used the carers' unique personal experience to improve my clinical performance. It is this combination of clinical expertise and understanding of client/carer perspective that is the cornerstone of my family-centred approach for children with autism.

The study has limitations; it does consider only a single case and so to generalise the findings would be inappropriate. It gives suggestions that other therapists may be able to transfer to their particular practice. It did not consider changes in play behaviour in the child's other environments, such as the Opportunity Playgroup. Although the child was not receiving any other therapy input, changes in her play behaviour could have been influenced by the experience of her playgroup.

Further research could be undertaken to extend the findings of this study:

- Parental perspectives on the application of therapeutic principles within the home
- An examination of change in play behaviours in all of a child's environments
- The relationship between play behaviour in the pre-school child and long-term outcomes
- A comparative study between the applications of the non-directive approach as provided by occupational therapists and speech and language therapists.

Conclusion

This study has confirmed for me the value of this approach when working with pre-school children with autism. It is an interdisciplinary approach and can be delivered by any experienced paediatric therapist. Interdisciplinary intervention programmes are a valuable and cost-effective method of ensuring comprehensive services that maximise professional expertise.

The findings of the study have implications for practising occupational therapists, in respect of the interventions provided for young children with autism. The study supports the growing body of professional opinion advocating parental inclusion in any intervention programme for young children.

The information gained may also be useful as a demonstration of clinical effectiveness that can be shared with fellow professionals and financing authorities.

References

Adams C, Sheslow T (1990) *Wide Range Assessment of Memory and Learning (WRAML)*. London: The Psychological Corporation.

Adams J (1996) Splinting the rheumatoid wrist and hand: evidence for its effectiveness. *British Journal of Therapy and Rehabilitation* 11: 621–624.

Adcock EW, Consolvo CA (1993) Fluid and electrolyte management. In: Merenstein GG, Gardner SL, eds, *Handbook of Neonatal Intensive Care*, 3rd edn. St Louis, MO: Mosby, pp 153–168.

Ainscough K, Telford R (1995) Conclusion. In: Kaplan C, Telford R (1998) *The Butterfly Children – An account of non-directive play therapy*. Edinburgh: Churchill Livingstone, pp 143–153.

Ainsworth MD (1978) *Patterns of Attachment: A psychological study of the strange situation*. New York: Halstead Press.

Alistair AH, Ross KR, Russell G (1979) The effect of posture on ventilation and lung mechanics in preterm and light-for-date infants. *Pediatrics* 64: 429–432.

Allen MC (1993) The high risk infant. *Pediatric Clinics of North America* 40: 479–490.

Als H (1982) Toward a synactive theory of development: promise for the assessment and support of infant individuality. *Infant Mental Health Journal* 3: 229–243.

Als H (1984) *Manual for the Naturalistic Observation of Newborn Behaviour (Preterm and Full-term Infants)*. Boston, MA: Children's Hospital.

Als H (1986) A synactive model of neonatal behavioural organisation: framework for the assessment of neurobehavioural development in the premature infant and for support of infants and parents in the Neonatal Intensive Care environment. *Physical and Occupational Therapy in Paediatrics* 6: 3–55.

Als H (1998) Developmental care in the newborn intensive care unit. *Current Opinion in Pediatrics* 10: 138–142.

Als H, Duffy FH (1989) Neurobehavioural assessment in the newborn period: Opportunity for early detection in later learning disabilities and for early intervention. *Birth Defects* 25: 127–152.

Als H, Lester BM (1982) Manual for the Assessment of preterm infants' behaviour (APIB). In: Fitzgerald HE, Lester BM, Yogman MW, eds, *Theory and Research in Behavioural Pediatrics*, vol 1. New York: Plenum, pp 65–132.

Als H, Lester BM, Tronich E, Brazelton TB (1982) Manual for the assessment of preterm infant behaviour (APIB). In: Fitzgerald HE, Lester BM, Yogman MW, eds, *Theory and Research in Behavioural Pediatrics*, vol II. New York: Plenum, pp 64–133.

Als H, Lawhon G, Browne E et al. (1986) Individualised behavioural and environmental care for the very low birth weight preterm infant at high risk for bronchopulmonary dysplasia: neonatal intensive care unit and developmental outcome. *Pediatrics* **78**: 1123–1132.

Alston J, Taylor J (1988) *The Handwriting File*. Wisbech, Cambs: LDA.

American Occupational Therapy Association (1988) *Efficacy Data Brief – Research supports efficacy of sensory integrative procedures*. Rockville, MD: AOTA.

American Occupational Therapy Association (1993) Knowledge and skills for occupational therapy practice in the neonatal intensive care unit. *American Journal of Occupational Therapy* **47**: 1100–1105.

American Occupational Therapy Association (1994) *Uniform Terminology*, 3rd edn. *American Journal of Occupational Therapy* **48**: 1047–1054.

American Psychiatric Association (1987) *Diagnostic and Statistical Manual of Mental Disorders*, 3rd edn revised. Washington, DC: American Psychiatric Association.

American Psychiatric Association (1994) *Diagnostic and Statistical Manual of Mental Disorders*, 4th edn. Washington, DC: American Psychiatric Association.

Amiel-Tison C, Grenier A (1986) *Neurological Assessment during the First Years of Life*. New York: Oxford University Press.

Amundson SJ (1995) *Evaluation Tool of Children's Handwriting*. Homer, AL: OT Kids.

Anderson G (2000) Applying the Bobath Concept in an underresourced and disadvantaged area – Lessons learned. *British Association of Bobath-Trained Therapists Newsletter* **35**: 34–37.

Anderson GM (1997) Studies on the neurochemistry of autism. In: Bauman ML, Kemper TL, eds, *The Neurobiology of Autism*. Baltimore, MD: Johns Hopkins University Press.

Anderson S (1992) Motor and sensory characteristics of fragile X. In: Schopmeyer BB, Lowe F (eds), *The Fragile X Child*. San Diego, CA: Singular Publishing Group, pp 59–70.

Anderson LJ, Anderson JM (1986) A positioning seat for the neonate and infant with high tone. *American Journal of Occupational Therapy* **40**: 186–190.

Andrews L (1995) Bathroom and toilet equipment for children. *British Journal of Therapy and Rehabilitation* **2**: 586 – 592.

Anzalone ME (1994) The issue is – occupational therapy in neonatology; what is our ethical responsibility? *American Journal of Occupational Therapy* **48**: 563–566.

Aram DM, Horwitz SJ (1983) Sequential and non-speech praxic abilities in developmental verbal apraxia. *Developmental Medicine and Child Neurology* **25**: 197–206.

Archer LA, Witelson SF (1988) Manual motor functions in developmental dysphasia. *Journal of Clinical and Experimental Neuropsychology* **10**: 47.

Arendt RE, Maclean WE, Baumeister AA (1988) Critique of sensory integration therapy and its application in mental retardation. *American Journal on Mental Retardation* **92**: 401–411.

Arthritis Research Campaign (1997) *Tim has Arthritis*. Chesterfield: ARC.

Arthritis Research Campaign (1998) *Diet and Arthritis*. Chesterfield: ARC.

Atkinson RL, Atkinson RC, Smith EE, Bem DJ, Hilgard ER (1990) *Introduction to Psychology*. Fort Worth: Harcourt Brace Jovanovich College Publishers.

Axline V (1947) *Play Therapy*. Edinburgh: Churchill Livingstone.

Axline V (1964) *Dibs in Search of Self*. Harmondsworth: Penguin.

Ayres AJ (1961) Development of body scheme in children. *American Journal of Occupational Therapy* **15**: 99–102.

Ayres AJ (1964) Tactile functions: their relation to hyperactive and perceptual-motor behaviour. *American Journal of Occupational Therapy* **18**: 6–11.

Ayres AJ (1965) A method of measurement of degree of sensorimotor integration. *Archives of Physical Medicine and Rehabilitation* **46**: 433–435.

Ayres AJ (1968) Sensory integrative processes and neuropsychological learning disabilities. *Learning Disorders* **3**: 41–58.

Ayres AJ (1972a) *Sensory Integration and Learning Disorders.* Los Angeles, CA: Western Psychological Services.

Ayres AJ (1972b) *Southern California Sensory Integration Tests – Manual.* Los Angeles, CA: Western Psychological Services.

Ayres AJ (1972c) Types of sensory integrative dysfunction among disabled learners. *American Journal of Occupational Therapy* **26**: 13–18.

Ayres AJ (1972d) Improving academic scores through sensory integration. *Journal of Learning Disabilities* **5**: 21–28.

Ayres AJ (1975) *Southern California Postrotary Nystagmus Test – Manual.* Los Angeles, CA: Western Psychological Services.

Ayres AJ (1976) *Interpreting the Southern California Sensory Integration Tests.* Los Angeles, CA: Western Psychological Services.

Ayres AJ (1979) *Sensory Integration and the Child.* Los Angeles, CA: Western Psychological Services.

Ayres AJ (1980) *Definition of Sensory Integrative Therapy – a position paper prepared for the California State Department of Special Education.* April, 1984.

Ayres AJ (1985) *Developmental Dyspraxia and Adult Onset Apraxia.* Torrance, CA: Sensory Integration International.

Ayres AJ (1989) *Sensory Integration and Praxis Tests (SIPT).* Los Angeles, CA: Western Psychological Services.

Ayres AJ, Mailloux Z (1981) Influence of sensory integration procedures on language development. *American Journal of Occupational Therapy* **35**: 383–390.

Ayres AJ, Mailloux ZK (1983) Possible pubertal effect on therapeutic gains in an autistic girl. *American Journal of Occupational Therapy* **37**: 535–540.

Ayres AJ, Marr DB (1991) Sensory Integration and Praxis Tests. In: Fisher AG, Murray EA, Bundy AC, Eds, *Sensory Integration: Theory and Practice.* Philadelphia, PA: FA Davis, Chapter 8.

Ayres AJ, Tickle LS (1980) Hyper-responsivity to touch and vestibular stimuli as a predictor of positive response to sensory integration procedures by autistic children. *American Journal of Occupational Therapy* **34**: 375–381.

Ayres AJ, Mailloux Z, Wendler CL (1987) Developmental dyspraxia: is it a unitary function? *Occupational Therapy Journal of Research* **7**: 93–110.

Badawi N, Watson L, Petterson B, Slee J, Haan E, Stanley F (1998) What constitutes cerebral palsy? *Developmental Medicine and Child Neurology* **40**: 520–527.

Bailey A, Bolton P, LeCouteur A et al. (1995) Fragile X in twins and multiplex families with autism. *Psychological Medicine* **25**: 63–67.

Bailey A, Phillips A, Rutter M (1996) Autism: towards an integration of clinical, genetic, neuropsychological, and neurobiological perspectives. *Journal of Child Psychology and Child Psychiatry* **1**: 89–126.

Baird TM, Paton JB, Fisher DE (1992) Improved oxygenation with prone positioning in neonates: Stability of increased transcutaneous Po. *Neonatal Intensive Care* July/August: 43–46.

Baranek GT, Foster LG, Berkson G (1997) Tactile defensiveness and stereotyped behaviors. *American Journal of Occupational Therapy* **51**: 91–95.

Baron-Cohen S (1989) The autistic child's theory of mind: a case of specific development delay. *Journal of Child Psychology and Psychiatry* **30**: 285–297.

Baron-Cohen S, Allen J, Gillberg C (1992) Can autism be detected at 18 months? The needle, the haystack and the CHAT. *British Journal of Psychiatry* **161**: 839–843.

Baron-Cohen S, Tager-Flusberg H, Cohen DIJ (1993) *Understanding Other Mind, Perspectives from Autism*, 2nd edn. Oxford: Oxford University Press.

Baron-Cohen S, Cox A, Baird G et al. (1996) Psychological markers in the detection of autism in infancy in a large population. *British Journal of Psychiatry* **168**: 158–163.

Barsch R (1968) *Achieving Perceptual–Motor Efficiency*. Seattle, WA: Special Child Publications.

Bartram J, Clewell WH (1989) Prenatal environment: impact on neonatal outcome. In: Merenstein GB, Gardner SL (eds), *Handbook of Neonatal Intensive Care*, 2nd edn. St Louis, MO: Mosby.

Basmajan JV, De Luca C (1985) *Muscles Alive. Their functions revealed by electromyography*. Baltimore, MD: Williams & Wilkins.

Bauman ML (1991) Microscopic neuroanatomic abnormalities in autism. *Pediatrics* **87**: 791–796.

Bauman ML, Kemper TL (1997) Observations of the brain in autism. In: Bauman ML, Kemper TL, eds, *The Neurobiology of Autism*. Baltimore, MD: Johns Hopkins University Press.

Baumgardner TL, Reiss AL, Freund LS, Abrams MT (1995) Specification of the neurobehavioural phenotype in males with Fragile X Syndrome. *Pediatrics* **95**: 744–752.

Bayley N (1991) *Bayley Scales of Infant Development, II*. Sidcup, Kent: Psychological Corporation.

Bear MF, Connors BW, Paradiso MA (1996) *Neuroscience, Exploring the Brain*. Baltimore, MD: Williams & Wilkins.

Becker PT, Grunwald PC, Moorman J, Stahr S (1991) Outcomes of developmentally supportive nursing care for very low birth weight infants. *Nursing Research* **40**: 150–155.

Becker PT, Grunwald PC, Moorman J, Stahr S (1993) Effects of developmental care on behavioural organisation in very low birth weight infants. *Nursing Research* **42**: 214–220.

Beckman PJ, Kohl FL (1984) The effects of social and isolate toys on the interactions and play of integrated and non-integrated groups of pre-schoolers. *Education and Training of the Mentally Retarded* **19**: 169–175.

Beery KE (1989) *Developmental Test of Visual Motor Integration*. London: The Psychological Corporation.

Beery KE, Buktenica NA (1989) *Developmental Test of Visual–Motor Integration*, 3rd revision. Cleveland, OH: Modern Curriculum Press.

Beery KE, Buktenica NA (1997) *The Beery–Buktenica Developmental Test of Visual–Motor Integration (VMI) Manual*. Parsippany, NJ: Modern Curriculum Press.

Bell V, Lyne S, Kolvin I (1989) Playgroup therapy with deprived children: community-based early secondary prevention. *British Journal of Occupational Therapy* **52**: 458–462.

Bennett SE, Karnes JL (1998) *Neurological Disabilities: Assessment and treatment.* Philadelphia, PA: Lippincott.

Bennetto L, Pennington BF (1996) The neuropsychology of Fragile X Syndrome. In: Hagerman RJ, Cronister JA, eds, *Fragile X Syndrome, Diagnosis, Treatment and Research*, 2nd edn. Baltimore, MD: Johns Hopkins University Press, pp 210–250.

Berk RA, DeGangi GA (1983*) DeGangi–Berk Test of Sensory Integration (TSI).* San Antonio, TX: Therapy Skill Builders.

Bernbaum JC, Pereria GR, Watkins JB, Peckham (1982) Non-nutritive sucking during gavage feeding enhances growth and maturation. *Pediatrics* 71: 41–45.

Berry J (1993) *Give Yourself a Hand – An Integrated Hand Skills Program.* Framingham, MA: Therapro Inc.

Bettleheim B (1967) *The Empty Fortress: Infantile autism and the birth of self.* New York: The Free Press.

Bishop D (1998) Development of the Children's Communication Checklist (CCC): a method of assessing qualitative aspects of communicative impairment in children. *Journal of Child and Adolescent Psychology and Psychiatry* 879–892.

Black S (1992) The genetics of fragile X syndrome. In: Schopmeyer BB, Lowe FF, eds, *The Fragile X Child.* San Diego, CA: Singular Publishing Group, pp 3–17.

Blackburn ST, VandenBerg KA (1993) Assessment and management of neonatal neurobehavioural development. In: Kenner C, Brueggemeyer A, Gunderson LP, eds, *Comprehensive Neonatal Nursing: A physiologic perspective.* Philadelphia, PA: WB Saunders, pp 1094–1130.

Blanchad Y (1991) Early intervention and stimulation of the hospitalized preterm infant. *Infants and Young Children* 4: 76–84.

Blanche EI (1997) Doing with – not doing to: play and the child with cerebral palsy. In: Parham LD, Fazio LS, eds, *Play in Occupational Therapy for Children.* St Louis, MO: Mosby.

Blanche EI (1998) Intervention for motor control and movement organization. In: Case-Smith J, ed., *Pediatric Occupational Therapy and Early Intervention*, 2nd edn. Oxford: Butterworth-Heinemann.

Blanche EI, Botticelli TM, Hallway MK (1995) *Combining Neuro-Developmental Treatment and Sensory Integration Principles. An approach to pediatric therapy.* . Harcourt, AZ Therapy Skill Builders.

Bloomer ML, Rose CC (1989a) Children with autism. In: Etheridge DA, ed., *Developmental Disabilities: A handbook for occupational therapists.* New York: The Haworth Press.

Bloomer ML, Rose CC (1989b) Frames of reference: guiding treatment for children with autism. *Occupational Therapy in Health Care* 6: 5–26.

Bloye D, Davies S (1999) *Psychiatry.* London: Mosby.

Bly L (1991) A historical and current view of the basis of NDT. *Pediatric Physical Therapy* 3: 131–5.

Bly L (1996) What is the role of sensation in motor learning? What is the role of feedback and feedforward? *NDTA Network* Sept/Oct: 1–7.

Bly L (1999) *Baby Treatment Based on NDT Principles.* Harcourt, AZ: Therapy Skill Builders.

Bly L (2000) Historical and current view of the basis of NDT. NDTA website: http://www.ndta.org 24/04/2000

Bly L, Whiteside A (1997) *Facilitation Techniques Based on NDT Principles*. San Antonio, TX: Therapy Skill Builders.

Bobath B (1972) Sensori-motor development. In: Course Notes. The Bobath Centre, London.

Bobath B (1997) Course Notes, Revised edn. The Bobath Centre, London.

Bobath B, Bobath K (1972) The neurodevelopmental approach to treatment. In: Pearson P, Williams C, eds, *Physical therapy services in the developmental disabilities.* Springfield, IL: Charles C. Thomas.

Bobath B, Bobath K (1975) *Motor Development of the Different Types of Cerebral Palsy*. Oxford: Butterworth–Heinemann.

Bobath Centre (1996) Advanced course on perception. In: *Course Notes*. London: The Bobath Centre.

Bobath Centre (1997) *Course Notes*. 1997 revised edn. London: The Bobath Centre.

Bobath Centre (2000) *Guide for Parents and Carers*. London: The Bobath Centre (http://www.bobath.org 08/05/2000).

Bobath K (1984) Cited in Bobath and Bobath (1984).

Bobath K, Bobath B (1984) The neuro-developmental treatment. In: Scrutton D, ed., *Management of Motor Disorders of Children with Cerebral Palsy*. Spastics International Publications. Oxford: Blackwell Scientific Publications Ltd.

Bochner S (1980) Sensory integration therapy and learning disabilities: a critique. *Journal of the Australian Association of Occupational Therapy* 27: 125–137.

Bolton P, Rutter M (1990) Genetic influences in autism. *International Review of Psychiatry* 2: 67–80.

Bolton P, Macdonald H, Pickles A et al. (1994) A case-controlled family history study of autism. *Journal of Child Psychology and Psychiatry* 35: 877–900.

Bottos M, Stafani D (1982) Letter. Postural and motor care of the premature baby. *Development Medicine and Child Neurology* 24: 706–707.

Bowlby J (1969) *Attachment and Loss Volume. 1 Attachment*. New York: Basic Books.

Boyd-Webb N (1993) *Helping Bereaved Children*. New York: Guilford Press.

Bracegirdle H (1992a) The use of play in occupational therapy for children: what is play? *British Journal of Occupational Therapy* 55: 107–108.

Bracegirdle H (1992b) The use of play in occupational therapy for children: how the therapist can help. *British Journal of Occupational Therapy* 55: 201–202.

Brackbill Y, Douthitt T, West H (1973) Psychophysiologic effects in the neonate of prone versus supine placement. *Journal of Pediatrics* 82: 82–83.

Bradlyn A, Himadi W, Crimmins D et al. (1983) Conversation skills training for retarded adolescents. *Behaviour Therapy* 14: 314–324.

Braun M, Palmer MM (1985) A pilot study of oral-motor dysfunction in 'at-risk' infants. *Physical and Occupational Therapy in Pediatrics* 5: 13–25.

Brazelton TB (1970) Effect of prenatal drugs on behaviour of the neonate. *American Journal of Psychiatry* 126: 1261–1266.

Brazelton TB (1973) The neonatal behavioural assessment scale. *Clinics in Developmental Medicine*, 50. Philadelphia, PA: JB Lippincott.

Brazelton TB (1979) Behavioural competence of the newborn infant. *Seminars in Perinatology* 3:35–44

Brazelton TB, Nugent JK (1995) *Neonatal Behavioural Assessment Scale*, 3rd edn. Cambridge: MacKeith Press.

Breathnach E (1996) The essence of play. *National Association of Paediatric Occupational Therapists Newsletter* Summer: 19–23.

Brenner CD (1992) Electric limbs for infants and pre-school children. *Journal of Prosthetics and Orthotics* 4: 184–190.

Brezman J, Kimberlin LVS (1993) Developmental outcome in extremely premature infants: Impact of surfactant. *Pediatric Clinics in North America* 40: 937–953.

British Institute of Mental Handicap (1981) *Ethical Implications of Behaviour Modification with Special Reference to Mental Handicap*. Kidderminster: British Institute of Mental Handicap.

British Psychological Society (1991) *Ethical Principles for Conducting Research with Human Participants*. Leicester: British Psychological Society.

Brooks VB (1986) *The Neural Basis for Motor Control*. Oxford: Oxford University Press.

Brown G (1996) Parents Experience of Learning about Their Child. Unpublished Master's Thesis. London: University of East London.

Brown MM (1999) Auditory integration training and autism: two case studies. *British Journal of Occupational Therapy* 62: 13–16.

Bruce MA, Borg B (1993) *Psychosocial Occupational Therapy Frames of Reference for Intervention*, 2nd edn. Thorofare, NJ: Slack.

Bruininks R (1978) *Bruininks–Oseretsky Test of Motor Proficiency*. Windsor, Berks: NFER-Nelson; Circle Pines, MN: American Guidance Service.

Bryce J (1991) Editorial – The Bobath Concept – where we are today. *British Association of Bobath-Trained Therapists Newsletter* 10: 1–6.

Bryze K (1997) Narrative Contributions to the Play History. In: Parham LD, Faxio LS, eds, *Play in Occupational Therapy for Children*. St Louis, MO: Mosby, pp 23–33.

Bu'Lock F, Woolridge MW, Baurn JD (1990) Development of co-ordination of sucking, swallowing and breathing: ultrasound study of term and preterm infants. *Developmental Medicine and Child Neurology* 32: 669–678.

Bundy A (1997) Test of Playfulness. In: Parnham LD, Faxio LS, eds, *Play in Occupational Therapy for Children*. St Louis, MO: Mosby, pp 57–65.

Bundy AC (1993) Assessment of play and leisure: delineation of the problem. *American Journal of Occupational Therapy* 47: 217–222.

Burke JP (1993) Play: the life role of the infant and young child. In: Case-Smith J, ed., *Pediatric Occupational Therapy and Early Intervention*. Stoneham: Heinemann.

Burke JP, Schaaf RC (1997) Family narratives and play assessment. In: Parham LD, Faxio LS, eds, *Play in Occupational Therapy for Children*. St Louis, MO: Mosby, pp 67–83.

Butler S, David A, Chalder T, Wesseley S (1989) Management of chronic fatigue syndrome. *Journal of the Royal College of General Practitioners* 39: 26–29.

Butler S, Chalder T, Ron M, Wesseley S (1991) Cognitive behaviour therapy in the chronic fatigue syndrome. *Journal of Neurology, Neurosurgery, and Psychiatry* 54: 153–158.

Byrnes M, Powers F (1989) Functional independence measure: its use in identifying rehabilitation needs in the head injured patient. *Journal of Neuroscience Nursing* 21: 61–63.

Cabay M, King LJ (1989) Sensory integration and perception: The foundation for concept formation. *Occupational Therapy Practice* 1: 18–27.

Cammisa KM, Hobbs SH (1993) Etiology of autism: A review of recent biogenic theories and research. *Occupational Therapy in Mental Health* 12: 36–67.

Carrasco RC, Lee CE (1993) Development of a teacher questionnaire on sensorimotor behaviour. *AOTA Sensory Integration Special Interest Section Newsletter* 16: 5–6.

Carte E (1984) Sensory integration therapy: a trial of a specific neurodevelopmental therapy for the remediation of learning disabilities. *Journal of Developmental and Behavioural Pediatrics* 5: 189–194.

Carter B, Dearman A (1995) *Child Health Care Nursing Concepts: Theory and practice.* Oxford: Blackwell Science.

Cartledge G, Milburn J (1980) *Teaching Social Skills for Children.* Oxford: Pergamon.

Casas MJ, Kenny DJ, McPherson KA (1994) Swallowing/ventilation interactions during oral swallow in normal children and children with cerebral palsy. *Dysphagia* 9: 40–46.

Case-Smith J (1989) Intervention strategies for promoting feeding skills in infants with sensory defects. *Occupational Therapy in Health Care* 6: 129–141.

Case-Smith J (1991) The family perspective. In Dunn W, ed., *Pediatric Occupational Therapy: Facilitating effective service delivery.* Thorofare, NJ: Slack.

Case-Smith J, ed. (1998) *Pediatric Occupational Therapy and Early Intervention*, 2nd edn. Oxford: Butterworth-Heinemann.

Case-Smith J, Allen AS, Pratt PN, eds (1996) *Occupational Therapy for Children*, 3rd edn. St Louis, MO: Mosby.

Cattanach A (1992) *Play Therapy with Abused Children.* London: Jessica Kingsley.

Cattanach A (1994) *Play Therapy: Where the sky meets the underworld.* London: Jessica Kingsley.

Cermak S (1988) The relationship between attention deficit and sensory integration disorders (Part I). *Sensory Integration Special Interest Section Newsletter* 11: 1–4.

Cermak SA (1985) Developmental dyspraxia. In: Roy EA, ed., *Neuropsychological Studies of Apraxia and Related Disorders.* Amsterdam, Netherlands: Elsevier (North-Holland), pp 115–248.

Cermak SA (1991) Somatodyspraxia. In: Fisher AG, Murray EA, Bundy AC, eds, *Sensory Integration – Theory and Practice.* Philadelphia, PA: FA Davis Co.

Cermak SA, Henderson A (1989) The efficacy of sensory integrative procedures – part I. *Sensory Integration Quarterly* XVII: 1–5.

Cermak SA, Henderson A (1990) The efficacy of sensory integrative procedures – part II. *Sensory Integration Quarterly* XVIII: 1–5.

Cermak SA, Coster W, Drake C (1980) Representational and non-representational gestures in boys with learning disabilities. *American Journal of Occupational Therapy* 34: 19–26.

Cermak SA, Ward EA, Ward LM (1986) The relationship between articulation disorders and motor coordination in children. *American Journal of Occupational Therapy* 40: 546–550.

Chandler LS, Andrews MS, Swanson MW (1980) *Movement Assessment of Infants (MAI).* Rolling Bay, WA: Infant Movement Research.

Charlton C, Kavanagh G (1994) An improved sloping desk-top: a controlled trial in South Australian school. *Handwriting Review* 1: 113–120.

Cheseldine S (1991) Gentle teaching for challenging behaviour. In: Waston J, ed., *Innovatory Practice and Severe Learning Difficulties*. Edinburgh: Murray House Publications.

Chia SH (1978) An introduction to the use of behaviour modification techniques in an occupational therapy activities of daily living (ADL) programme for mentally handicapped children. *British Journal of Occupational Therapy* **41**: 299–301.

Chia SH (1987) Occupational therapy and mental handicap. In: Bumphrey EE, ed., *Occupational Therapy in the Community*. Cambridge: Woodhead Faulkner.

Chia SH (1995) Evaluating groups in learning disabilities. *Nursing Standard* **10**: 25–27.

Chia SH (1996a) A survey of practice among occupational therapists working with children. Unpublished. Norwich: University of East Anglia.

Chia SH (1996b) The use of non-standardised assessments in occupational therapy with children with disabilities: a perspective. *British Journal of Occupational Therapy* **59**: 363–364.

Chia SH (1997a) Occupational therapists' assessment practices with children who have disabilities. *British Journal of Therapy and Rehabilitation* **4**: 123–128.

Chia SH (1997b) Occupational therapy and children with learning disabilities. In: Fawcus M, ed., *Children with Learning Difficulties*. London: Whurr.

Chia SH, St John C, Gabriel H (1996) *Sensory Motor Activities for Early Development*. Oxford: Winslow.

Chow SMK (1989) Assessment practices of paediatric occupational therapists. Unpublished MSc Dissertation. Southampton: University of Southampton.

Christiansen C (1994) *Ways of Living – Self-Care Strategies for Special Needs*. Rockville, MD: American Occupational Therapy Association.

Chu S (1990) Misconceptions in the theory and practice of sensory integrative therapy. *National Association of Paediatric Occupational Therapists Newsletter* Autumn: 13–17.

Chu S (1993) Clinical observations for evaluation in sensory integration. In: *Manual of Advanced Workshop I, The Treatment of Sensory Integrative Dysfunctions*. London: British Institute for Sensory Integration.

Chu S (1996) Evaluating the sensory integrative functions of mainstream school children with specific developmental disorders. *British Journal of Occupational Therapy* **59**: 465–474.

Chu S (1997) Developing sensory-perceptual-motor skills in children with autistic spectrum disorder: an occupational therapist's perspective. *National Association of Paediatric Occupational Therapists Newsletter* Summer: 19–23.

Chu S (1998a) Developmental dyspraxia 1: The diagnosis. *British Journal of Therapy and Rehabilitation* **5**: 131–138.

Chu S (1998b) Developmental dyspraxia 2: Evaluation and treatment. *British Journal of Therapy and Rehabilitation* **5**: 176–180.

Chu S (1999) *Course Handbook – Assessment and Treatment of Children with Handwriting Difficulties*, 11th edn. London.

Clancy H, Clark MJ (1990) *Occupational Therapy with Children*. Melbourne: Churchill Livingstone.

Clark FA, Pierce A (1986) Synopsis of pediatric occupational therapy effectiveness: studies on sensory integrative procedures, controlled vestibular stimulation, other sensory stimulation approaches, and perceptual-motor training. *Proceedings of the*

Occupational Therapy for Maternal and Child Health Conference. Vol. 1 – Leadership, Practice, Research. Santa Monica, CA, January 13–14, pp 226–244.

Cogher L, Savage E, Smith MF (1992) *Cerebral Palsy*. London: Chapman & Hall.

Cohen L, Manion L (1994) *Research Methods in Education*, 4th edn. London: Routledge.

Cohn ES, Cermak SA (1998) Including the family perspective in sensory integration outcomes research. *American Journal of Occupational Therapy* **52**: 540–546.

Colangelo CA (1999) Biomechanical frame of reference. In: Kramer P, Hinojosa J, eds, *Frames of Reference for Pediatric Occupational Therapy*, 2nd edn. Baltimore, MD: Williams & Wilkins.

Colarusso R, Hammill D (1995a) *Motor Free Visual Perception Test*. Novato, CA: Academic Therapy Publications.

Colarusso RP, Hammill DD (1995b) *Motor Free Visual Perception Test – Revised*. Novato, CA: Academic Therapy Publications.

Colarusso RP, Hammill DD (1996) *Motor-Free Test of Visual Perception – Revised (MVPT-R) Manual*. Novato, CA: Academic Therapy Publications.

Cole KN, Harris SR, Eland SF, Mills PE (1989) Comparisons of two service delivery models: In-class and out-of-class therapy approaches. *Pediatric Physical Therapy* **1**: 49–54.

Cole JG (1985) Infant stimulation re-examined: an environmental and behavioural based approach. *Neonatal Network* **3**: 24–31.

Coleman M, Gillberg C (1990) *The Biology of Autistic Syndromes*. New York: Praeger.

College of Occupational Therapists (2000, updated regularly) *Code of Professional Conduct*. London: British Association of Occupational Therapists.

College of Occupational Therapists' Research and Development Group (1998) *Occupational Therapy for People with Learning Disabilities Living in the Community*. London: College of Occupational Therapists.

Collin MF, Havey CL, Anderson CL (1991) Emerging developmental sequelae in the 'normal' extremely low birth weight infant. *Pediatrics* **88**: 115–120.

Comrie JD, Helm JM (1997) Common feeding problems in the intensive care nursery: maturation, organisation, evaluation and management strategies. *Seminars in Speech and Language* **18**: 239–261.

Connally BH, Montgomery PC, eds (1987) *Therapeutic Exercise in Developmental Disabilities*. Chattanooga, TN: Chattanooga Corporation.

Cook DG (1996) The impact of having a child with autism: Developmental disabilities. *American Journal of Occupational Therapy* **19**: 1–4.

Cornish K (1996) The relationship between cognitive functioning and molecular characteristics. *Fragile X Society Newsletter* **14**: 32–34.

Correll H, Dodd K (2000) Neuro-Developmental Therapy to improve motor function in treatment in children with cerebral palsy. Research which concludes that NDT is effective. *Australian Bobath Neuro-Developmental Therapy Association (Inc) Newsletter* May 2000:6.

Corrigan J, Smith-Knapp K, Granger C (1997) Validity of FIM for persons with traumatic brain injury. *Archives of Physical Medicine and Rehabilitation* **78**: 828–834.

Coster W, Deeney T, Haltiwanger, Haley S (1998) *School Function Assessment Manual*. San Antonio, TX: Therapy Skill Builders.

Cratty BJ (1986) *Perceptual and Motor Development in Infants and Children*. Englewood Cliffs, NJ: Prentice-Hall.

Creger PJ, Browne JV (1989) *Developmental Interventions for Preterm and High-risk Infants: Self-study modules for professionals*. Tucson, AZ: Therapy Skill Builders.

Cronin AF (1989) Children with emotional and behavioural disorders. In: Pratt PN, Allen AS, eds, *Occupational Therapy for Children*, 2nd edn. St Louis, MO: Mosby.

Cummins RA (1991) Sensory integration and learning disabilities: Ayres' factor analysis reappraised. *Journal of Learning Disabilities* 24: 160–168.

Cupps B (1997) Postural control: a current view. *NDTA Network* Jan/Feb: 1–7.

Curran B, Hambrey R (1991) The prosthetic treatment of upper limb deficiency. *Prosthetics and Orthotics International* 15: 82–87.

David R, Deuel R, Ferry P et al. (1981) Proposed nosology of disorders of higher cerebral function in children. Task Force on Nosology of Disorders of Higher Cerebral Function in Children. Child Neurology Society. Unpublished Manuscript.

Davies P, Gavin W (1993) Comparison of individual and group/consultation treatment methods for pre-school children with developmental delays. *American Journal of Occupational Therapy* 48: 155–161.

Dawdy SC (1981) Pediatric neuropsychology: caring for the developmentally dyspraxic child. *Clinical Neuropsychology* 3: 30–37.

Dawson G, Adams A (1984) Imitation and social responsiveness in autistic children. *Journal of Abnormal Child Psychology* 12: 209–224.

Dawson G, Galpert L (1990) Mothers use of imitative play for facilitating social responsiveness and toy play in young children. *Development and Psychopathology* 2: 151–162.

Dawson G, Meltzoff Osterling J, Rinaldi J, Brown E (1998) Children with autism fail to orient to naturally occurring social stimuli. *Journal of Autism and Developmental Disorder* 28: 479–485.

De-Clive Lowe S (1996) Outcome measurement, cost-effectiveness and clinical audit: the importance of standardised assessment to occupational therapists in meeting these new demands. *British Journal of Occupational Therapy* 59: 357–362.

DeGangi GA, Greenspan SI (1989) *Test of Sensory Functions in Infants (TSFI)*. Los Angeles, CA: Western Psychological Services.

DeGangi GA, Porges SW (1991) Lesson 5 – Attention/Alertness/Arousal. In: Royeen CB, ed., *AOTA Self-Study Series – Neuroscience Foundations of Human Performance*. Bethesda, MD: The American Occupational Therapy Association.

DeGangi GA, Royeen CB (1994) Current practice among Neuro-Developmental Treatment Association members. *American Journal of Occupational Therapy* 48: 803–809.

DeMatteo C, Law M, Russell D, Pollock N, Rosenbaum P, Walter S (1992) Quality of Upper Extremity Skills Test Manual. Available from Mary Law, Neurodevelopmental Clinical Research Unit, McMaster University, Rm 126, Bldg T-16, 1280 Main Street, Hamilton, West Ontario L83 4J9, Canada.

Denckla MB, Roeltgen DP (1992) Disorders of motor function and control. In: Rapin I, Segalowitz L, eds, *Handbook of Neuropsychology*, vol. 6. *Child Neuropsychology*. Amsterdam: Elsevier Science.

Densem JF (1989) Effectiveness of a sensory integrative therapy program for children with perceptual–motor deficits. *Journal of Learning Disabilities* 22: 221–229.

Department of Health and Social Security (1978) *Health Services Development: Court report on child health services*. Circular HC(78) 5 London: DHSS.

De Sanctis S (1906) On some varieties of dementia praecox. In: Howells JG (1969) *Modern Perspectives in International Psychiatry*. Edinburgh: Oliver & Boyd.

Deuel PK, Doar BP (1992) Developmental manual dyspraxia: a lesson in mind and brain. *Journal of Child Neurology* 7: 99–103.

Dewey D (1995) What is developmental dyspraxia? *Brain and Cognition* 29: 254–274.

Dewey D, Roy EA, Square-torer PA, Hayden D (1988) Limb and oral praxic abilities in children with verbal sequencing deficits. *Developmental Medicine and Child Neurology* 30: 743–751.

Dietz V (1992) Spasticity: exaggerated reflexes or movement disorder. *Medical Sports Science* 36: 1–6.

Dobbins JG, Randall B, Reyes M, Reeves WC (1997) The prevalence of chronic fatigue illnesses among adolescents in the United States. *Journal of Chronic Fatigue Syndrome* 3(2): 15–27.

Dolan J (1995) The challenge of community integration for people with learning difficulties. In: Bumphrey EE, ed., *Community Practice*. Hemel Hempstead: Prentice-Hall/Harvester Wheatsheaf.

Doverty N (1992) The therapeutic use of play in hospital. *British Journal of Nursing* 1: 77–80.

Drotar D, Baskiewics A, Irwin A, Kennel J, Klaus M (1975) The adaptation of parents to the birth of an infant with a congenital malformation: a hypothetical model. *Pediatrics* 56: 710–717.

Dubignon JM et al. (1969) The development of non-nutritive sucking in premature infants. *Biology of the Neonate* 14: 270–278.

Dubowitz L, Dubowitz V (1981) Neurological assessment of the preterm and full term newborn infant. Clinics in developmental medicine, no. 70. London: Heinemann.

Dubowitz L, Dubowitz V, Meruri E (1999) *Clinics in Developmental Medicine*, No. 18. Cambridge: MacKeith Press/Cambridge University Press.

Duncombe L, Howe M (1994) Group treatment: goals, tasks and economic implications. *American Journal of Occupational Therapy* 49: 199–205.

Dunn W (1990) A comparison of service provision models in school-based occupational therapy services; a pilot study. *Occupational Therapy Journal of Research* 10: 300–319.

Dunn W (1994) Performance of typical children on the sensory profile: an item analysis. *American Journal of Occupational Therapy* 48: 967–974.

Dunn W (1997) The sensory profile: a discriminatory measure of sensory processing in daily life. *AOTA Sensory Integration Special Interest Section Quarterly* 20: 1–3.

Dunn W (1999) *Sensory Profile – User's Manual*. San Antonio, TX: The Psychological Corporation.

Dunn W (2000) *Best Practice Occupational Therapy in Community Service with Children and Families*. Thorofare, NJ: Slack Inc.

Dunn W, Brown C (1997) Factor analysis on the sensory profile from a national sample of children without disabilities. *American Journal of Occupational Therapy* 51: 490–495.

Dunn W, Campbell PH (1991) Designing pediatric service provision. In: Dunn W, ed, *Pediatric Occupational Therapy – Facilitating Effective Service Provision*. Thorofare, NJ: Slack Inc.

Dunn W, Westman K (1997) The sensory profile: the performance of a national sample of children without disabilities. *American Journal of Occupational Therapy* 51: 25–34.

Edwards S, ed. (2001) *Neurological Physiotherapy – a Problem Solving Approach*, 2nd edn. Edinburgh: Churchill Livingstone.

Edwards SJ, Yuen HK (1990) An intervention programme for a fraternal twin with Down Syndrome. *American Journal of Occupational Therapy* 44: 454–458.

Elenko BK (1999) Case study: Neurodevelopmental treatment frame of reference. In: Kramer P, Hinojosa J, eds, *Frames of Reference for Pediatric Occupational Therapy*, 2nd edn. Baltimore, MD: Williams & Wilkins.

Ellis R, Whittington D (1993) *Quality Assurance in Health Care: A handbook*. London: Edward Arnold.

Emery AEH (1994) *Muscular Dystrophy: The facts*. Oxford: Oxford University Press.

Emery JR, Peabody JL (1983) Head position affects intracranial pressure in newborn infants. *Journal of Pediatrics* 103: 950–953.

Emunah R (1995) From adolescent trauma to adolescent drama. In: Jennings S, ed., *Dramatherapy with Children and Adolescents*. London: Routledge.

Engvall J (1996) Innovative approaches for teaching children with chronic conditions. *Journal of Paediatric Health Care* 5: 239–242.

Erhardt RP (1982) *Developmental Hand Dysfunction: Theory, assessment and treatment*. Amapolis, MD: RAMSCO Publishing Co.

Erhardt RP, ed. (1999) *Parent Articles about NDT*. Harcourt, AZ: Therapy Skill Builders.

Ermer J, Dunn W (1998) The sensory profile: a discriminant analysis of children with and without disabilities. *American Journal of Occupational Therapy* 52: 283–290.

Escobar G, Littenberg B, Pettittl D (1991) Outcome among surviving very low birth weight infants. A meta-analysis. *Archives of Diseases in Childhood* 66: 204–211.

Ethridge DA (1970) Behavioural modification techniques in occupational therapy. Occupational therapy today and tomorrow. *Proceedings 5th International Congress, World Federation of Occupational Therapists*, Zurich, pp 215–219.

Evans D, Thakker Y, Donnai D (1991) Hereditary and dysmorphic syndromes in congenital limb deficiencies. *Prosthetics and Orthotics International* 15: 70–77.

Falk-Kessler J, Momich C, Perel S (1991) Therapeutic factors in occupational therapy groups. *American Journal of Occupational Therapy* 45: 59–66.

Farrington K, Pruzansky C (1999) Case study: Combined sensory integration and neuro-developmental treatment frames of reference. In: Kramer P, Hinojosa J, eds, *Frames of Reference for Pediatric Occupational Therapy*, 2nd edn. Baltimore, MD: Williams & Wilkins.

Ferri R, Musumeci SA, Elia M, Del Gracco S, Scuderi C, Bergonzi P (1994) BIT-mapped somatosensory evoked potentials in the fragile x syndrome. *Neurophysiology Clinics* 24: 413–426.

Ferrier LJ, Bashir AS, Meryash DL, Johnston J, Wolff P (1991) Conversational skills of individuals with Fragile-X Syndrome: a comparison with autism and own syndrome. *Developmental Medicine and Child Neurology* 33: 776–788.

Fink BE (1989) *Sensory–Motor Integration Activities*. Tucson, AZ: Therapy Skill Builders.

Finlay L (1999) When action speaks louder: group work in occupational therapy. *Group Work* 11: 19–29.

Finnie NR (1997) *Handling the Young Child with Cerebral Palsy at Home*, 3rd edn. Oxford: Butterworth-Heinemann.

Fiorentino M (1965) *Reflex Testing Methods for Evaluating CNS Development*, 2nd edn. Springfield, IL: Charles Thomas.

Firth U (1992) Cognitive development and cognitive deficit. *The Psychologist* **5**: 13–19.

Fisher AG (1995) *AMPS Manual*. Fort Collins, CO: Three Star Press.

Fisher AG, Bundy AC (1991) The interpretation process. In: Fisher AG, Murray EA, Bundy AC, eds, *Sensory Integration: Theory and practice*. Philadelphia, PA: FA Davis, Chapter 9.

Fisher AG, Murray EA (1991) Introduction to sensory integration theory. In: Fisher AG, Murray EA, Bundy AC, eds, *Sensory Integration: Theory and practice*. Philadelphia, PA: FA Davis, Chapter 1.

Fisher AG, Murray EA, Bundy AC, eds (1991) *Sensory Integration: Theory and practice*. Philadelphia, PA: FA Davis.

Folio R, Fewell R (1984) *Peabody Developmental Motor Scales*. Allen, TX: Developmental Language Materials.

Folstein SE, Rutter ML (1977) Infantile autism: a genetic study of 21 twin pairs. *Journal of Child Psychology and Psychiatry* **18**: 297–321.

Forrai J (1999) Memoirs of the Beginnings of Conductive Pedagogy and Andras Petö. Budapest: Uj Aranhyid.

Fox (1985) Good Grief: Helping groups of children when a friend dies. Boston, MA: New England Association for the Education of Young Children.

Fox AM, Polatajko HJ (1994) *'The London Consensus' – from Children and Clumsiness: An International Consensus Meeting*. London, Ontario, Canada, 11–14 October 1994.

Fox M, Molesky M (1990) The effects of prone and supine positioning on arterial oxygen pressure. *Neonatal Network* **8**: 25–29.

Fraser WI, MacGillivray RC, Green AM (1995) *Hallas' Caring for People with Mental Handicaps*. Oxford: Butterworth-Heinemann.

Freeman JE (1995) Treatment of hand dysfunction in the child with cerebral palsy. In: Henderson A, Pehoski C, eds, *Hand Function in the Child. Foundations for Remediation*. St Louis, MO: Mosby.

Frith U (1989) *Autism: Explaining the enigma*. Oxford: Blackwell.

Frostig M, Horne D (1973) *The Frostig Programme for the Development of Visual Perception*. Chicago: Follett.

Frostig MR (1982) *Move. Grow. Learn – Movement education activities*. Chicago: Follett.

Gallahue DL (1982) *Understanding Motor Development in Children*. New York: John Wiley.

Gardner M (1986) *Test of Visual Motor Skills (TVMS)*. Burlingame, CA: Psychological and Educational Publications.

Gardner MF (1982) *Test of Visual–Perceptual Skills (Non-Motor)*. Burlingame, CA: Psychological and Educational Publications.

Gardner-Medwin D (1999) *Duchenne Muscular Dystrophy: Medical Factsheet*. London: Muscular Dystrophy Campaign.

Garner C, Callias M, Turk J (1999) The executive function and theory of mind performance of young men with Fragile X syndrome. *Journal of Intellectual Disability Research* **43**: 466–474.

Gates B, ed. (1997) *Learning Disabilities*, 3rd edn. New York: Churchill Livingstone.

Gelman R (1978) Cognitive development. *Annual Review of Psychology* **29**: 297–332.

Getman G (1965) The visuomotor complex in the acquisition of learning skills. In: Hellmath J, ed., *Learning Disorders*. Seattle, WA: Special Child Publications.

Giangreco ME, Edelman SW, MacFarland S, Luiselli TE (1997) Attitudes about educational and related service provision for students with deaf-blindness and multiple disabilities. *Exceptional Children* **63**: 329–342.

Gibb C (1996) The switched off gene. *Special Children* September 12–16.

Gibson H, Carroll N, Clague JE, Edwards RM (1993) Exercise performance and fatiguability in patients with chronic fatigue syndrome. *Journal of Neurology, Neurosurgery, and Psychiatry* **56**: 993–998.

Gillberg C (1995) *Clinical Child Neuropsychiatry*. Cambridge: Cambridge University Press, pp 203–208.

Gilroy PJ (1985) *Kids in Motion – an Early Childhood Movement Education Program*. Tucson, AZ: Communication Skill Builders.

Gilroy PJ (1989a) *Discovery in Motion – Movement Exploration for Problem-Solving and Self-Concept*. Tucson, AZ: Communication Skill Builders.

Gilroy PJ (1989b) *Kids in Action – Developing Body Awareness in Young Children*. Tucson, AZ: Communication Skill Builders.

Goggin C (1997) To what extent and in what ways do occupational therapists use play therapy with children with mental health needs? Unpublished dissertation. Norwich: University of East Anglia.

Golding R, Goldsmith L (1986) *The Caring Person's Guide to Handling the Severely Multiply Handicapped*. Basingstoke: Macmillan.

Goldstein H, Kaczmarek L, Pennington R, Shafer K (1992) Peer mediated intervention: acknowledging, attending to and commenting on the behaviour of pre-schoolers with autism. *Journal of Applied Behaviour Analysis* **25**: 289–305.

Goldstein PK (1978) Defining disciplinary roles with the learning disabled child. Tel Aviv: *Proceedings of the 7th International Congress of the World Federation of Occupational Therapists*.

Goodenough FL, Harris DB (1963) *Goodenough–Harris Drawing Test*. Sidcup, Kent: The Psychological Corporation.

Goodgold-Edwards SA, Cermak SA (1990) Interpreting motor control and motor learning concepts with neuropsychological perspectives on apraxia and developmental dyspraxia. *American Journal of Occupational Therapy* **44**: 431–439.

Gordon CH, Schanzenbacher KE, Case-Smith J, Carrasco RC (1996) Diagnostic problems in pediatrics. In: Case-Smith J, Allen AS, Pratt PN, eds, *Occupational Therapy for Children*. St Louis, MO: Mosby.

Gorga D (1994) Nationally speaking: the evolution of occupational therapy practice for infants in the neonatal intensive care unit. *American Journal of Occupational Therapy* **48**: 487–489.

Gorman PA (1997) Sensory dysfunction in dual diagnosis: mental retardation/mental illness and autism. *Occupational Therapy in Mental Health* **13**: 3–22.

Gottfried AW, Gaiter JC (1985*) Infant Stress under Intensive Care: Environmental neonatology*. Baltimore, MD: University Park Press

Graham P (1998) *Cognitive Behaviour Therapy for Children and Families*. Cambridge: Cambridge University Press.

Grandin T (1986) *Emergence Labelled Autistic*. London: Athena Press.

Granger C, Divan N, Fielder R (1995) Functional Assessment Scales. A study of persons after traumatic brain injury. *American Journal of Physical Medicine and Rehabilitation* **74**: 107–113.

Graven S, Bowen F, Brooten D et al. (1992) The high-risk infant environment, Part 1. *Journal of Perinatology* **12**: 164–172.

Green D (1997) Social Behaviour Scale. Research Edition. Unpublished. London: Guy's and St Thomas' NHS Trust.

Grunwald PC, Becker PT(1990) Developmental enhancement: Implementing a program for the NICU. *Neonatal Network* **9**: 29–45.

Gryboski JD (1969) Suck and swallow in premature infants. *Pediatrics* **43**: 96–102.

Gubbay SS (1975) *The Clumsy Child*. New York: WB Saunders.

Gunn SL (1975) Play as occupation: implications for the handicapped. *American Journal of Occupational Therapy* **29**: 222–225.

Hack M, Klein NK, Taylor HG (1995a) Long term developmental outcomes of low birth weight infants. *Future of Children* **5**: 176.

Hack M, Wright LL, Shankaran S et al. (1995b) Very low birth weight outcomes of the national institute of child health and human development neonatal network, November 1989–October 1990. *American Journal of Obstetrics and Gynecology* **172**: 457–468.

Hackett J, Johnson B, Parkin A, Southwood T (1996) Physiotherapy and occupational therapy for juvenile chronic arthritis: custom and practice in 5 centres in the UK, USA and Canada. *British Journal of Rheumatology* **35**: 695–699.

Hagberg B, Hagberg G, Olow I, von Wendt L (1989) The changing panorama of cerebral palsy in Sweden V. The birth year period 1979–82. *Acta Paediatrica Scandinavica* **78**: 283–290.

Hagberg B, Hagberg G, Olow I (1993) The changing panorama of cerebral palsy in Sweden VI. Prevalence and origin during birth year period 1983–1986. *Acta Paediatrica Scandinavica* 82:387–393.

Hagberg B, Hagberg G, Olow I, von Wendt L (1996) The changing panorama of cerebral palsy in Sweden VII. Prevalence and origin in the birth year period 1987–90. *Acta Paediatrica Scandinavica* **85**: 954–960.

Hagedorn R (1992) *Occupational Therapy: Foundations for practice*. Edinburgh: Churchill Livingstone.

Hagedorn R (1997) *Foundations for Practice in Occupational Therapy*, 2nd edn. Edinburgh: Churchill Livingstone.

Hagerman RJ (1991a) Fragile X Syndrome. *Encyclopedia of Human Biology* **3**: 709–717.

Hagerman RJ (1991b) Issues of diagnosis and treatment report on Family Day Conference, 28 Sept 1991. The Fragile X Society, UK.

Hagerman RJ (1996) Physical and behavioural phenotype. In: Hagerman RJ, Cronister A, eds, *Fragile X Syndrome, Diagnosis, Treatment and Research*, 2nd edn. Baltimore, MD: Johns Hopkins University Press, pp 3–87.

Hagerman RJ, Cronister A, eds (1996) *Fragile X Syndrome, Diagnosis, Treatment and Research*, 2nd edn. Baltimore, MD: Johns Hopkins University Press.

Haley SM, Coster WJ, Ludlow LH, Haltiwanger JT, Andrellos PJ (1992) *Paediatric Evaluation of Disability Inventory*. London: Psychological Corporation.

Hammill DD, Pearson NA, Voress JK (1993) *Developmental Test of Visual Perception*. Windsor, Berks: NFER-Nelson.

Hansen RA, Atchison B (2000*) Conditions in Occupational Therapy – Effect on Occupational Performance*. Philadelphia, PA: Lippincott Williams & Wilkins.

Happé F (1994) *Autism: An introduction to psychological theory*. London: University College London Press.

Hari M, Akos K (1988) *Conductive Education*. London: Routledge.

Harpin P (1997) *Mobile Stair Climbers: Factsheet*. London: Muscular Dystrophy Campaign.

Harpin P (1999a) *Information Leaflets on Equipment and Adaptations, Adaptations Manual – a Guide for Parents, Carers and Professionals*. London: Muscular Dystrophy Group.

Harpin P (1999b) *Wheelchairs for Children and Adults with Muscular Dystrophy and Allied Neuromuscular Conditions: Factsheet*. London: Muscular Dystrophy Campaign.

Harpin P (2000) *Adaptations Manual*. London: Muscular Dystrophy Campaign.

Harris DB (1963) *Goodenough–Harris Drawing Test*. New York, NY: Harcourt Brace Jovanovich.

Harris M, Jones D, Brooks S, Grant J (1986) Relations between the non-verbal context of maternal speech and rate of language development. *British Journal of Developmental Psychology* 4: 261–268.

Hashimoto T, Hiura K, Endo S, Fukuda K, Mori A, Tayama M (1983) Postural effects on behavioural states of newborn infants: A sleep polygraphic study. *Brain Development* 5: 286–291.

Hayley SM, Coster WJ, Ludlow LH, Haltiwanger JT, Andrellos PJ (1992) *Pediatric Evaluation of Disability Inventory (PEDI) Manual*. Boston, MA: PEDI Research Group.

Hebdon K (1998) Unpublished. Poster presentation at Paediatric Rheumatology Conference.

Henderson A, Llorens L, Gilfoyle E, Myers C, Prevel S (1974) *The Development of Sensory Integrative Theory and Practice: A collection of works by A. Jean Ayres*. Dubuque, IL: Kendall/Hunt Publishing Company.

Henderson SE (1993) Motor development and minor handicap. In: Kalverboer AF, Hopkins B, Geuze R, eds, *Motor Development in Early and Later Childhood: Longitudinal approaches*. Cambridge: Cambridge University Press.

Henderson SE, Sugden D (1992) *Movement Assessment Battery for Children (Movement ABC)*. London: The Psychological Corporation.

Hewett D (1998) Challenging behaviour is normal. In: Lacey P, Ouvry, C, eds, *People with Profound and Multiple Learning Disabilities: A collaborative approach to meeting complex needs*. London: David Fulton Publishers.

Hewitt V (1976) Effect of posture on the presence of fat in tracheal aspirate in neonates. *Australian Paediatric Journal* 12: 267.

Hickling A (2000) Education and therapy needs of children with multiple disabilities. *British Journal of Therapy and Rehabilitation* 7: 334–338.

Hickman L (1989) Fragile X syndrome and sensory integrative therapy. *Sensory Integration International News* 17: 14–15.

Higgins K (1999) Bobath approach: Theory and practice. Series of essays. Bachelor of Occupational Therapy (Hons) course. School of Occupational Therapy, Otago Polytechnic, New Zealand (Unpublished).

Hobson PR (1987) On acquiring knowledge about people and the capacity to pretend: response to Leslie 1987. *Psychological Review* 97: 114–121.

Hoehn TP, Baumeister AA (1994) A critique of the application of Sensory Integrative Therapy to children with learning disabilities. *Journal of Learning Disabilities* **27**: 338–350.

Holmes GP, Kaplan JE, Gantz NM et al. (1988) Chronic fatigue syndrome: a working case definition. *Archives of Internal Medicine* **108**: 115–21.

Holt KS (1975) Importance of movement in child development. In: Holt KS, ed., *Movement and Child Development, Clinics in Developmental Medicine*, No. 55. Spastics International Medical Publications. London: William Heinemann Medical.

Howard L (1994a) Multidisciplinary quality assessment: the case of a child development team Part 1. *British Journal of Occupational Therapy* **57**: 345–348.

Howard L (1994b) Multidisciplinary quality assessment: the case of a child development team Part 2. *British Journal of Occupational Therapy* **57**: 393–397.

Howard L (1994c) Multidisciplinary quality assessment: the case of a child development team Part 3. *British Journal of Occupational Therapy* **57**: 437–440.

Howard L (1997) Developmental co-ordination disorder: can we measure our intervention? *British Journal of Occupational Therapy* **60**: 219–220.

Howard L (2000) The clinical practice patterns of British paediatric Occupational Therapists. Unpublished survey, Norwich: University of East Anglia.

Howard L, Leeson, J (1999) Conducting a service review *British Journal of Occupational Therapy* **62**: 249–251.

Howe M, Swartzberg S (1986) *A Functional Approach to Group Work in Occupational Therapy*. Philadelphia, PA: Lippincott.

Howe S, Levinson J, Shear E et al. (1991) Development of a disability measurement tool for JRA. *Arthritis and Rheumatism* **7**: 873–880.

Howlin P (1981) The effectiveness of operant language training with autistic children. *Journal of Autism and Developmental Disorders* **11**: 89–106.

Howlin P (1998) *Children with Autism and Asperger Syndrome.* Chichester: John Wiley.

Hughes C, Russell J (1993) Autistic children's difficulty with mental disengagement from an object: its implications for theories of autism. *Developmental Psychology* **29**: 498–510.

Humphrey GM (1962) *The Wild Boy of Aveyon.* Translation from Itard JM (1801). New York: Appleton Century Crofts.

Hunter J, Mullen J, Varga Dallas D (1994) Medical considerations and practice. Guidelines for the neonatal occupational therapist. *American Journal of Occupational Therapy* **48**: 546–560.

Hunter JG (1996) The neonatal intensive care unit. *Occupational Therapy for Children* **22**: 583–631.

Hyde S (1993) *Duchenne Muscular Dystrophy: A parent's guide to physiotherapy.* London: Muscular Dystrophy Campaign.

Inglis S (1990) Are there schoolchildren in Lewisham who are experiencing practical difficulties at home and/or at school? *British Journal of Occupational Therapy* **53**: 151–154.

Ingram TTS (1962) Clinical significance of the infantile feeding reflexes. *Developmental Medicine and Child Neurology* **4**: 159–169.

Jacobs PA, Bullman H, MacPherson J et al. (1993) Population studies of the fragile X: a molecular approach. *Journal of Medical Genetics* **30**: 454–459.

Jain L, Sivieri E, Abassi S, Bhutani V (1987) Energetics and mechanics of nutritive sucking in the preterm and term neonate. *Journal of Pediatrics* **6**: 894–898.

Janeschild ME (1996) Integrating the dynamical systems theory with the neurodevelopmental approach. Developmental Disabilities. *AOTA's Special Interest Section Newsletter* March 19:1.

Jeffrey LIH (1982) Occupational therapy in child and adolescent psychiatry: the future. *Occupational Therapy* **44**: 330–334.

Jeffrey LIH (1990) Play therapy. In Creek J, ed., *Occupational Therapy and Mental Health*. Edinburgh: Churchill Livingstone.

Jenkins J, Sells C (1984) Physical and occupational therapy: effects relating to treatment, frequency and motor delay. *Journal of Learning Disabilities* **17**: 89–95.

Jennet B, Teaside G, Braakman R, Minderhoud J, Heiden J, Kurtze T (1979) Prognosis of patients with severe head injury. *Neurosurgery* **4**: 283–289.

Jenni OG, Vonshieventhal K, Woy M, Keel M, Duc G, Bucher HU (1997) Effect of nursing in the head elevated tilt position (15°) on the incidence of bradycardic and hypoxemic episodes in preterm infants. *Pediatrics* **100**: 622–625.

Jennings S (1990) *Dramatherapy with Families, Groups and Individuals Waiting in the Wings*. London: Jessica Kingsley.

Jennings S (1993) *Playtherapy with Children: A practitioner's guide*. Oxford: Blackwell Scientific.

Jones D (1995) Learning disabilities; an alternative frame of reference. *British Journal of Occupational Therapy* **58**: 423–426.

Jordan KM, Kolak AM, Jason LA (1997) Research with children and adolescents with chronic fatigue syndrome, methodologies, designs and special considerations. *Journal of Chronic Fatigue Syndrome* **3**: 3–13.

Jordan R (1993) The nature of communication and linguistic difficulties of children with autism. In: Meser DJ, Turner GJ, eds, *Critical Influences on Child Language Acquisition and Development*. New York: St Martin's Press.

Jupp S (1992) *Making the Right Start*. Cheshire: Opened Eye Publications.

Kandel ER, Schwartz JH, Jessell TM (1991) *Principles of Neural Science*, 3rd edn. International edition. London: Prentice-Hall International.

Kanner L (1943) Autistic disturbances of affective contact. *Nervous Child* **2**: 217–250.

Kaplan BJ (1993) Reexamination of sensory integration treatment: a combination of two efficacy studies. *Journal of Learning Disabilities* **26**: 342–347.

Kaplan C, Telford R (1998) *The Butterfly Children: An account of non-directive play therapy*. Edinburgh: Churchill Livingstone.

Kaplan M (1994) Motor learning: Implication for occupational therapy and neurodevelopmental treatment. Developmental Disabilities. *AOTA's Special Interest Section Newsletter* September 17: 3.

Kawar M (1973) The effects of sensori-motor therapy on dichotic listening in children with learning disabilities. *American Journal of Occupational Therapy* **27**: 226–231.

Kelly D (1995) *Central Auditory Processing Disorder*. San Antonio, TX: Communication Skill Builders.

Kephart NC (1960) *The Slow Learner in the Classroom*. Columbus, OH: Merrill Publishing.

Kid Source Online (Update August 1994) *A Parent's Guide to Accessing Programs for Infants, Toddlers and Pre-schoolers with Disabilities*.

Kielhofner G (1992) *Conceptual Foundations of Occupational Therapy*. Philadelphia, PA: FA Davis.

Kielhofner GK (1997) *Conceptual Foundations of Occupational Therapy*, 2nd edn. Philadelphia, PA: FA Davis Co.

Kientz M, Dunn W (1997) A comparison of children with autism and typical children using the sensory profile. *American Journal of Occupational Therapy* **51**: 530–537.

Kiernan C, Jones MC (1982) *Behaviour Assessment Battery*. Windsor, Berks: NFER-Nelson.

Kimball JG (1988) The emphasis is on integration, not sensory. *American Journal on Mental Retardation* **92**: 423–424.

Kimball JG (1993) Sensory integrative frame of reference. In: Kramer P, Hinojosa J, eds, *Frames of Reference for Paediatric Occupational Therapy*. Baltimore, MD: Williams & Wilkins.

King LJ (1992) Sensory integration: an effective approach to therapy and education. *Sensory Integration Quarterly* **XX**: 3–4.

King LJ, Grandin T (1990) Attention deficits in Learning Disorder and Autism: A Sensory Integrative Treatment Approach. Madison, Wisconsin: Workshop presented at Conference Proceedings of the Continuing Education Programs of America.

Kinnealey M, Miller LJ (1993) Sensory integration and learning disabilities. In: Hopkins HM, Smith HD, eds, *Willard and Spackman: Occupational Therapy*. Unit VI, Section 4. Philadelphia, PA: JB Lippincott Co., pp 474–489.

Kjerland L, Kovach J (1990) Family-Staff Collaboration for Tailored Infant Assessment. In: Gibbs ED, Teti DM, eds, *Interdisciplinary Assessment of Infants: A guide for early intervention professionals*. Baltimore, MD: Paul H Brookes.

Klein MD (1983) *Pre-dressing Skills*. Tucson, AZ: Communication Skill Builders.

Knickerbocker BM (1980) *A Holistic Approach to the Treatment of Learning Disorders*. Thorofare, NJ: Slack.

Knox S (1997) Revised Knox Preschool Play Scale. In: Parham LD, Faxio LS, eds, *Play in Occupational Therapy for Children*. St Louis, MO: Mosby, pp 47–49.

Knox SH (1996) Play and playfulness in pre-school children. In: Zemke R, Clark F, eds, *Occupational Science – the Evolving Discipline*. Philadelphia, PA: Davis & Co.

Knox V (2000) Gross motor function classification system. *British Association of Bobath Trained Therapists Newsletter* **36**: 12–14.

Koomar JA, Bundy AC (1991) The art and science of creating direct intervention from theory. In: Fisher AG, Murray EA, Bundy AC, eds, *Sensory Integration: Theory and practice*. Philadelphia, PA: FA Davis, Chapter 10.

Kortman B (1995) The eye of the beholder: models in occupational therapy. *British Journal of Occupational Therapy* **58**: 532–536.

Kramer P, Hinojosa J, eds (1993) *Frames of Reference for Pediatric Occupational Therapy*. Baltimore, MD: Williams & Wilkins.

Kramer P, Hinojosa J, eds (1999) *Frames of Reference for Pediatric Occupational Therapy*, 2nd edn. Baltimore, MD: Williams & Wilkins.

Krefting L (1990) Rigor in qualitative research; the assessment of trustworthiness. *American Journal of Occupational Therapy* **45**: 214–222.

Krementz J (1988) *How it Feels when a Parent Dies*. London: Victor Golancz.

Kubler-Ross E (1969) *On Death and Dying*. New York: Macmillan.

Kubler-Ross E (1982) *On Death and Dying*, 2nd edn. London: Tavistock.

Lacey P (1998) Meeting complex needs through collaborative multidisciplinary teamwork. In: Lacey P, Ouvry C, eds, *People with Profound and Multiple Learning Disabilities: A collaborative approach to meeting complex needs*. London: David Fulton Publishers.

Lachiewicz AM, Spiridgliozzi GA, Guillion CM, Ransford SN, Rao K (1994) Aberrant behaviours of young boys with fragile X syndrome. *American Journal of Mental Retardation* **98**: 567–579.

LaCroix J, Johnson C, Parham LD (1997) The development of a new sensory history: the evaluation of sensory process. *AOTA Sensory Integration Special Interest Section Quarterly* **20**: 3–4.

Landy R (1992) One-on-one. In: Jennings S, ed., *Dramatherapy Theory and Practice 2*. London: Tavistock/Routledge.

Lane A, Ziviani J (1999) Children's computer access: analysis of the visual-motor demands of software designed for children. *British Journal of Occupational Therapy* **62**: 19–25.

Larrington GG (1987) A sensory integration based program with a severely retarded/autistic teenager: an occupational therapy case report. *Occupational Therapy in Health Care* **4**: 101–117.

Larson RA (1982) The sensory history of developmentally delayed children with and without tactile defensiveness. *American Journal of Occupational Therapy* **36**: 590–596.

Laslow J, Bairstow P (1985) Kinesthetic sensitivity test. In: Laslow J, Bairstow P, eds, *Perceptual Motor Behaviour*. London: Holt, Rinehart & Winston.

Laszlo JI, Bairstow PJ, eds (1989) *Perceptual–Motor Behaviour – development, assessment and therapy*. London: Holt, Rinehart & Winston.

Laufer L (1995) *Callirobics*. Charlottesville, VA: Callirobics.

Law M, ed. (1998) *Client Centred Occupational Therapy*. Thorofare, NJ: Slack.

Law M, Polatajko HL, Schaffer R, Miller J, Macnab J (1991) The effect of a Sensory Integration Program on academic achievement, motor performance, and self-esteem in children identified as learning disabled: results of a clinical trial. *Occupational Therapy Journal of Research* **11**: 155–176.

Law M, Baptiste S, Carswell A, McColl MA, Polatajko H, Pollock N (1994) *Canadian Occupational Performance Measure*, 2nd edn. ACE, Canada: CAOT Publications.

Law M, Russell D, Pollock N, Rosenbaum P, Walter S, King G (1997) A comparison of intensive neurodevelopmental therapy plus casting and a regular occupational therapy program for children with cerebral palsy. *Developmental Medicine and Child Neurology* **39**: 664–670.

Law M, Darrah J, Pollock N, King G et al. (1998) Family-centred functional therapy for children with cerebral palsy: An emerging practice model. *Physical and Occupational Therapy in Paediatrics* **18**: 83–102.

Lawlor M, Henderson A (1989) A descriptive study of the clinical practice patterns of occupational therapists working with infants and young children. *American Journal of Occupational Therapy* **43**: 755–764.

Lawton S (1994) *National Association of Paediatric Occupational Therapists Newsletter*, Spring edition.

LDA (2000) *Write from the Start*. Wisbech: LDA.

Le Couteur A, Bailey A, Goode S et al. (1996) A broader phenotype of autism: the clinical picture in twins. *Journal of Child Psychology and Psychiatry* **37**: 785–802.

Lefrak-Okikawa L, Lund CH (1993) Nursing practice in the neonatal intensive care unit. In: Klaus MH, Fanaroff AA, eds, *Care of the High Risk Neonate*, 4th edn. Philadelphia, PA: Saunders, pp 212–227.

Leiner HC, Leiner AL, Dow RS (1986) Does the cerebellum contribute to mental skills? *Behavioral Neuroscience* **100**: 443–54.

Lennox L, Cermak SA, Koomer J (1988) Praxis and gesture comprehension in 4-, 5- and 6-year-olds. *American Journal of Occupational Therapy* **42**: 99–104.

Lesny LA (1980) Developmental dyspraxia-dysgnosia as a cause of congenital children's clumsiness. *Brain and Development* **2**: 69–71.

Levine KJ (1991) *Fine Motor Dysfunction – Therapeutic Strategies in the Classroom*. Tucson, AZ: Therapy Skill Builders.

Lewis V, Boucher J (1995) Generativity in the play of young people with autism. *Journal of Autism and Developmental Disorders* **25**: 105–121.

Lewy AL, Dawson G (1992) Social stimulation and joint attention in young autistic children. *Journal of Abnormal Child Psychology* **20**: 555–566.

Light CM, Chappell PH, Kyberd PJ, Ellis BS (1999) A critical review of functionality assessment in natural and prosthetic hand. *British Journal of Occupational Therapy* **1**: 7–12.

Lilly LA, Powell NJ (1990) Measuring the effects of neuro-developmental treatment on the daily living skills of two children with cerebral palsy. *American Journal of Occupational Therapy* **44**: 139–145.

Lindsay WR, Michie AM (1995) Teaching new skills. In: Fraser WI, MacGillivray RC, Green AM, eds, *Hallas' Caring for People with Mental Handicaps*. Oxford: Butterworth-Heinemann, pp 48–63.

Lonetto R (1980) *Children's Conceptions of Death*. New York: Springer.

Lord C, Rutter M, DiLavore P, Risi S (2000) *Autism Diagnostic Observation Schedule*. Los Angeles, CA: Western Psychological Services.

Lott J (1989) Developmental care of the preterm infant. *Neonatal Network* **7**: 21–28.

Lovaas OI (1977) *The Autistic Child: Language development through behaviour modification*. New York: Halstead Press.

Lovaas OI (1987) Behavioural treatment and normal educational and intellectual functioning in young autistic children. *Journal of Consulting and Clinical Psychology* **55**: 3–9.

Lovaas OI, Newson C, Hickman C (1987) Self stimulatory behaviour and perceptual reinforcement. *Journal of Applied Behaviour Analysis* **20**: 45–48.

Lowenfeld M (1951) Questions of therapeutic technique. In: Urwin C, Hood-Williams J, eds (1988) *Child Psychotherapy, War and the Normal Child*. London: Free Association Books.

Lowenfeld M (1979) *Understanding Children's Sandplay*. Lowenfeld Trust, Brudenell House, Quainton, Aylesbury, Bucks HP22 4AW.

Lowenfeld M (1993) *Understanding Children's Sandplay. Lowenfeld's World Technique*. Cambridge: Margaret Lowenfeld Trust.

Luebben AJ, Hinojosa J, Kramer P (1999) Legitimate tools of pediatric occupational therapy. In: Kramer P, Hinojosa J, eds, *Frames of Reference for Pediatric Occupational Therapy*, 2nd edn. Baltimore, MD: Williams & Wilkins.

McCall SA, Schneck CM (2000) Parents' perceptions of occupational therapy services for their children with developmental disabilities. *Developmental Disabilities Special Interest Section Quarterly* **23**: 1–3.

McCettrick BJ (1999) Conductive Education Forum, London.

McClennon S (1991) *Cognitive Skills for Community Living: Teaching students with moderate to severe disabilities*. Austin, TX: PRO-ED.

McClennon S (1992) Cognitive characteristics, assessment and intervention. In: Schopmeyer BB, Lowe F, eds, *The Fragile X Child*. San Diego, CA: Singular Publishing Group, pp 33–58.

McClure M, Holtz-Yotz M (1991) The effects of sensory stimulatory treatment on an autistic child. *American Journal of Occupational Therapy* 45: 1138–1142.

McConnell D (1995) Processes underlying clumsiness: a review of perspectives. *Physical and Occupational Therapy in Paediatrics* 15: 33–52.

McCue M (1993) Helping with behavioural problems. In: Shanley E, Starrs TA, eds, *Learning Disabilities: A Handbook of Care*, 2nd edn. Edinburgh: Churchill Livingstone, pp 149–210.

McEvoy RE, Rogers SJ, Pennington BF (1993) Executive function and social communication deficits in young autistic children. *Journal of Child Psychology and Psychiatry* 34: 563–578.

McGee JJ (1992) Gentle teaching: assumptions and paradigm. *Journal of Applied Behaviour Analysis* 25: 869–872.

McGee JJ, Menolascino FJ, Hobbs DC (1987) *Gentle Teaching: A nonaversive approach for helping persons with mental retardation*. New York: Human Sciences Press.

McIntosh DN, Miller LJ, Shyu V, Hagerman RJ (1999) Sensory-modulation disruption, electrodermal responses, and functional behaviors. *Developmental Medicine and Child Neurology* 41: 608–615.

MacKay G (1993) Helping with learning difficulties. In: Shanley E, Starrs TA, eds, *Learning Disabilities. A Handbook of Care*, 2nd edn. Edinburgh: Churchill Livingstone, pp 119–134.

MacKeith R (1973) The feelings and behaviour of parents of handicapped children. *Developmental Medicine and Child Neurology* 15: 524–527.

McMahon L (1992) *Handbook of Play Therapy*. London: Routledge.

Magrun WM (1989) *Evaluating Movement and Posture Disorganisation in Dyspraxic Children*. Syracuse, NY: Advanced Therapeutics.

Magrun WM (1990) *A Neuro-postural Approach to Movement and Posture disorganisation in Learning Disabilities*. Syracuse, NY: Advanced Therapeutics.

Magrun WM, McCue S, Keefe R, Ottenbacher K (1981) Effects of vestibular stimulation on spontaneous use of verbal language in developmentally delayed children. *American Journal of Occupational Therapy* 35: 101–104.

Mailloux Z (1990) An overview of the sensory integration and praxis tests. *American Journal of Occupational Therapy* 44: 589–94.

Manjiviona J, Prior M (1995) Comparison of Asperger Syndrome and high functioning autistic children on a test of motor impairment. *Journal of Autism and Developmental Disorders* 25: 23–40.

Martin JP, Bell J (1943) A pedigree of mental defect showing sex-linkage. *Journal of Neurology and Psychiatry* 6: 154–157.

Martin RJ, Herrell N, Rubin D, Fanaroff A (1979) Effects of supine and prone positioning on arterial oxygen tension in the preterm infant. *Pediatrics* 63: 528–531.

Marvin C (1999) Teaching and learning for children with profound and multiple learning difficulties. In: Lacey P, Ouvry, C, eds, *People with Profound and Multiple Learning Disabilities*. London: David Fulton, pp 117–129.

Masterson J, Zucker C, Shulze K (1987) Prone and supine positioning effects on energy expenditure and behaviour of low birthweight infants. *Pediatrics* **80**: 689–692.

Matson JL, Ollendick TH, Adkins J (1980) A comprehensive dining program for mentally retarded adults. *American Journal on Mental Deficiency* **86**: 533–542.

Maudsley H (1867) *The Physiology and Pathology of the Mind*. London: Macmillan.

Mayston M (1995) Some aspects of the physiological basis for intervention techniques. *Association of Paediatric Chartered Physiotherapists Journal* November: 15–21.

Mayston M (1996) Tone influencing patterns. In: *Course Notes*. Revised edn (1997). London: The Bobath Centre.

Mayston MJ (1992) The Bobath concept – evolution and application. In: Forssberg H, Hirschfield H, eds, *Movement Disorders in Children. Medical Sport Science*, vol. 36. Basel, Switzerland: Karger, pp 1–6.

Mayston MJ (2000a) Motor learning now needs meaningful goals. *Physiotherapy* **86**: 492–493.

Mayston MJ (2000b) Inhibition. Notes to accompany 5.4 of the Bobath course notes (1997, paediatrics). *British Association of Bobath Trained Therapists Newsletter* **37**: 7–11.

Mayston MJ (2001) Setting the scene. In: Edwards S., ed., *Neurological Physiotherapy – A Problem Solving Approach*, 2nd edn. Edingburgh: Churchill Livingstone.

Mayston MJ, Barber CB, Stern G, Bryce J (1997) The Bobath Concept – Will it stand the test of time? *British Association of Bobath Trained Therapists Newsletter* **28**: 3–9.

Mazzocco MM (1998) A process approach to describing mathematics difficulties in girls with Turner syndrome. *Pediatrics* **102**(suppl): 492–496.

Mazzocco MM, Pennington BF, Hagerman RJ (1994) Social cognition skills among females with Fragile X. *Journal of Autism and Developmental Disabilities* **24**: 473–485.

Medhust A, Ryan S (1996) Clinical reasoning in local authority paediatric Occupational Therapy: Planning a major adaptation for the child with a degenerative condition. Parts 1 and 2. *British Journal of Occupational Therapy* **59**: 203–206; **59**: 269–272.

Melton J (1998) Occupational therapy for adults with learning disabilities and other complex needs. *British Journal of Therapy and Rehabilitation* **5**: 461–464.

Mendoza J, Roberts J, Cook L (1991) Postural effects on pulmonary function and heart rate of preterm infants with lung disease. *Journal of Pediatrics* **118**: 445–448.

Menken C, Cermak SA, Fisher A (1987) Evaluating visual-perceptual skills of children with cerebral palsy. *American Journal of Occupational Therapy* **41**: 646–650.

Mental Health Foundation (1993) *Learning Disabilities: The fundamental facts*. London: Mental Health Foundation.

Meredith J, Vellendahl, Keagy R (1993) Successful voluntary grasp and release using the cookie crusher myoelectric hand in two year olds. *American Journal of Occupational Therapy* **47**: 825–829.

Merril SC (1990) *Environment: Implications for Occupational Therapy Practice – A Sensory Integrative Perspective*. Rockville, MD: American Occupational Therapy Association.

Meyers WF, Herbst JJ (1982) Effectiveness of position therapy for gastroesophageal reflux. *Pediatrics* **69**: 768–772.

Michealman S (1971) The importance of creative play. *American Journal of Occupational Therapy* **25**: 285–290.

Miller L, McIntosh DN (1998) The diagnosis, treatment and etiology of sensory modulation disorder. *Sensory Integration Special Interest Section Quarterly* **21**: 1–3.

Miller LJ (1988) *The Miller Assessment for Preschoolers*. Sidcup, Kent: The Psychological Corporation.

Miller LJ, Kinnealey M (1993) Research the effectiveness of sensory integration. *Sensory Integration Quarterly* **XXI**: 1–7.

Miller LJ, Roid GH (1994) *The Toddler Infant Motor Evaluation Manual*. Tucson, AZ: Therapy Skill Builders.

Miller LJ, McIntosh DN, McGrath J et al. (1999) Electrodermal responses to sensory stimuli in individuals with Fragile X syndrome: a preliminary report. *American Journal of Medical Genetics* **83**: 268–279.

Miller N (1986) *Dyspraxia and its Management*. Rockville, MD: Aspen Publishers.

Miller S (1968) *The Psychology of Play*. Harmondsworth: Penguin.

Minuchin S (1974) *Families and Family Therapy*. Cambridge, MA: Harvard University Press.

Missiuna C, Polatajko HJ (1995) Developmental Dyspraxia by any other name: are they all just clumsy children? *American Journal of Occupational Therapy* **49**: 619 – 627.

Miyahara M, Mobs I (1995) Developmental dyspraxia and developmental coordination Disorder. *Neuropsychology Review* **5**: 245–268.

Morris MK (1997) Developmental dyspraxia. In: Rothi LJG, Heilman KM , eds, *Apraxia: The neuropsychology of action*. East Sussex: Psychology Press Publishers.

Morris EE, Klein MD (1987) *Pre-feeding Skills*. Tucson, AZ: Therapy Skill Builders.

Morrison CD, Metzger P, Pratt PN (1996) Play. In: Case-Smith J, Allen AS, Pratt PN, eds, *Occupational Therapy for Children*, 3rd edn. St Louis, MO: Mosby.

Mosey AC (1986) *Psychosocial Components of Occupational Therapy*. New York: Raven Press.

Mosey AC (1993) Introduction to cognitive rehabilitation – working taxonomies. In: Royeen CB, ed., *AOTA. Self Study Series: Cognitive Rehabilitation*. Rockville, MD: American Occupational Therapy Association.

Mountain G (2000) *Occupational Therapy in Social Service Departments: A Review of the Current Literature*. London: College of Occupational Therapists.

Mouradian LE, Als H (1994) The influence of neonatal intensive care unit caregiving practices on motor functioning of preterm infants. *American Journal of Occupational Therapy* **48**: 527–33.

Muscular Dystrophy Campaign (1994) *Surgical Correction of Spinal Deformity in Muscular Dystrophy and other Neuromuscular Disorders: Factsheet*. London: Leaflet prepared with the assistance of a number of orthopaedic surgeons.

Nihira K, Leland H, Lambert N (1993) *AAMR Adaptive Behaviour Scales*. Windsor, Berks: NFER-Nelson.

Norton Y (1979) Neurodevelopment and sensory integration for the profoundly retarded multiply handicapped child. *American Journal of Occupational Therapy* **29**: 93–100.

Oaklander V (1988) *Windows to Our Children*. New York: The Gestalt Journal Press.

O'Brien J (1987) A guide to lifestyle planning. In: Wilcox B, Bellamy GT, eds, *A Comprehensive Guide to the Activities Catalogue: An alternative curriculum for youth and adults with severe disabilities*. Baltimore, MD: Paul H Brookes.

Oetter P, Richter EW, Frick SM (1995) *M.O.R.E. Integrating the Mouth with Sensory and Postural Functions*, 2nd edn. Hugo, MN: PDP Press.

Oldman C, Beresford B (1998) *Removing Barriers for Disabled Children: Inspection of services to disabled children and their families*. London: Department of Health.

Olsen JZ (1980) *Handwriting without Tears*. Brookfield, IL: Fred Sammons.

Olson LJ (1999) Psychosocial frame of reference. In: Kramer P. Hinojosa J, eds, *Frames of Reference of Pediatric Occupational Therapy*, 2nd edn. Philadelphia, PA: Lippincott Williams & Wilkins.

O'Rafferty J (1998) A study of occupational therapy interventions, particularly sensory integration for children with pervasive developmental disorders. *National Association of Paediatric Occupational Therapists Journal*: 27–32.

Orenstein W, Whitington P, Ornstein D (1983) The infant seat as treatment for gastroesophageal reflux. *New England Journal of Medicine* 309: 760–763.

Ornitz E (1985) Neurophysiology of infantile autism. *Journal of American Academy of Child Psychiatry* 24: 251–262.

Orton ST (1937) *Reading, Writing and Speech Problems in Children*. New York: Norton.

Ottenbacher K (1982a) Sensory integration therapy: affect or effect. *American Journal of Occupational Therapy* 36: 571–578.

Ottenbacher K (1982b) Vestibular processing dysfunction in children with severe emotional and behavior disorders: a review. *Physical and Occupational Therapy in Paediatrics* 2: 3–12.

Ottenbacher K (1988) Sensory integration – myth, method, and imperative. *American Journal on Mental Retardation* 92: 425–426.

Ottenbacher K (1991) Research in sensory integration: empirical perceptions and progress. In: Fisher AG, Murray EA, Bundy AC, eds, *Sensory Integration – Theory and Practice*. Philadelphia, PA: FA Davis.

Palisano R, Rosenbaum P, Walter S, Russell D, Wood E, Galuppi B (1997) Development and reliability of a system to classify gross motor function in children with cerebral palsy. *Developmental Medicine and Child Neurology* 39: 214–223.

Paneth NS (1995) The problem of low birth weight. *Future of Children* 5: 19.

Parham LD (1986) Assessment: The preschooler with suspected dyspraxia. *AOTA's Sensory Integration Special Interest Section Newsletter* 9: 1–4.

Parham LD, Fazio LS (1997) *Play in Occupational Therapy for Children*. St Louis, MO: Mosby.

Parham LD, Mailloux Z (1996) Sensory integration. In: Case-Smith J, Allen AN, Pratt PN, eds, *Occupational Therapy for Children*, 3rd edn. St Louis, MO: Mosby, Chapter 13.

Parks S (1994) *Hawaii Early Learning Profile – HELP*. Palo Alto, CA: VORT.

Parry A (1991) A universe of stories. *Family Process* 30: 37–54.

Payne A (1999) Children's bathing and showering adaptations: an evaluation. *Occupational Therapy News* 7: 17.

Peck C, Hong CS (1994) *Living Skills for Mentally Handicapped People*. London: Chapman & Hall.

Penso DE (1987) *Occupational Therapy for Children with Disabilities*. London: Croom Helm.

Penso DE (1990) *Keyboard, Graphic and Handwriting Skills: Helping people with motor disabilities*. London: Chapman & Hall.

Penso DE (1993) *Perceptuo-Motor Difficulties: Theory and Strategies to Help Children, Adolescents and Adults*. London: Chapman & Hall.

Peterson BS (1995) Neuroimaging in child and adolescent neuropsychiatric disorders. *Journal of American Academic Child and Adolescent Psychiatry* **34**: 1560–1576.

Piaget J (1969) *The Psychology of the Child*. New York: Basic Books.

Piven J, Folstein S (1997) The genetics of autism. In: Bauman ML, Kemper TL, eds, *The Neurobiology of Autism*. Baltimore, MD: The Johns Hopkins University Press.

Polatajko HJ, Kaplan BJ, Wilson BN (1992) Sensory integration treatment for children with learning disabilities: its status 20 years later. *Occupational Therapy Journal of Research* **12**: 323–341.

Polatajko HJ, Macnab JJ, Anstett B, Malloy-Miller T, Murphy K, Noh S (1995) A clinical trial of the process-oriented treatment approach for children with developmental co-ordination disorder. *Developmental Medicine and Child Neurology* **37**: 310–319.

Pratt PN (1989) Play and recreational activities. In: Pratt PN, Allen AS, eds, *Occupational Therapy for Children*, 2nd edn. St Louis, MO: Mosby.

Pratt PN, Allen AS (1989) *Occupational Therapy for Children*. St Louis, MO: Mosby.

Pratt PN, Florey LA, Clark F (1989) Developmental principles and theories. In: Pratt PN, Allen AS, eds, *Occupational Therapy for Children*, 2nd edn. St Louis, MO: Mosby.

Prechtl HFR (1990) Qualitative changes of spontaneous movements in fetus and preterm infants are a marker of neurological dysfunction. *Early Human Development* **23**: 151–159.

Prechtl HFR, Bos AF, Cioni G, Ferrari F, Enspieler C (1997) Spontaneous motor activity as a diagnostic tool. Functional assessments of the young nervous system. A specific illustration of Prechtl's method. Video guide. From the GM Trust, Dept of Physiology, University of Graz, Harrachgasse 21, A-8010 Graz, Austria.

Presland JL (1989) *Overcoming Difficult Behaviours – A Guide and Source Book for Helping People with Severe Mental Handicap*. Kidderminster: British Institute of Mental Handicap.

Price A (1978) ISG-P vs CSSID? The role of sensory-based therapy systems. *International Study Group for Perception* **2**: 2–3.

Prior M, Hoffman W (1990) Brief report: neuropsychological testing of autistic children through an exploration with frontal lobe tests. *Journal of Autism and Developmental Disorders* **20**: 581–590.

Priven J, Arndt S, Bailey J, Andreasen N (1996) Regional brain enlargement in autism: a magnetic resonance imaging study. *Journal of the American Academy of Child and Adolescent Psychiatry* **35**: 530–536.

Pruzansky C, Farrington K (1999) Case study: combined sensory integration and neuro-developmental treatment frames of reference. In: Kramer P, Hinojosa J, eds, *Frames of Reference for Pediatric Occupational Therapy*, 2nd edn. Baltimore, MD: Williams & Wilkins.

Quirk NJ, DiMatties ME (1990) *The Relationship of Learning Problems and Classroom Performance to Sensory Integration*. Cherry Hill, NJ: Quirk.

Rab S (1997) Brain Impairment. Conference, Brisbane.

Read DL (1996) Play as a phenomenon in occupational therapy literature: a literature review. *New Zealand Journal of Occupational Therapy* **47**: 15–17.

Recordon A (1998) Evaluation of motor control theory in relation to the Bobath Concept. Lecture/course notes. Functional Problem Solving Workshop, November 13–14. New Zealand Bobath Association (NZBA Inc.).

Reed KL, Sanderson SR (1983) *Concepts of Occupational Therapy*. Baltimore, MD: Williams & Wilkins.

Reed KL, Sanderson SN (1992) *Concepts of Occupational Therapy*, 3rd edn. Baltimore, MD: Williams & Wilkins.

Reid D, Drake S (1990) A comparative study of visual perceptual skills in normal children and children with diplegic cerebral palsy. *Canadian Journal of Occupational Therapy* June: 141–146.

Reilly M (1974) *Play as Exploratory Learning Studies of Curiosity Behaviour*. London: Sage Publications.

Reinecke MA, Dattilio FM, Freeman A (1995) *Cognitive Therapy with Children and Adolescents – A Case Book for Clinical Practice*. New York: The Guilford Press.

Reisman J, Hanschu B (1992) *Sensory Integration Inventory Revised for Adults with Developmental Disabilities – User's Manual*. St Paul, MN: PDP Press.

Resnick MB, Eyler FD, Nelson RM, Eitzman DV, Bucciarelli RL (1987) Developmental intervention for low birth weight infants: Improved early developmental outcome. *Pediatrics* **80**: 68–74.

Restall G, Magill-Evans J (1994) Play and pre-school children with autism. *American Journal of Occupational Therapy* **48**: 113–120.

Reuben RN, Bakwin H (1968) Developmental clumsiness. *Pediatric Clinics of North America* **15**: 601–610.

Robson C (1993) *Real World Research*. Oxford: Blackwell.

Rodger S (1994) A survey of assessments used by paediatric occupational therapists. *Australian Occupational Therapy Journal* **41**: 137–142.

Romano L, Dodd, K (2000) Abstract: Does neuro-developmental therapy improve motor function in children with cerebral palsy? An analysis of the research concluding the Neuro-Developmental Therapy is not effective. *Australian Bobath Neuro-Developmental Therapy Association Newsletter* May: 5.

Rosenbloom L (1975) The consequences of impaired movement – a hypothesis and review. In: Holt KS, ed., *Movement and Child Development. Clinics in Developmental Medicine*, No. 55. Spastic International Medical Publications. London: William Heinemann Medical.

Royeen CB (1989) Commentary on 'Tactile function in learning disabled and normal children: reliability and validity considerations'. *Occupational Therapy Journal of Research* **9**: 16–23.

Royeen CB (1991) TIE: Tactile Inventory for School-Aged Children. In: Fisher A, Murray E, Bundy A, eds, *Sensory Integration: Theory and practice*. Philadelphia, PA: FA Davis, pp 134–136.

Royeen CB (1997) Lesson 5 – Sensory Modulation: a theoretical exploration of the construct. In: Royeen CB, ed., *AOTA Self-Paced Clinical Course – Neuroscience and Occupational: links to practice*. Bethesda, MD: American Occupational Therapy Association.

Royeen CB, Duncan M (1999) Acquisition frame of reference. In: Kramer P, Hinojosa J, eds, *Frames of Reference for Pediatric Occupational Therapy*. Baltimore, MD: Lippincott Williams & Wilkins.

Royeen CB, Lane SJ (1991) Tactile processing and sensory defensiveness. In: Fisher A, Murray E, Bundy AC, eds, *Sensory Integration: Theory and practice*. Philadelphia, PA: FA Davis, pp 108–131.

Russell D, Rosenbaum P, Gowland C et al. (1993) *Gross Motor Function Measure Manual*, 2nd edn. Ontario: Gross Motor Measures Group.

Rydell PJ, Mirenda P (1994) Effects of high and low constraint utterances on the production of immediate and delayed echolalia in young children with autism. *Journal of Autism and Developmental Disorders* **24**: 719–735.

Safire W (1989) Rethinking reclaim. *The New York Times Magazine* 20.

Sanders D (1993) Selected literature and case studies supporting the effectiveness of a sensorimotor and behavior modification approach to autism. *Sensory Integration Special Interest Section Newsletter* **16**: 3–6.

Sasad C (1998) Research articles pertaining to the efficacy of neurodevelopmental treatment. Developmental Disabilities. *AOTA's Special Interest Section Quarterly* **21**: 1–2.

Schaffer R (1984) Sensory integration therapy with learning disabled children: a critical review. *Canadian Journal of Occupational Therapy* **51**: 73–77.

Scharfenaker S, O'Connor R, Stackhouse T, Braden M, Hickman L, Gray K (1996) An integrated approach to intervention. In: Hagerman RJ, Cronister A, eds, *Fragile X Syndrome, Diagnosis, Treatment and Research*, 2nd edn. Baltimore, MD: Johns Hopkins University Press, pp 349–411.

Scheerer CR (1997) *Sensorimotor Groups – Activities for School and Home*. Tucson, AZ: Therapy Skill Builders.

Schleichkorn J (1988) *The Bobaths: A biography of Berta and Karel Bobath*. Tucson, AZ: Therapy Skill Builders.

Schneck CM (1998) Lesson 5: interventions for visual perception problems. In: Case-Smih J, ed., *AOTA Self-Paced Clinical Course – Making a Difference in School System Practice*. Bethesda, MD: American Occupational Therapy Association.

Schoen S, Anderson J (1999) Neurodevelopmental treatment frame of reference. In: Kramer P, Hinojosa J, eds, *Frames of Reference for Pediatric Occupational Therapy*, 2nd edn. Baltimore, MD: Williams & Wilkins.

Schopler E, Olley JG (1982) Comprehensive educational services for children. The TEACCH Model. In: Reynolds CR, Gurkin TR, eds, *Handbook of Social Psychology*. New York: Wiley.

Schopler E, Mesibow GB, Shigley RH, Bashford A (1984) Helping autistic children through their parents – the TEACCH Model. In: Schopler E, Mesibov GB, eds, *The Effects of Autism on the Family*. New York: Plenum, pp 65–81.

Schopmeyer BB, Lowe F, eds (1992) *The Fragile X Child*. San Diego, CA: Singular Publishing Group.

Scrutton D (1984) Aim-oriented management. In: Scrutton D, ed., *Management of Motor Disorders of Children with Cerebral Palsy*. Spastics International Publications. Oxford: Blackwell Scientific Publications Ltd.

Seifert A (1973) Sensory-motor stimulation for the young handicapped child. *Occupational Therapy* **36**: 559–566.

Seigel I (1997) *Hey, I'm Here Too!* London: Muscular Dystrophy Campaign.

Sensory Integration International (1991) *A Parent's Guide to Understanding Sensory Integration*. Torrance, CA: Sensory Integration International.

Shanley E, Starrs TA (1995) *Learning Disabilities: A handbook of care*. Edinburgh: Churchill Livingstone.

Sheridan MD (1993) *Spontaneous Play in Early Childhood*. London: Routledge.

Shumway-Cook A, Woollacott M (1995) *Motor Control. Theory and practical applications*. Baltimore, MD: Williams & Wilkins.

Sigman M, Mundy P, Sherman T, Ungerer J (1986) Social interactions of autistic mentally retarded and normal children and their caregivers. *Journal of Child Psychology and Psychiatry* **27**: 647–656.

Simeonsson RJ, Bailey DB, Huntington GS, Comfort M (1986) Testing the concept of goodness of fit in early intervention. *Infant Mental Health Journal* **7**: 81–91.

Simmons Carlsson CE (1997) Sensory and motor – two sides of the same coin. *British Association of Bobath Trained Therapists Newsletter* **28**: 3–9.

Simmons Carlsson CE (1999a) Addressing aspects of sensation and sensory processing in children with cerebral palsy. Lecture/course notes. New Zealand eight-week paediatric basic Bobath course. Unpublished, New Zealand Bobath Association Inc.

Simmons Carlsson CE (1999b) Introduction to perception and cognition: The child with cerebral palsy. Lecture/course notes. New Zealand eight-week paediatric basic Bobath course. Unpublished, New Zealand Bobath Association Inc.

Simmons Carlsson CE, Recordon A (2000) Development of a Bobath clinical reasoning tool. Unpublished.

Simmons Carlsson CE, Savage S (1995) Occupational therapy: Working in a Bobath Centre. OT News. *British Association of Occupational Therapists Newsletter* 3/10: 8–19.

Simon GB (1981) *The Next Step on the Ladder*. Worcester: British Institute of Mental Handicap.

Sims A, Owens D (1993) *Psychiatry*. London: Baillière Tindall.

Singh G, Athreya B, Fries J, Goldsmith D (1994) Measurement of health status in children with JRA. *Arthritis and Rheumatism* **12**: 1761–1769.

Slavik B, Kitsuna LJ, Danner P, Green J, Ayres A J (1984) Vestibular stimulation and eye contact in autistic children. *Neuropaediatrics* **15**: 33–36.

Sloman L (1991) Use of medication in pervasive developmental disorder. *Pediatric Clinics of North America* **14**: 165–182.

Smith B (1991) Introduction and background to interactive approaches. In: Smith B, ed., *Interactive Approaches to Teaching the Core Subjects*. Bristol: Lame Duck Publishing.

Smith P, Turner B (1990) The physiological effect of positioning premature infants in car seats. *Neonatal Network* **9**: 11–15.

Sobesky WE, Porter D, Pennington BF, Hagerman RJ (1995) Dimensions of shyness in fragile X females. *Developmental Brain Dysfunction* **8**: 280–292.

Social Services Inspectorate and Department of Health (1998) *Removing Barriers for Disabled Children: Inspection of services to disabled children and their families*. London: Stationery Office.

Sonuga-Barke EJS (1994) Annotation: on dysfunction and function in psychological theories of childhood disorder. *Journal of Child Psychology and Psychiatry* **35**: 801–815.

Southwood T (1992) Kids like us. A disease education video for children with chronic arthritis.

Southwood T, Malleson P, eds (1993) Arthritis in children and adolescents. *Ballière's Clinical Paediatrics*. London: Baillière Tindall.

Sparrow SS, Balla DA, Cicchettic DV (1984) *Vineland Adaptive Behaviour Scales*. Circle Pines, MN: American Guidance Corp.

Spence S (1980) *Social Skills Training with Children and Adolescents*. Windsor, Berks: NFER-Nelson.

Spitzer SL (1999) Dynamic systems theory: relevance to the theory of Sensory Integration and the study of occupation. American Occupational Therapy Association (AOTA) *Sensory Integration Special Interest Section Quarterly* 22: 1–4.

Stackhouse T (1994) Sensory integration concepts and Fragile X syndrome. *SISIS Newsletter* 17 March: 2–6.

Stahmer AC, Schreibman L (1992) Teaching children with autism appropriate play in unsupervised environments using a self management treatment package. *Journal of Applied Behaviour Analysis* 25: 447–459.

Stancliff B (1996) Autism: defining the OT's role in treating this confusing disorder. *OT Practice* July: 18–29.

Stanley FJ (1987) The changing face of cerebral palsy? *Developmental Medicine and Child Neurology* 29: 263–265.

Stanley FJ, Watson L (1992) Trends in perinatal mortality and cerebral palsy in Western Australia, 1967–1985. *British Medical Journal* 304: 1658–63.

Stein F, Cutler SK (1998) *Psychosocial Occupational Therapy: A Holistic Approach*. San Diego, CA: Singular Publishing Group.

Stephens TM (1992) *Social Skills in the Classroom*, 2nd edn. Odessa, FL: Psychological Assessment Resources.

Stevens B, Petryshen P, Hawkins J, Smith B, Taylor P (1996): Developmental versus conventional care: A comparison of clinical outcomes for very low birth weight infants. *Canadian Journal of Nursing Research* 28: 97–113.

Stewart S, Neyerlin-Beale J (2000) The impact of community paediatric occupational therapy on children with disabilities and their carers. *British Journal of Occupational Therapy* 63: 373–379.

Stow BM (1946) Occupational therapy for children. *Occupational Therapy* 24: 11–12.

Strupp H, Bergin A (1972) *Changing Frontiers in the Science of Psychotherapy*. Chicago: Aldine.

Sudhalter V, Cohen IL, Silverman W, Wolf-Schein EG (1990) Conversational analyses of males with fragile X, Down syndrome and autism: a comparison of the emergence of deviant language. *American Journal of Mental Retardation* 94: 431–441.

Sugden D, Wann C (1987) The assessment of motor impairment in children with moderate learning difficulties. *British Journal of Educational Psychology* 37: 225–236.

Sugden DA, Keogh JF (1990) *Problems in Movement Skill Development*. Columbia, SC: University of South Carolina.

Sumsion T, ed., (1999) *Client-centred Practice in Occupational Therapy*. London: Churchill Livingstone.

Sumsion T (2000) A revised occupational therapy definition of client-centred practice. *British Journal of Occupational Therapy* 63: 304–309.

Swain J, Gillman M, Heyman B (1999) Challenging questions. In: Swain J, French S, eds, *Therapy and Learning Difficulties: Advocacy, participation and partnership*. Oxford: Butterworth-Heinemann, pp 202–212.

Sweeney JK, Chandler LS (1990) Neonatal physical therapy: medical risks and professional education. *Infants and Young Children* 2: 59–68.

Szatmani P, Bartolucci G, Bremmer RS, Bond S, Rich S (1989) A follow-up study of high functioning autistic children. *Journal of Autism and Developmental Disorders* 19: 213–226.

Takata N (1969) The play history. *American Journal of Occupational Therapy* 23: 314–318.

Thal D, Tobias S, Morrison D (1991) Language and gesture in late talkers: a 1-year follow-up. *Journal of Speech and Hearing Research* **34**: 604–612.

Thomson ME, Watkins EJ (1990) *Dyslexia – A Teaching Handbook*. London: Whurr Publications.

Thornton S (1971) *Laban's Theory of Movement – A New Perspective*. Boston, MA: Plays.

Thress-Suchy L, Roantee E, Pfeffer N, Reese K, Jennings T (1999) Mothers', fathers' and teachers' perceptions of direct and consultative occupational therapy services. *School System* **6**(3): 1–3.

Tiegerman E, Primavera L (1984) Imitating the autistic child: facilitating communication and gaze behaviour. *Journal of Autism and Developmental Disorders* **11**: 427–438.

Todd VR (1993) Visual Perceptual frame of reference: an information processing approach. In: Kramer P, Hinojosa J, eds, *Frame of Reference for Pediatric Occupational Therapy*. Baltimore, MD: Williams & Wilkins, Chapter 7.

Torode IP, Gillespie R (1991) The classification and treatment of proximal femoral deficiencies. *Journal of the International Society for Orthotics and Prosthetics* **15**: 117–126.

Touwen BCL (1979) *Examination of the Child with Minor Neurological Dysfunction*, 2nd edn. London: Heinemann Medical Books.

Townsend E, Stanton S, Law M et al. (1997) *Enabling Occupation. An Occupational Therapy Perspective*. Ottawa: Canadian Association of Occupational Therapists.

Trafford G (1997) Case study: play therapy with children in Saudi Arabia. *British Journal of Therapy and Rehabilitation* **4**: 34–36.

Trahey P (1991) A comparison of the cost effectiveness of two types of occupational therapy services. *American Journal of Occupational Therapy* **45**: 397–400.

Trevarthen C (1986) Form, significance and psychological potential of hand gestures in infants. In: Nespoulos P, Perronland AR, eds, *The Biological Foundation of Gestures: Motor and Semiotic Aspects*. Cambridge, MA: MIT Press.

Trevarthen C, Aitken KJ (1994) Brain development, infant communication and empathy disorders: intrinsic factors in child mental health. *Development and Psychopathology* **6**: 599–635.

Trevarthen C, Aitken K, Papoudi D, Robarts J (1996) *Children with Autism: Diagnosis and interventions to meet their needs*, 2nd edn. London: Jessica Kingsley Publishers.

Turk J (1998) Fragile X syndrome and attentional deficits. *Journal of Applied Research in Intellectual Disabilities* **11**: 175–191.

Turk J, Cornish KM (1998) Face recognition and emotion perception in boys with Fragile-X syndrome. *Journal of Intellectual Disability Research* **42**: 490–499.

Turk J, Graham P (1997) Fragile X syndrome, autism and autistic features. *Autism* **1**: 175–197.

Turnbull A, Turnbull HR (1991) *Families, Professionals and Exceptionalities: A special partnership*, 2nd edn. Columbus, OH: Charles E Merrill.

Turnbull AP, Summers JA, Brotherson MJ (1986) Family life cycle: theoretical and empirical implications and future directions of families with mentally retarded members. In: Gallagher JJ, Vietze PM, eds, *Family of Handicapped Persons: Research, programs and policy issues*. Baltimore, MD: Paul H Brookes.

Turner A, Forster M, Johnson S (1996a) *Occupational Therapy and Physical Dysfunction: Principles, Skills and Practice*, 4th edn. London: Churchill Livingstone.

Turner G, Webb T, Wake S, Robinson H (1996b) Prevalence of Fragile X syndrome. *American Journal of Medical Genetics* 64: 196–197.

Tyerman R, Tyerman A, Howard P, Hadfield C (1986) *The Chessington Occupational Therapy Neurological Assessment Battery.* Nottingham: Nottingham Rehabilitation.

UDS Data Management Services (1991) *Guide for Use of the Uniform Data Set for Medical Rehabilitation including the Functional Independence Measure for Children – (WeeFIM).* Buffalo, NY: Uniform Data System for Medical Rehabilitation.

VandenBerg KA (1990) Nippling management of the sick neonate in the NICU: the disorganised feeder. *Neonatal Network* 9: 9–16.

Vargas S, Camilli G (1999) A meta-analysis of research on sensory integration treatment. *American Journal of Occupational Therapy* 53: 189–198.

Vereker M (1992) Chronic fatigue syndrome. A joint paediatric-psychiatric approach. *Archives of Disease in Childhood* 4: 550–555.

Vergara E (1993) *Foundations of Practice in the Neonatal Intensive Care Unit and Early Intervention: A self-guided practice manual.* Rockville, MD: American Occupational Therapy Association.

Verral T, Kulkani J (1995) Driving appliances for upper limb amputees. *Prosthetics and Orthotics International* 19: 124–127.

Vollmer TR, Iwata BA, Smith RG, Rodgers TA (1992) Reduction of multiple aberrant behaviours and concurrent development of self-care skills with differential reinforcement. *Research in Developmental Disabilities* 13: 287–299.

Volpe JJ, Hill H (1981) Disorders of sucking and swallowing in the newborn infant: clinicopathological correlations. In: Korofiken R, Guilleminault C, eds, *ProgressiIn Perinatal Neurology*, Vol 1. Baltimore, MD: Williams & Wilkins, pp 157–181.

Wacker DP, Steege MW, Northup J (1990) A component analysis of functional communication teaching across three topographies of severe behaviour problems. *Journal of Applied Behaviour Analysis* 23: 417–429.

Wagaman MJ, Shutack JG, Moomjian AS, Schwartz JG, Shaffer TH, Foz WW (1979) Improved oxygenation and lung compliance with prone positioning of neonates. *Journal of Pediatrics* 94: 787–791.

Ware J (1996) Creating a responsive environment for people with profound and multiple learning difficulties. In: Lacey P, Ouvry C, eds, *People with Profound and Multiple Learning Disabilities.* London: David Fulton.

Watson DE (1997) *Task Analysis: An occupational performance approach.* Bethesda, MD: American Occupational Therapy Association.

Weaver S, Lange L, Vogts V (1988) A comparison of myoelectric and conventional prostheses for adolescent amputees. *American Journal of Occupational Therapy* 42: 87–91.

Wehman P, Karan O, Rettie C (1976) Developing independent play in three severely retarded women. *Psychological Reports* 39: 995–998.

Weick KE (1968) Systematic observational methods. In: Lindsey G, Aronson E, eds, *The Handbook of Social Psychology*, Vol 2, 2nd edn. Reading, MA: Addison-Wesley.

Weidmer-Mikhail W, Sheldon S, Ghaziuddin M (1998) Chromosomes in autism and related pervasive developmental disorders: a cytogenetic study. *Journal of Intellectual Disability Research* 42: 8–12.

Wessely S (1990) Old wine in new bottles: neurasthenia and ME. *Psychological Medicine* 20: 35–53.

West J (1992) *Child-centred Play Therapy*. London: Edward Arnold.

Westrup B, Kleberg A, Wallin L, Lagercrantz H, Wikblad K, Stjernqvist K (1997) Evaluation of the newborn individualised developmental care and assessment program (NIDCAP) in a Swedish setting. *Prenatal and Neonatal Medicine* 2: 366–375.

Wetherbee L, Neil M (1989) *Educational Rights for Children with Arthritis. A Manual for Parents*. Atlanta, GA: American Arthritis Foundation.

White M, Bungay C, Gabriel H (1994) *Guide to Early Movement Skills*. Windsor, Berks: NFER-Nelson.

Whiting S, Lincoln N, Bhavnani G, Cockburn J (1984) *Rivermead Perceptual Assessment Battery*. Windsor, Berks: NFER-Nelson.

WHO (1992) *International Classification of Diseases*, 10th edn. *Diagnostic Criteria for Research. Geneva: World Health Organization.*

Wilbarger P (1995) The sensory diet: activity programs based on sensory processing theory. *AOTA Sensory Integration Special Interest Section Newsletter* 18: 2.

Wilbarger P, Wilbarger J (1991) *Sensory Defensiveness in Children aged 2–12: An intervention guide for parents and other caretakers*. Santa Barbara, CA: Avanti Educational Programmes.

Willett L (1986) Risk of hypoventilation in premature infants in car seats. *Journal of Pediatrics* 109: 245–248.

Williams D (1996) *Autism: An inside out approach*. London: Kingsley.

Williams HG (1983) *Perceptual and Motor Development*. Englewood Cliffs, NJ: Prentice-Hall.

Williams MS, Shellenberger S (1992) *How does your engine run? A Leader's Guide Regulation to the Alert Program for Self*. Albuquerque, NM: Therapy Works.

Willson M (1996) *Occupational Therapy in Short-term Psychiatry*. London: Churchill Livingstone.

Wilson BA, Cockburn J, Baddeley A (1985) *The Rivermead Behavioural Memory Test*. London: Thames Valley Test Company.

Wilson BN, Kaplan BJ, Fellows S, Gruchy C, Faris P (1992) The efficacy of sensory integration treatment compared to tutoring. *Physical and Occupational Therapy in Paediatrics* 12: 1–36.

Wilson BN, Pollock N, Kaplan BJ, Law M (1994) *Clinical Observations of Motor and Postural Skills (COMPS)*. San Antonio, TX: The Psychological Corporation.

Wilson K, Kendrick P, Ryan V (1992) *Play Therapy: A Non Directive Approach for Children and Adolescents*. London: Baillière Tindall.

Wilson Howle JM (1999a) Description, assessment and treatment progression of a child with ataxic cerebral palsy: A single subject case study: Part I. *NDTA Network* March–April 1, 3, 4, 19.

Wilson Howle JM (1999b) Description, assessment and treatment progression of a child with ataxic cerebral palsy: A single subject case study: Part II. *NDTA Network*, May–June 1, 3, 12, 19.

Wing L (1981) Asperger's syndrome: a clinical account. *Psychological Medicine* 11: 115–129.

Wing L (1988) The continuum of autistic characteristics. In: Scholer E, Mesibov GB, eds, *Diagnosis and Assessment in Autism*. New York: Plenum Press.

Winnicott DN (1971) *Play and Reality*. Harmondsworth: Penguin.

Winnicott DW (1964) *The Child, the Family and the Outside World*. Harmondsworth: Penguin.

Wolfberg PJ, Schuler AL (1993) Integrated playgroups: a model for promoting the social and cognitive dimensions of play in children in autism. *Journal of Autism and Developmental Disorders* **23**: 467–489.

Wolfsenberger W (1983) Social role valorisation: a proposed new term for the principle of normalisation. *Mental Retardation* **21**: 234–9.

Wolke D (1987) Environmental neonatology. *Archives of Disease in Childhood* **62**: 987–988.

Wood E, Rosenbaum P (2000) The Gross Motor Function classification system for cerebral palsy: A study of reliability and stability over time. *Developmental Medicine and Child Neurology* **42**: 292–296.

Wood W (1996) The value of studying occupation: an example with primate play. *American Journal of Occupational Therapy* **50**: 327–337.

Woolf S (1973) *Children Under Stress*. Harmondsworth: Penguin.

Wright C, Whittington D (1992) *Quality Assurance: An Introduction for Health Care Professionals*. Edinburgh: Churchill Livingstone.

Wright-Strawderman C, Watson BL (1992) The prevalence of depressive symptoms in children with learning disabilities. *Journal of Learning Disabilities* **25**: 258–264.

Wrisley D (1996) *A Day with Sam*. London: Arthritis Care.

Yalom I (1985) *The Theory and Practice of Group Psychotherapy*, 3rd edn. New York: Basic.

Young A, Harvais V, Joy D, Chesson R (1995) *Occupational Therapy: Made to measure, a study of the feasibility of goal attainment scaling in the treatment of children with learning disabilities*. Aberdeen: The Robert Gordon University.

Yule W, Carr J (1990) *Behaviour Modification for People with Mental Handicaps*, 2nd edn. London: Chapman & Hall.

Zisserman L (1992) The effects of deep pressure on self-stimulating behaviors in a child with autism and other disabilities. *American Journal of Occupational Therapy* **46**: 547–551.

Further reading

Chapter 4

Akos K (1991) *Dina: A mother practises conductive education (Petö system)*. Birmingham: Foundation for Conductive Education.

Bairstow PJ (1993) *Evaluation of Conductive Education for Children with Cerebral Palsy Final Report*. Part 1. London: HMSO.

Bairstow PJ (1993) *Evaluation of Conductive Education for Children with Cerebral Palsy Final Report*. Part 2. London: HMSO.

Cottam PJ, Sutton A (1986) *Conductive Education: A system for overcoming motor disorder*. London: Croom Helm.

Read J (1992) *Conductive Education 1987–1992: The transitional years*. Birmingham: Foundation for Conductive Education.

Chapter 5

Adams J (1997) Until disabled people get consulted. The role of occupational therapy in meeting housing needs. *British Journal of Occupational Therapy* 60: 115–122.

Barker P, ed (1995) *Building Sight*. Peterborough: Royal National Institute for the Blind.

Care and Repair England (1997) *Adaptations for Disabled Children: The impact of the Disabled Facilities Grant test of resources*. Nottingham: Care and Repair.

Gateshead Access Panel (1997) *Designing to Enable*. Gateshead: Gateshead Access Panel.

Goldsmith S (1984) *Designing for the Disabled*. London: RIBA Publications Ltd.

Heywood F, Smart G (1996) *Funding Adaptations: The need to co-operate*. Bristol: The Policy Press.

Heywood F (1994) *Adaptations: Finding ways to say yes*. Bristol: SAUS Publications.

Holmes-Siedle J (1996) *Barrier Free Design*. London: Butterworth.

Joseph Rowntree Fund (1999) *Adaptations to Housing*. York: Family Fund Trust.

Joseph Rowntree Foundation (1997) *Lifetime Homes*. York: Joseph Rowntree Foundation.

Macdonald EM, ed. (1974) *Occupational Therapy in Rehabilitation*, 4th edn. London: Baillière Tindall.

Mandelstram M (1997) *Equipment for Older or Disabled People and the Law*. London: Jessica Kingsley Publishers.

Mandelstram M (1998) *An A–Z of Community Care Law*. London: Jessica Kingsley Publishers.

Mandelstram M (1999) *Community Care Practice and the Law*, 2nd edn. London: Jessica Kingsley Publishers.

National Back Exchange (Essex Group) (1996) *Paediatric Moving and Handling*. Essex: NBE.

Chapter 13

AMRS (1997) *Congenital Limb Deficiency. Recommended Standards of Care*. London: Amputee Medical Rehabilitation Society (11 St Andrew's Place, Regents Park, London).

Atkins D, Meier R, eds (1989) *Comprehensive Management of the Upper Limb Amputee*. New York: Springer-Verlag.

Clinical Interest Group in Orthotics Prosthetics and Wheelchairs (CIGOPW) (1995) *Occupational Therapy in the Rehabilitation of Upper Limb Amputees and Limb Deficient Children, Standards and Guidelines*. Manchester: CIGOPW.

Day H, Kulkarni J, Datta D (1993) *Prescribing Upper Limb Prostheses*. London: Amputee Medical Rehabilitation Society.

Robertson E (1978) *Rehabilitation of Arm Amputees and Limb Deficient Children*. London: Baillière Tindall.

Chapter 14

Anon (1997) *Children Have Arthritis Too*. Blackmore Press.

Ansell B (1990) *When Your Child Has Arthritis*. Chesterfield: Arthritis Research Campaign.

Arthritis Research Campaign (1993) *When a Young Person has Arthritis*. Chesterfield: ARC.

Lady Hoare Trust (1997) *Living with Juvenile Chronic Arthritis*. London: LHT.

The Arthritis and Rheumatism Council have a variety of booklets available to teach patients. These include: *When Your Child Has Arthritis, Diet and Arthritis, When A Child Has Arthritis – a guide for teachers* and *Tim Has Arthritis* – a booklet specially written for young children. Many more titles are available and are free of charge from the ARC. The Lady Hoare Trust, Arthritis Care and the Children's Chronic Arthritis Association also produce a helpful booklet entitled *Children Have Arthritis Too*.

Chapter 17

Pincus L (1976) *Death and the Family*. London: Faber.

Wells R (1989) *Helping Children Cope with Grief*. London: Sheldon Press.

Index